M000210597

Ferri's
DIFFERENTIAL DIAGNOSIS

Ferri's DIFFERENTIAL DIAGNOSIS

A Practical Guide to the Differential Diagnosis of Symptoms, Signs, and Clinical Disorders

Edition 2

Fred F. Ferri, MD, FACP
Clinical Professor
Alpert Medical School
Brown University
Providence, Rhode Island

MOSBY

ELSEVIER

MOSBY
ELSEVIER

1600 John F. Kennedy Blvd.
Ste 1800
Philadelphia, PA 19103-2899

FERRI'S DIFFERENTIAL DIAGNOSIS   ISBN: 978-0-323-07699-9

Notice

Neither the Publisher nor the author assumes any responsibility for any loss or injury and/or damage to persons or property arising out of or related to any use of the material contained in this book. It is the responsibility of the treating practitioner, relying on independent expertise and knowledge of the patient, to determine the best treatment and method of application for the patient.

The Publisher

Library of Congress Cataloging-in-Publication Data

Ferri, Fred F.
  Ferri's differential diagnosis : a practical guide to the differential diagnosis of symptoms, signs, and clinical disorders / Fred F. Ferri.—2nd ed.
     p. ; cm.
  Includes bibliographical references and index.
  ISBN 978-0-323-07699-9
1. Diagnosis, Differential—Handbooks, manuals, etc.   I. Title.   II. Title: Differential diagnosis.
  [DNLM: 1. Diagnosis, Differential—Handbooks. WB 39 F388f 2011]
  RC71.5.F47 2011
  616.07′5—dc22
                                                                  2010011153

Acquisitions Editor: Jim Merritt
Developmental Editor: Lora Sickora
Publishing Services Manager: Linda Van Pelt
Design Direction: Lou Forgione

Printed in China

Last digit is the print number   9   8   7   6   5

Preface

The purpose of this handbook is to provide the clinician with a quick reference to the differential diagnosis, etiology, and classification of clinical disorders, signs, and symptoms. These various differential diagnoses are readily available in general medical texts, but the information is often scattered and difficult to find. The second edition of this manual has been significantly expanded and now contains the differential diagnosis of over 1500 signs, symptoms, and clinical disorders, yet its small size easily fits in a lab coat pocket. To facilitate its use, each condition is listed alphabetically. Differential diagnoses are listed in order of decreasing frequency.

This book differs from other differential diagnosis books because it lists not only the differential diagnosis of signs, symptoms, and laboratory abnormalities but also the differential diagnosis of more than 600 clinical disorders. For example, its user can rapidly locate the differential diagnosis of "Calcifications on Chest X-ray" and further identify the differential diagnosis of "Silicosis," "Tuberculosis," and other diseases that can cause calcifications on chest x-ray, thus narrowing down the correct diagnosis.

This book is intended for use by medical students, physicians, and allied health professionals in need of a practical rapid reference covering nearly every possible sign, symptom, and clinical disorder that will be encountered in the daily practice of both in-patient and out-patient medicine.

Fred F. Ferri, MD, FACP

Acknowledgments

The author wishes to acknowledge the following physicians for their contribution to the creation of this handbook: Ruben Alvero, Michael Benetar, Jeffrey Borkan, George Danakas, Michael Dobbs, Mitchell Feldman, Glen Fort, Joseph Masci, Lonnie Mercier, Dennis Mikolich, Peter Petropoulos, Iris Tong, and Wen-Chih Wu.

COMMENTS

Comments from readers regarding this manual are always welcome and can be forwarded to Dr. Ferri at Fred_Ferri@brown.edu.

Contents

Abdominal Distention

NONMECHANICAL OBSTRUCTION
* Excessive intraluminal gas
* Intra-abdominal infection
* Trauma
* Retroperitoneal irritation (renal colic, neoplasms, infections, hemorrhage)
* Vascular insufficiency (thrombosis, embolism)
* Mechanical ventilation
* Extra-abdominal infection (sepsis, pneumonia, empyema, osteomyelitis of spine)
* Metabolic/toxic abnormalities (hypokalemia, uremia, lead poisoning)
* Chemical irritation (perforated ulcer, bile, pancreatitis)
* Peritoneal inflammation
* Severe pain
* Pain medications

MECHANICAL OBSTRUCTION
* Neoplasm (intraluminal, extraluminal)
* Adhesions, endometriosis
* Infection (intra-abdominal abscess, diverticulitis)
* Gallstones
* Foreign body, bezoars
* Pregnancy
* Hernias
* Volvulus
* Stenosis at surgical anastomosis, radiation stenosis
* Fecaliths
* Inflammatory bowel disease (IBD)
* Gastric outlet obstruction
* Hematoma
* Other: parasites, superior mesenteric artery (SMA) syndrome, pneumatosis intestinalis, annular pancreas, Hirschsprung's disease, intussusception, meconium

Abdominal Pain, Adolescence[27]

- Irritable bowel syndrome
- Acute gastroenteritis
- Appendicitis
- Inflammatory bowel disease (IBD)
- Peptic ulcer disease
- Cholecystitis
- Neoplasm
- Other: functional abdominal pain, pelvic inflammatory disease, pregnancy, pyelonephritis, renal stone, trauma, anxiety

Abdominal Pain, Childhood[27]

- Acute gastroenteritis
- Appendicitis
- Constipation
- Anxiety
- Cholecystitis, acute
- Intestinal obstruction
- Pancreatitis
- Neoplasm
- Inflammatory bowel disease (IBD)
- Other: functional abdominal pain, pyelonephritis, pneumonia, diabetic ketoacidosis (DKA), heavy metal poisoning, sickle cell crisis, trauma

Abdominal Pain, Chronic Lower[39]

ORGANIC DISORDERS

Common
- Gynecologic disease
- Lactase deficiency
- Diverticulitis
- Crohn's disease
- Intestinal obstruction

Uncommon
- Chronic intestinal pseudo-obstruction
- Mesenteric ischemia
- Malignant neoplasm (e.g., ovarian carcinoma)

- Abdominal wall pain
- Spinal disease
- Testicular disease
- Metabolic diseases (e.g., diabetes mellitus [DM], familial Mediterranean fever, C1 esterase deficiency [angioneurotic edema], porphyria, lead poisoning, tabes dorsalis, renal failure)

FUNCTIONAL DISORDERS

Common
- Irritable bowel syndrome
- Functional abdominal bloating

Uncommon
- Functional abdominal pain

Abdominal Pain, Diffuse

- Early appendicitis
- Aortic aneurysm
- Gastroenteritis
- Intestinal obstruction
- Diverticulitis
- Peritonitis
- Mesenteric insufficiency or infarction
- Pancreatitis
- Inflammatory bowel disease (IBD)
- Irritable bowel
- Mesenteric adenitis
- Metabolic: toxins, lead poisoning, uremia, drug overdose, diabetic ketoacidosis (DKA), heavy metal poisoning
- Sickle cell crisis
- Pneumonia (rare)
- Trauma
- Urinary tract infection, pelvic inflammatory disease (PID)
- Other: acute intermittent porphyria, tabes dorsalis, periarteritis nodosa, Henoch-Schönlein purpura, adrenal insufficiency

Abdominal Pain, Epigastric

- Gastric: peptic ulcer disease (PUD), gastric outlet obstruction, gastric ulcer
- Duodenal: PUD, duodenitis

- Biliary: cholecystitis, cholangitis
- Hepatic: hepatitis
- Pancreatic: pancreatitis
- Intestinal: high small bowel obstruction, early appendicitis
- Cardiac: angina, myocardial infarction (MI), pericarditis
- Pulmonary: pneumonia, pleurisy, pneumothorax
- Subphrenic abscess
- Vascular: dissecting aneurysm, mesenteric ischemia
- Other: gastroenteritis, anxiety

Abdominal Pain, Infancy[27]

- Acute gastroenteritis
- Appendicitis
- Intussusception
- Volvulus
- Meckel's diverticulum
- Other: colic, trauma

Abdominal Pain, Left Lower Quadrant

- Intestinal: diverticulitis, intestinal obstruction, perforated ulcer, inflammatory bowel disease (IBD), perforated descending colon, inguinal hernia, neoplasm, appendicitis, adhesions
- Reproductive: ectopic pregnancy, ovarian cyst, torsion of ovarian cyst, tubo-ovarian abscess, mittelschmerz, endometriosis, seminal vesiculitis
- Renal: renal or ureteral calculi, pyelonephritis, neoplasm
- Vascular: leaking aortic aneurysm
- Psoas abscess
- Trauma

Abdominal Pain, Left Upper Quadrant

- Gastric: peptic ulcer disease (PUD), gastritis, pyloric stenosis, hiatal hernia
- Pancreatic: pancreatitis, neoplasm, stone in pancreatic duct or ampulla
- Cardiac: myocardial infarction (MI), angina pectoris

- Splenic: splenomegaly, ruptured spleen, splenic abscess, splenic infarction
- Renal: calculi, pyelonephritis, neoplasm
- Pulmonary: pneumonia, empyema, pulmonary infarction
- Vascular: ruptured aortic aneurysm
- Cutaneous: herpes zoster
- Trauma
- Intestinal: high fecal impaction, perforated colon, diverticulitis

Abdominal Pain, Nonsurgical Causes

- Irritable bowel syndrome
- Urinary tract infection, pyelonephritis, salpingitis, pelvic inflammatory disease (PID)
- Gastroenteritis, gastritis, peptic ulcer
- Diverticular spasm
- Hepatitis, mononucleosis
- Pancreatitis
- Inferior wall myocardial infarction
- Basilar pneumonia, pulmonary embolism
- Diabetic ketoacidosis (DKA)
- Strain or hematoma of rectus muscle
- Ruptured graafian follicle
- Herpes zoster
- Nerve root compression
- Sickle cell crisis
- Acute adrenal insufficiency
- Other: acute porphyria, familial Mediterranean fever, tabes dorsalis

Abdominal Pain, Periumbilical

- Intestinal: small bowel obstruction or gangrene, early appendicitis
- Vascular: mesenteric thrombosis, dissecting aortic aneurysm
- Pancreatic: pancreatitis
- Metabolic: uremia, diabetic ketoacidosis (DKA)
- Trauma
- Irritable bowel, anxiety

Abdominal Pain, Poorly Localized[27]

EXTRA-ABDOMINAL
- Metabolic: diabetic ketoacidosis (DKA), acute intermittent porphyria, hyperthyroidism, hypothyroidism, hypercalcemia, hypokalemia, uremia, hyperlipidemia, hyperparathyroidism
- Hematologic: sickle cell crisis, leukemia or lymphoma, Henoch-Schönlein purpura
- Infectious: infectious mononucleosis, Rocky Mountain spotted fever, acquired immunodeficiency syndrome (AIDS), streptococcal pharyngitis (in children), herpes zoster
- Drugs and toxins: heavy metal poisoning, black widow spider bites, withdrawal syndromes, mushroom ingestion
- Referred pain:
  - Pulmonary: pneumonia, pulmonary embolism, pneumothorax
  - Cardiac: angina, myocardial infarction, pericarditis, myocarditis
  - Genitourinary: prostatitis, epididymitis, orchitis, testicular torsion
  - Musculoskeletal: rectus sheath hematoma
- Somatization disorder, malingering, hypochondriasis, Munchausen's syndrome, functional

INTRA-ABDOMINAL
- Early appendicitis, gastroenteritis, peritonitis, pancreatitis, abdominal aortic aneurysm, mesenteric insufficiency or infarction, intestinal obstruction, volvulus, ulcerative colitis

Abdominal Pain, Pregnancy[27]

GYNECOLOGIC (GESTATIONAL AGE IN PARENTHESES)
- Miscarriage (<20 wk; 80% <12 wk)
- Septic abortion (<20 wk)
- Ectopic pregnancy (<14 wk)
- Corpus luteum cyst rupture (<12 wk)
- Ovarian torsion (especially <24 wk)
- Pelvic inflammatory disease (<12 wk)
- Chorioamnionitis (>16 wk)
- Abruptio placentae (>16 wk)

NONGYNECOLOGIC
- Appendicitis (throughout)
- Cholecystitis (throughout)
- Hepatitis (throughout)
- Pyelonephritis (throughout)
- Preeclampsia (>20 wk)

Abdominal Pain, Right Lower Quadrant

- Intestinal: acute appendicitis, regional enteritis, incarcerated hernia, cecal diverticulitis, intestinal obstruction, perforated ulcer, perforated cecum, Meckel's diverticulitis
- Reproductive: ectopic pregnancy, ovarian cyst, torsion of ovarian cyst, salpingitis, tubo-ovarian abscess, mittelschmerz, endometriosis, seminal vesiculitis
- Renal: renal and ureteral calculi, neoplasms, pyelonephritis
- Vascular: leaking aortic aneurysm
- Psoas abscess
- Trauma
- Cholecystitis

Abdominal Pain, Right Upper Quadrant

- Biliary: calculi, infection, inflammation, neoplasm
- Hepatic: hepatitis, abscess, hepatic congestion, neoplasm, trauma
- Gastric: peptic ulcer disease (PUD), pyloric stenosis, neoplasm, alcoholic gastritis, hiatal hernia
- Pancreatic: pancreatitis, neoplasm, stone in pancreatic duct or ampulla
- Renal: calculi, infection, inflammation, neoplasm, rupture of kidney
- Pulmonary: pneumonia, pulmonary infarction, right-sided pleurisy
- Intestinal: retrocecal appendicitis, intestinal obstruction, high fecal impaction, diverticulitis
- Cardiac: myocardial ischemia (particularly involving the inferior wall), pericarditis
- Cutaneous: herpes zoster
- Trauma
- Fitz-Hugh–Curtis syndrome (perihepatitis)

Abdominal Pain, Suprapubic

- Intestinal: colon obstruction or gangrene, diverticulitis, appendicitis
- Reproductive system: ectopic pregnancy, mittelschmerz, torsion of ovarian cyst, pelvic inflammatory disease (PID), salpingitis, endometriosis, rupture of endometrioma
- Cystitis, rupture of urinary bladder

Abdominal Wall Masses[39]

LUMPS ARISING IN THE SKIN AND SUBCUTANEOUS FAT (THAT COULD OCCUR ANYWHERE ON THE BODY)
- Lipoma
- Sebaceous cyst

LUMPS ARISING IN THE SKIN AND SUBCUTANEOUS FAT (SPECIFIC TO THE ANTERIOR ABDOMINAL WALL)
- Tumor nodule of the umbilicus (secondary to intraperitoneal malignant neoplasm, also called Sister Mary Joseph nodule)

LUMPS ARISING IN THE FASCIA AND MUSCLE
- Rectus sheath hematoma (usually painful)
- Desmoid tumor (associated with Gardner's syndrome)

HERNIA
- Incisional: It has an overlying scar. The sac may be very much larger than the neck of the hernia.
- Umbilical: The hernia is through the umbilical scar. Those presenting at birth commonly resolve in the first years of life.
- Paraumbilical: The neck is just lateral to the umbilical scar. Patients usually present later in life.
- Epigastric: It occurs in the midline between the xiphoid process and the umbilicus. They are usually small (<2 cm). They result when a knuckle of extraperitoneal fat extrudes through a small defect in the linea alba. Commonly irreducible and without an expansile cough impulse.
- Spigelian: A rare hernia found along the linea semilunaris at the lateral edge of the rectus sheath, most commonly a third of the way between the umbilicus and the pubis.

DIVARICATION OF THE RECTI
- Supraumbilical elliptical swelling of attenuated linea alba (no cough impulse)

Abortion, Recurrent

- Congenital anatomic abnormalities
- Adhesions (uterine synechiae)
- Uterine fibroids
- Endometriosis
- Endocrine abnormalities (luteal phase insufficiency, hypothyroidism, uncontrolled diabetes mellitus [DM])
- Parental chromosome abnormalities
- Maternal infections (cervical *Mycoplasma, Ureaplasma, Chlamydia* infection)
- Diethylstilbestrol (DES) exposure, heavy metal exposure
- Thrombocytosis
- Allogenic immunity, autoimmunity, lupus anticoagulant

Abruptio Placentae

- Placenta previa
- Cervical or vaginal trauma
- Labor
- Cervical cancer
- Rupture of membranes

Abscess, Brain

- Other parameningeal infections: subdural empyema, epidural abscess, thrombophlebitis of the major dural venous sinuses and cortical veins
- Embolic strokes in patients with bacterial endocarditis
- Mycotic aneurysms with leakage
- Viral encephalitis (usually resulting from herpes simplex)
- Acute hemorrhagic leukoencephalitis
- Parasitic infections: toxoplasmosis, echinococcosis, cysticercosis
- Metastatic or primary brain tumors
- Cerebral infarction

- Central nervous system (CNS) vasculitis
- Chronic subdural hematoma

Abscess, Breast

- Sebaceous cyst with infection
- Inflammatory carcinoma
- Advanced carcinoma with erythema, edema, or ulceration
- Hidradenitis of breast skin
- Tuberculous abscess (rare)

Abscess, Liver

- Cholangitis
- Cholecystitis
- Diverticulitis
- Appendicitis
- Perforated viscus
- Mesentery ischemia
- Pulmonary embolism
- Pancreatitis

Abscess, Lung

- Bacterial (anaerobic, aerobic, infected bulla, empyema, actinomycosis, tuberculosis)
- Fungal (histoplasmosis, coccidioidomycosis, blastomycosis, aspergillosis, cryptococcosis)
- Parasitic (amebiasis, echinococcosis)
- Malignant neoplasm (primary lung carcinoma, metastatic lung disease, lymphoma, Hodgkin's disease)
- Wegener's granulomatosis, sarcoidosis, endocarditis, septic pulmonary emboli

Abscess, Pelvic

- Pelvic neoplasms, such as ovarian tumors and leiomyomas
- Inflammatory masses involving adjacent bowel or omentum, such as ruptured appendicitis or diverticulitis

- Pelvic hematomas, as may occur after cesarean section or hysterectomy

Abscess, Perirectal

- Pilonidal disease
- Crohn's disease (inflammatory bowel disease [IBD])
- Hidradenitis suppurativa
- Tuberculosis or actinomycosis; Chagas' disease
- Cancerous lesions
- Chronic anal fistula
- Rectovaginal fistula
- Proctitis—often STD associated—including syphilis, gonococcal, chlamydial, chancroid, condylomata acuminata
- AIDS associated: Kaposi's sarcoma, lymphoma, cytomegalovirus (CMV)
- Neutropenic enterocolitis

Abuse, Child

In all categories, accidental injury is the most common entity to be distinguished from abuse. Accidental injuries are most common over bone prominences: forehead, elbows, knees, shins; soft, fleshy areas are more common for inflicted injury: buttocks, thighs, upper arms.

BRUISING
- Bleeding disorder (idiopathic thrombocytopenic purpura, hemophilia, leukemia, hemorrhagic disease of the newborn, von Willebrand disease)
- Connective tissue disorder (Ehlers-Danlos syndrome, vasculitis)
- Pigments (mongolian spots)
- Dermatitis (phytophotodermatitis, nickel allergy)
- Folk treatment (coining, cupping)

BURNS
- Chemical burn
- Impetigo
- Folk treatment (moxibustion)
- Dermatitis (phytophotodermatitis)

INTRACRANIAL HEMORRHAGE
- Bleeding disorder
- Perinatal trauma (should resolve by 4 wk)
- Arteriovenous malformation rupture
- Glutaric aciduria

FRACTURES
- Osteogenesis imperfecta
- Rickets
- Congenital syphilis
- Very low birth weight (osteopenia of prematurity)

SEXUAL ABUSE
- Normal variants
- Lichen sclerosus et atrophicus
- Congenital abnormalities
- Urethral prolapse
- Hemangioma
- Non–sexually acquired infection (group A streptococcus, *Shigella*)

Abuse, Elder

- Advancing dementia
- Depression or other psychiatric disorder
- Malnutrition from intrinsic causes
- Conscious nonadherence
- Financial hardship
- Falling

Acanthosis Nigricans

- Seborrheic keratosis
- Hyperpigmented nevus (Becker's nevus), linear epidermal nevus
- Pemphigus vegetans
- Lichen simplex chronicus
- Confluent and reticulated papillomatosis

Achalasia

- Angina
- Bulimia

- Anorexia nervosa
- Gastritis
- Peptic ulcer disease
- Postvagotomy dysmotility
- Esophageal disease: gastroesophageal reflux disease (GERD), sarcoidosis, amyloidosis, esophageal stricture, esophageal webs and rings, scleroderma, Barrett's esophagus, Chagas' disease, esophagitis
- Diffuse esophageal spasm
- Malignant neoplasm: esophageal cancer, infiltrating gastric cancer, lung cancer, lymphoma
- Gastric bezoar

Aches and Pains, Diffuse[25]

- Postviral arthralgias/myalgias
- Bilateral soft tissue rheumatism
- Overuse syndromes
- Fibrositis
- Hypothyroidism
- Metabolic bone disease
- Paraneoplastic syndrome
- Myopathy (polymyositis, dermatomyositis)
- Rheumatoid arthritis (RA)
- Sjögren's syndrome
- Polymyalgia rheumatica
- Hypermobility
- Benign arthralgias/myalgias
- Chronic fatigue syndrome
- Hypophosphatemia

Achilles Tendon Rupture

- Incomplete (partial) tendo Achillis rupture
- Partial rupture of gastrocnemius muscle, often medial head (previously thought to be "plantaris tendon rupture")

Acidosis, Lactic

TISSUE HYPOXIA
- Shock (hypovolemic, cardiogenic, endotoxic)
- Respiratory failure (asphyxia)
- Severe congestive heart failure (CHF)
- Severe anemia
- Carbon monoxide (CO) or cyanide poisoning

ASSOCIATED WITH SYSTEMIC DISORDERS
- Neoplastic diseases (e.g., leukemia, lymphoma)
- Liver or renal failure
- Sepsis
- Diabetes mellitus (DM)
- Seizure activity
- Abnormal intestinal flora
- Alkalosis
- HIV infection

SECONDARY TO DRUGS OR TOXINS
- Salicylates
- Ethanol, methanol, ethylene glycol
- Fructose or sorbitol
- Biguanides (phenformin, metformin [usually occurring in patients with renal insufficiency])
- Isoniazid
- Streptozocin
- Nucleoside reverse transcriptase inhibitors (e.g., zidovudine, didanosine, stavudine)

HEREDITARY DISORDERS
- Glucose-6-phosphate dehydrogenase (G6PD) deficiency and others

Acidosis, Metabolic

METABOLIC ACIDOSIS WITH INCREASED ANION GAP
(ANION GAP ACIDOSIS)
- Lactic acidosis
- Ketoacidosis (diabetes mellitus [DM], alcoholic ketoacidosis)

Addison's Disease (Primary Adrenocortical Insufficiency)

- Sepsis
- Hypovolemic shock
- Acute abdomen
- Apathetic hyperthyroidism in the elderly
- Myopathies
- GI malignant neoplasm
- Major depression
- Anorexia nervosa
- Hemochromatosis
- Salt-losing nephritis
- Chronic infection

Adnexal Mass[27]

- Ovary (neoplasm, endometriosis, functional cyst)
- Fallopian tube (ectopic pregnancy, neoplasm, tubo-ovarian abscess, hydrosalpinx, paratubal cyst)
- Uterus (fibroid, neoplasm)
- Retroperitoneum (neoplasm, abdominal wall hematoma or abscess)
- Urinary tract (pelvic kidney, distended bladder, urachal cyst)
- Inflammatory bowel disease (IBD)
- GI tract neoplasm
- Diverticular disease
- Appendicitis
- Bowel loop with feces

Adrenal Masses[37]

UNILATERAL ADRENAL MASS
- Functional lesions: adrenal adenoma; adrenal carcinoma; pheochromocytoma; primary aldosteronism, adenomatous type
- Nonfunctional lesions: incidentaloma of adrenal, ganglioneuroma, myelolipoma, hematoma, adenolipoma, metastasis

BILATERAL ADRENAL MASS

- Functional lesions: adrenocorticotropic hormone (ACTH)–dependent Cushing's syndrome; congenital adrenal hyperplasia; pheochromocytoma; Conn's syndrome, hyperplastic variety; micronodular adrenal disease; idiopathic bilateral adrenal hypertrophy
- Nonfunctional lesions: infection (tuberculosis, fungi), infiltration (leukemia, lymphoma), replacement (amyloidosis), hemorrhage, bilateral metastases

Adynamic Ileus[27]

- Abdominal trauma
- Infection (retroperitoneal, pelvic, intrathoracic)
- Laparotomy
- Metabolic disease (hypokalemia)
- Renal colic
- Skeletal injury (rib fracture, vertebral fracture)
- Medications (e.g., narcotics)

Aerophagia (Belching, Eructation)

- Anxiety disorders
- Rapid food ingestion
- Carbonated beverages
- Nursing infants (especially when nursing in horizontal position)
- Eating or drinking in supine position
- Gum chewing
- Poorly fitting dentures, orthodontic appliances
- Hiatal hernia, gastritis, nonulcer dyspepsia
- Cholelithiasis, cholecystitis
- Ingestion of legumes, onions, peppers

Agoraphobia

- Medical conditions: arrhythmias, hyperthyroidism, hyperparathyroidism, seizure disorders, respiratory diseases, pheochromocytoma

- Therapeutic (theophylline, steroids) and recreational (cocaine, amphetamine, caffeine) drugs and drug withdrawal (alcohol, barbiturates, benzodiazepines)
- Phobias (e.g., specific phobia or social phobia)
- Obsessive-compulsive disorder (cued by exposure to the object of the obsession)
- Post-traumatic stress disorder (cued by recall of a stressor)

Airway Obstruction, Pediatric Age[20]

CONGENITAL CAUSES
- Craniofacial dysmorphism
- Hemangioma
- Laryngeal cleft/web
- Laryngoceles, cysts
- Laryngomalacia
- Macroglossia
- Tracheal stenosis
- Vascular ring
- Vocal cord paralysis

ACQUIRED INFECTIOUS CAUSES
- Acute laryngotracheobronchitis
- Diphtheria
- Epiglottitis
- Laryngeal papillomatosis
- Membranous croup (bacterial tracheitis)
- Mononucleosis
- Retropharyngeal abscess
- Spasmodic croup

ACQUIRED NONINFECTIOUS CAUSES
- Anaphylaxis
- Angioneurotic edema
- Foreign body aspiration
- Supraglottic hypotonia
- Thermal/chemical burn
- Trauma
- Vocal cord paralysis

Akinetic/Rigid Syndrome[1]

- Parkinsonism (idiopathic, drug induced)
- Catatonia (psychosis)
- Progressive supranuclear palsy
- Multisystem atrophy (Shy-Drager syndrome, olivopontocerebellar atrophy)
- Diffuse Lewy body disease
- Toxins (MPTP, manganese, carbon monoxide [CO])
- Huntington's disease and other hereditary neurodegenerative disorders

Aldosteronism, Primary

- Diuretic use
- Hypokalemia from vomiting, diarrhea
- Renovascular hypertension
- Other endocrine neoplasm (pheochromocytoma, deoxycorticosterone-producing tumor, renin-secreting tumor)

Alkalosis, Metabolic

CHLORIDE RESPONSIVE
- Vomiting
- Nasogastric (NG) suction
- Diuretics
- Post hypercapnic alkalosis
- Stool losses (laxative abuse, cystic fibrosis, villous adenoma)
- Massive blood transfusion
- Exogenous alkali administration

CHLORIDE RESISTANT
- Hyperadrenocorticoid states (Cushing's syndrome, primary hyperaldosteronism, secondary mineralocorticoidism [licorice, chewing tobacco])
- Hypomagnesemia
- Hypokalemia
- Bartter's syndrome

Alkalosis, Respiratory

- Hypoxemia (pneumonia, pulmonary embolism, atelectasis, high-altitude living)
- Drugs (salicylates, xanthines, progesterone, epinephrine, thyroxine, nicotine)
- CNS disorders (tumor, cerebrovascular accident [CVA], trauma, infections)
- Psychogenic hyperventilation (anxiety, hysteria)
- Hepatic encephalopathy
- Gram-negative sepsis
- Hyponatremia
- Sudden recovery from metabolic acidosis
- Assisted ventilation

Alopecia[14,29]

SCARRING ALOPECIA
- Congenital (aplasia cutis)
- Tinea capitis with inflammation (kerion)
- Bacterial folliculitis
- Discoid lupus erythematosus
- Lichen planopilaris
- Folliculitis decalvans
- Neoplasm
- Trauma

NONSCARRING ALOPECIA
- Cosmetic treatment
- Tinea capitis
- Structural hair shaft disease
- Trichotillomania (hair pulling)
- Anagen arrest
- Telogen arrest
- Alopecia areata
- Androgenic alopecia

Alopecia, Androgenic

- Iron deficiency
- Malnutrition

- Hypothyroidism
- Telogen effluvium
- Trichotillomania
- Traction alopecia
- Alopecia areata
- Anagen effluvium
- Tinea capitis

Alopecia Areata

- Androgenic alopecia
- Trichotillomania
- Secondary syphilis
- Telogen effluvium
- Tinea capitis

Altitude Sickness

- Dehydration
- Carbon monoxide (CO) poisoning
- Hypothermia
- Infection
- Substance abuse
- Congestive heart failure (CHF)
- Pulmonary embolism
- Cerebrovascular accident

Alveolar Consolidation

- Infection
- Neoplasm (bronchoalveolar carcinoma, lymphoma)
- Aspiration
- Trauma
- Hemorrhage (Wegener's granulomatosis, Goodpasture's syndrome, bleeding diathesis)
- Acute respiratory distress syndrome (ARDS)
- Congestive heart failure (CHF)
- Renal failure
- Eosinophilic pneumonia

- Bronchiolitis obliterans
- Pulmonary alveolar proteinosis

Alveolar Hemorrhage[29]

- Hematologic disorders (coagulopathies, thrombocytopenia)
- Goodpasture's syndrome (anti–basement membrane antibody disease)
- Wegener's vasculitis
- Immune complex–mediated vasculitis
- Idiopathic pulmonary hemosiderosis
- Drugs (penicillamine)
- Lymphangiographic contrast medium
- Mitral stenosis

Alzheimer's Disease (AD)

- Normal aging memory loss
- Multi-infarct dementia
- Depression
- Cancer (brain tumor, meningeal neoplasia)
- Infection (AIDS, neurosyphilis, progressive multifocal leukoencephalopathy [PML])
- Metabolic (alcohol, hypothyroidism, vitamin B_{12} deficiency)
- Organ failure (dialysis dementia, Wilson's disease)
- Vascular disorder (chronic subdural hematoma [SDH])
- Normal-pressure hydrocephalus
- Lewy body dementia, Pick's disease, Creutzfeldt-Jakob disease, Huntington's dementia

Amaurosis Fugax

- Retinal migraine: In contrast to amaurosis, the onset of visual loss develops more slowly, usually during a period of 15 to 20 minutes.
- Transient visual obscurations (TVOs) occur in the setting of papilledema; intermittent rises in intracranial pressure briefly compromise optic disc perfusion and cause transient visual loss lasting 1 to 2 seconds, and the episodes may be binocular.

- If the visual loss persists at the time of evaluation (i.e., vision has not yet recovered), the differential diagnosis should be broadened to include
  - Anterior ischemic optic neuropathy—arteritic (classically giant cell arteritis [GCA]) or nonarteritic
  - Central retinal vein occlusion

Amblyopia

- CNS disease (brainstem)
- Optic nerve disorders
- Corneal or other eye diseases

Amebiasis

- Ulcerative colitis
- Infectious enterocolitis syndromes, such as those caused by *Shigella*, *Salmonella*, *Campylobacter*, or invasive *Escherichia coli*
- Ischemic bowel in elderly patients

Amenorrhea

- Pregnancy
- Early menopause
- Hypothalamic dysfunction: defective synthesis or release of luteinizing hormone–releasing hormone (LH-RH), anorexia nervosa, stress, exercise
- Pituitary dysfunction: neoplasm, postpartum hemorrhage, surgery, radiotherapy
- Ovarian dysfunction: gonadal dysgenesis, 17α-hydroxylase deficiency, premature ovarian failure, polycystic ovarian disease, gonadal stromal tumors
- Uterovaginal abnormalities
  - Congenital: imperforate hymen, imperforate cervix, imperforate or absent vagina, müllerian agenesis
  - Acquired: destruction of endometrium with curettage (Asherman's syndrome), closure of cervix or vagina caused by traumatic injury, hysterectomy

- Other: metabolic diseases (liver, kidney), malnutrition, rapid weight loss, exogenous obesity, endocrine abnormalities (Cushing's syndrome, Graves' disease, hypothyroidism)

Amnesia

- Degenerative diseases (e.g., Alzheimer's disease, Huntington's disease)
- Cerebrovascular accident (CVA) (especially when involving thalamus, basal forebrain, and hippocampus)
- Head trauma
- Postsurgical (e.g., mammillary body surgery, bilateral temporal lobectomy)
- Infections (herpes simplex encephalitis, meningitis)
- Wernicke-Korsakoff syndrome
- Cerebral hypoxia
- Hypoglycemia
- CNS neoplasms
- Creutzfeldt-Jakob disease
- Medications (e.g., midazolam and other benzodiazepines)
- Psychosis
- Malingering

Amyloidosis

Differential variable, depending on the organ involvement
- Renal involvement (toxin- or drug-induced necrosis, glomerulonephritis, renal vein thrombosis)
- Interstitial lung disease (sarcoidosis, connective tissue disease, infectious etiologies)
- Restrictive cardiac (endomyocardial fibrosis, viral myocarditis)
- Carpal tunnel (rheumatoid arthritis, hypothyroidism, overuse)
- Mental status changes (multi-infarct dementia)
- Peripheral neuropathy (alcohol abuse, vitamin deficiencies, diabetes mellitus [DM])

Amyotrophic Lateral Sclerosis (ALS)

- Multifocal motor neuropathy (MMN) with conduction block
- Cervical spondylotic myelopathy with polyradiculopathy

- Spinal stenosis with compression of lumbosacral nerve roots
- Chronic inflammatory demyelinating polyneuropathy with CNS lesions
- Syringomyelia
- Syringobulbia
- Foramen magnum tumor
- Spinal muscular atrophy
- Late-onset hexosaminidase A deficiency
- Polyglucosan body disease
- Bulbospinal muscular atrophy (Kennedy's disease)
- Monomelic amyotrophy
- ALS-like syndromes have been reported in the setting of lead intoxication, HIV infection, hyperparathyroidism, hyperthyroidism, lymphoma, and vitamin B_{12} deficiency

Anaerobic Infections

- Primary differential possibility is an aerobic bacterial infection without the presence of anaerobic bacteria.
- Ischemic necrosis without accompanying anaerobic infection (or "dry" gangrene [noninfected necrosis] vs. "wet" gangrene [infected tissue with anaerobic infection])

Anal Abscess and Fistula[39]

- Primary anal gland infection
- Secondary abscess
  - Inflammatory bowel disease (IBD)
  - Crohn's disease—ulcerative colitis
  - Infection
  - Tuberculosis
  - Actinomycosis
  - Threadworm
  - Trauma
  - Leukopenia
  - Immunosuppression
  - HIV infection
  - Drugs
  - Rectal cancer
  - Diabetes mellitus (DM)

Anal Fissure

- Proctalgia fugax
- Thrombosed hemorrhoid

Anal Fistula

- Hidradenitis suppurativa
- Pilonidal sinus
- Bartholin's gland abscess or sinus
- Infected perianal sebaceous cysts

Anal Incontinence[27]

- Traumatic: nerve injured in surgery, spinal cord injury, obstetric trauma, sphincter injury
- Neurologic: spinal cord lesions, dementia, autonomic neuropathy (e.g., diabetes mellitus [DM])
- Obstetrics: pudendal nerve stretched during surgery, Hirschsprung's disease
- Mass effect: carcinoma of anal canal, carcinoma of rectum, foreign body, fecal impaction, hemorrhoids
- Medical: procidentia, inflammatory disease, diarrhea, laxative abuse
- Pediatric: congenital, meningocele, myelomeningocele, spina bifida, after corrective surgery for imperforate anus, sexual abuse, encopresis

Anaphylaxis[22]

- Pulmonary: laryngeal edema, epiglottitis, foreign body aspiration, pulmonary embolus, asphyxiation, hyperventilation
- Cardiovascular: myocardial infarction, arrhythmia, hypovolemic shock, cardiac arrest
- CNS: vasovagal reaction, cerebrovascular accident (CVA), seizure disorder, drug overdose
- Endocrine: hypoglycemia, pheochromocytoma, carcinoid syndrome, catamenial (progesterone-induced anaphylaxis)
- Psychiatric: vocal cord dysfunction syndrome, Munchausen's disease, panic attack/globus hystericus

- Other: hereditary angioedema, cord urticaria, idiopathic urticaria, mastocytosis, serum sickness, idiopathic capillary leak syndrome, sulfite exposure, scombroid poisoning (tuna, bluefish, mackerel)

Androgen Excess, Reproductive-Age Woman

- Polycystic ovary syndrome
- Idiopathic
- Medications (e.g., anabolizing agents, testosterone, danazol)
- Pregnancy (luteoma, hyperreactio luteinalis)
- Sertoli-Leydig ovarian neoplasm
- Adrenal adenoma or hyperplasia
- Cushing's syndrome
- Glucocorticoid resistance
- Hypothyroidism
- Hyperprolactinemia

Anemia, Aplastic

- Bone marrow infiltration from lymphoma, carcinoma, myelofibrosis
- Severe infection
- Hypoplastic acute lymphoblastic leukemia in children
- Hypoplastic myelodysplastic syndrome or hypoplastic acute myeloid leukemia in adults
- Hypersplenism
- Hairy cell leukemia

Anemia, Autoimmune, Hemolytic

- Hemolytic anemia caused by membrane defects: paroxysmal nocturnal hemoglobinuria, spur cell anemia, Wilson's disease
- Nonimmune mediated: microangiopathic hemolytic anemia, hypersplenism, cardiac valve prosthesis, giant cavernous hemangiomas, march hemoglobinuria, physical agents, infections, heavy metals, drugs (nitrofurantoin, sulfonamides)

Anemia, Drug Induced[18]

- Drugs that may interfere with red cell production by inducing marrow suppression or aplasia: alcohol, antineoplastic drugs, antithyroid drugs, antibiotics, oral hypoglycemic agents, phenylbutazone, azidothymidine (AZT)
- Drugs that interfere with vitamin B_{12}, folate, or iron absorption or utilization: nitrous oxide, anticonvulsant drugs, antineoplastic drugs, isoniazid, cycloserine
- Drugs capable of promoting hemolysis: immune mediated, penicillins, quinine, methyldopa, procainamide, mitomycin C, oxidative stress, antimalarials, sulfonamide drugs, nalidixic acid
- Drugs that may produce or promote blood loss: aspirin, alcohol, nonsteroidal anti-inflammatory agents, corticosteroids, anticoagulants

Anemia, Hypochromic[21]

- Decreased body iron stores
  - Iron deficiency anemia
- Normal or increased body iron stores
  - Impaired iron metabolism
  - Anemia of chronic disease
  - Defective absorption, transport, or use of iron
  - Disorders of globin synthesis
  - Thalassemia
  - Other microcytic hemoglobinopathies
  - Disorders of heme synthesis: sideroblastic anemias
  - Hereditary
  - Acquired

Anemia, Iron Deficiency

- Anemia of chronic disease
- Sideroblastic anemia
- Thalassemia trait
- Lead poisoning

Anemia, Low Reticulocyte Count[1]

- Microcytic anemia (mean corpuscular volume [MCV] < 80): iron deficiency, thalassemia minor, sideroblastic anemia, lead poisoning
- Macrocytic anemia (MCV > 100): megaloblastic anemias, folate deficiency, vitamin B_{12} deficiency, drug-induced megaloblastic anemia, nonmegaloblastic macrocytosis, liver disease, hypothyroidism
- Normocytic anemia (MCV 80–100): early iron deficiency, aplastic anemia, myelophthisic disorders, endocrinopathies, anemia of chronic disease, uremia, mixed nutritional deficiency

Anemia, Megaloblastic[37]

COBALAMIN (Cbl) DEFICIENCY
- *Nutritional Cbl deficiency* (insufficient Cbl intake): vegetarians, vegans, breast-fed infants of mothers with pernicious anemia
- *Abnormal intragastric events* (inadequate proteolysis of food Cbl): atrophic gastritis, partial gastrectomy with hypochlorhydria
- *Loss or atrophy of gastric oxyntic mucosa* (deficient intrinsic factor [IF] molecules): total or partial gastrectomy, pernicious anemia, caustic destruction (lye)
- *Abnormal events in small bowel lumen:* inadequate pancreatic protease (R-Cbl not degraded, Cbl not transferred to IF)
  - Insufficiency of pancreatic protease: pancreatic insufficiency
  - Inactivation of pancreatic protease: Zollinger-Ellison syndrome
  - Usurping of luminal Cbl (inadequate Cbl binding to IF)
  - By bacteria; stasis syndromes (blind loops, pouches of diverticulosis, strictures, fistulas, anastomoses); impaired bowel motility (scleroderma, pseudo-obstruction); hypogammaglobulinemia
  - By *Diphyllobothrium latum*
- *Disorders of ileal mucosa/IF receptors* (IF-Cbl not bound to IF receptors)
  - Diminished or absent IF receptors: ileal bypass, resection, or fistula
  - Abnormal mucosal architecture/function: tropical or nontropical sprue, Crohn's disease, TB ileitis, infiltration by lymphomas, amyloidosis

- IF/post IF receptor defects: Imerslund-Graesbeck syndrome, transcobalamin (TC) II deficiency
- Drug-induced effects (Slow-K, biguanides, cholestyramine, colchicine, neomycin, *p*-aminosalicylic acid [PAS])
- *Disorders of plasma Cbl transport* (TC II–Cbl not delivered to TC II receptors)
  - Congenital TC II deficiency, defective binding of TC II–Cbl to TC II receptors (rare)
- *Metabolic disorders* (Cbl not used by cell)
  - Inborn enzyme errors (rare)
- *Acquired disorders*: N_2O inhalation

FOLATE DEFICIENCY

Nutritional Causes

- Decreased dietary intake: poverty and famine (associated with kwashiorkor, marasmus), institutionalized individuals (psychiatric/nursing homes), chronic debilitating disease/goat's milk (low in folate), special diets (slimming), cultural/ethnic cooking techniques (food folate destroyed) or habits (folate-rich foods not consumed)

Decreased Diet and Increased Requirements

- Physiologic: pregnancy and lactation, prematurity, infancy
- Pathologic: intrinsic hematologic disease (autoimmune hemolytic disease), drugs, malaria; hemoglobinopathies (Sjögren's syndrome, thalassemia), red blood cell (RBC) membrane defects (hereditary spherocytosis, paroxysmal nocturnal hemoglobinopathy); abnormal hematopoiesis (leukemia/lymphoma, myelodysplastic syndrome, agnogenic myeloid metaplasia with myelofibrosis); infiltration with malignant disease; dermatologic (psoriasis)

Folate Malabsorption

- With normal intestinal mucosa
  - Some drugs (controversial)
  - Congenital folate malabsorption (rare)
- With mucosal abnormalities: tropical and nontropical sprue, regional enteritis
- Defective cellular folate uptake: familial aplastic anemia (rare)
- Inadequate cellular utilization: folate antagonists (methotrexate), hereditary enzyme deficiencies involving folate

- Drugs (multiple effects on folate metabolism): alcohol, sulfasalazine, triamterene, pyrimethamine, trimethoprim-sulfamethoxazole, diphenylhydantoin, barbiturates

MISCELLANEOUS MEGALOBLASTIC ANEMIAS (NOT CAUSED BY Cbl OR FOLATE DEFICIENCY)
- Congenital disorders of DNA synthesis (rare): orotic aciduria, Lesch-Nyhan syndrome, congenital dyserythropoietic anemia
- Acquired disorders of DNA synthesis: thiamine-responsive megaloblastosis (rare); malignant neoplasia, erythroleukemia, refractory sideroblastic anemias; all antineoplastic drugs that inhibit DNA synthesis; toxic alcohol

Anemia, Pernicious

- Nutritional vitamin B_{12} deficiency
- Malabsorption
- Chronic alcoholism (multifactorial)
- Chronic gastritis related to *Helicobacter pylori* infection
- Folic acid deficiency
- Myelodysplasia

Anemia, Sideroblastic

- Iron deficiency anemia
- Thalassemia
- Anemia of chronic disease
- Lead poisoning
- Blood loss

Anergy, Cutaneous[37]

- Immunologic
  - Acquired (AIDS, acute leukemia, carcinoma, chronic lymphocytic leukemia [CLL], Hodgkin's lymphoma, non-Hodgkin's lymphoma)
  - Congenital (ataxia-telangiectasia, DiGeorge syndrome, severe combined immunodeficiency, Wiskott-Aldrich syndrome)
- Infections: bacterial (bacterial pneumonia, brucellosis), disseminated mycotic infections, mycobacterial (lepromatous

leprosy, TB), viral (varicella, hepatitis, influenza, mononucleosis, measles, mumps)
- Immunosuppressive medications: systemic corticosteroids, methotrexate, cyclophosphamide, rifampin
- Other: alcoholic cirrhosis, biliary cirrhosis, sarcoidosis, rheumatic disease, diabetes, Crohn's disease, uremia, anemia, pyridoxine deficiency, sickle cell anemia, burns, malnutrition, pregnancy, old age, surgery

Aneurysms, Thoracic Aorta

- Trauma
- Infection
- Inflammatory (syphilis, Takayasu's disease)
- Collagen-vascular disease (rheumatoid arthritis, ankylosing spondylitis)
- Annuloaortic ectasia (Marfan syndrome, Ehlers-Danlos syndrome)
- Congenital
- Coarctation
- Cystic medial necrosis

Angina Pectoris

- Pulmonary diseases: pulmonary hypertension, pulmonary embolism, pleurisy, pneumothorax, pneumonia
- GI disorders: peptic ulcer disease, pancreatitis, esophageal spasm or spontaneous esophageal muscle contraction, esophageal reflux, cholecystitis, cholelithiasis
- Musculoskeletal conditions: costochondritis, chest wall trauma, cervical arthritis with radiculopathy, muscle strain, myositis
- Acute aortic dissection
- Herpes zoster

Angioedema

- Cellulitis
- Arthropod bite
- Hypothyroidism
- Contact dermatitis

- Atopic dermatitis
- Mastocytosis
- Granulomatous cheilitis
- Bullous pemphigoid
- Urticaria pigmentosa
- Anaphylaxis
- Erythema multiforme
- Epiglottitis
- Peritonsillar abscess

Angioma (Cherry Angioma)

- Petechiae
- Telangiectasia
- Bacillary angiomatosis
- Melanoma
- Benign pigmented purpura
- Insect bite
- Pyogenic granuloma
- Angiokeratoma

Angular Cheilitis (Perlèche)

- Impetigo
- Contact dermatitis (lip balms, mouthwash, toothpaste)
- Lip smacking dermatitis

Anhidrosis

- Drugs (anticholinergics)
- Dehydration
- Hysteria
- Obstruction of sweat ducts (e.g., inflammation, miliaria)
- Local radiant heat or pressure
- CNS lesions (medulla, hypothalamus, pons)
- Spinal cord lesions
- Lesions of sympathetic nerves
- Congenital sweat gland disturbances

Anion Gap, Decrease

- Hypoalbuminemia
- Severe hypermagnesemia
- IgG myeloma
- Lithium toxicity
- Laboratory error (falsely decreased sodium or overestimation of bicarbonate or chloride)
- Hypercalcemia of parathyroid origin, antibiotics (e.g., polymyxin)

Anion Gap, Increase

- Uremia
- Ketoacidosis (diabetic, starvation, alcoholic)
- Lactic acidosis
- Ethylene glycol poisoning
- Salicylate overdose
- Methanol poisoning

Anisocoria

- Mydriatic or miotic drugs
- Prosthetic eye
- Inflammation (keratitis, iridocyclitis)
- Infections (herpes zoster, syphilis, meningitis, encephalitis, TB, diphtheria, botulism)
- Subdural hemorrhage
- Cavernous sinus thrombosis
- Intracranial neoplasm
- Cerebral aneurysm
- Glaucoma
- CNS degenerative diseases
- Internal carotid ischemia
- Toxic polyneuritis (alcohol, lead)
- Adie's syndrome
- Horner's syndrome
- Diabetes mellitus (DM)
- Trauma
- Congenital

Ankle Fracture

- Ankle sprain
- Avulsion fracture of hindfoot or metatarsal

Ankle Sprain

- Fracture of the ankle or foot, particularly involving the distal fibular growth plate in the immature patient
- Avulsion fracture of the fifth metatarsal base

Anorectal Fissure

- Proctalgia fugax
- Thrombosed hemorrhoid
- Anorectal abscess
- Fistula

Anorexia Nervosa

- Depression with loss of appetite
- Schizophrenia
- Conversion disorder
- Occult carcinoma, lymphoma
- Endocrine disorders: Addison's disease, diabetes mellitus (DM), hypothyroidism or hyperthyroidism, panhypopituitarism
- GI disorders: celiac disease, Crohn's disease, intestinal parasitosis
- Infectious disorders: AIDS, TB

Anovulation

- Anorexia and bulimia
- Strenuous exercise
- Weight loss/malnutrition
- Empty sella syndrome
- Pituitary disorders (infarction, infection, trauma, irradiation, surgery, microadenomas, macroadenomas)
- Idiopathic hypopituitarism
- Drug induced
- Thyroid dysfunction (hypothyroidism, hyperthyroidism)

- Systemic diseases (e.g., liver disease)
- Adrenal hyperfunction (Cushing's syndrome, congenital adrenal hyperplasia)
- Polycystic ovary syndrome
- Isolated gonadotropin deficiency

Anthrax

- Inhalation anthrax must be distinguished from influenza-like illness (ILI) and tularemia. Most cases of ILI are associated with nasal congestion and rhinorrhea, which are unusual in inhalation anthrax. An additional distinguishing factor is the usual absence of an abnormal chest radiograph in ILI.
- Cutaneous anthrax should be distinguished from staphylococcal disease, ecthyma, ecthyma gangrenosum, plague, brown recluse spider bite, and tularemia.
- The differential diagnosis of gastrointestinal anthrax includes viral gastroenteritis, shigellosis, and yersiniosis.

Antinuclear Antibody (ANA) Positive

- Systemic lupus erythematosus (SLE) (more significant if titer >1:160)
- Drugs (e.g., phenytoin, ethosuximide, primidone, methyldopa, hydralazine, carbamazepine, penicillin, procainamide, chlorpromazine, griseofulvin, thiazides)
- Autoimmune hepatitis
- Age older than 60 years (particularly age older than 80 years)
- Rheumatoid arthritis (RA)
- Scleroderma
- Mixed connective tissue disease
- Necrotizing vasculitis
- Sjögren's syndrome

Antiphospholipid Antibody Syndrome (APS)

- Other hypercoagulable states (inherited or acquired)
- Inherited: ATIII, protein C and S deficiencies, factor V Leiden, prothrombin gene mutation

- Acquired: heparin-induced thrombopathy, myeloproliferative syndromes, cancer, hyperviscosity
- Homocystinemia
- Nephrotic syndrome

Anxiety

- Wide range of psychiatric and medical conditions; however, for a diagnosis of generalized anxiety disorder (GAD) to be made, a person must experience anxiety with coexisting physical symptoms the majority of the time continuously for at least 6 months.
- Cardiovascular or pulmonary disease
- Hyperthyroidism
- Parkinson's disease
- Myasthenia gravis
- Consequence of recreational drug use (e.g., cocaine, amphetamine, and PCP) or withdrawal (e.g., alcohol or benzodiazepines)

Aortic Dissection

- Acute myocardial infarction (MI)
- Aortic insufficiency
- Nondissecting aortic aneurysm
- Pulmonary embolism
- Rib fracture
- Esophageal spasm
- Esophagitis
- Cholelithiasis, cholecystitis
- Pancreatitis

Aortic Stenosis

- Hypertrophic cardiomyopathy
- Mitral regurgitation
- Ventricular septal defect
- Aortic sclerosis. Aortic stenosis is distinguished from aortic sclerosis by the degree of valve impairment. In aortic sclerosis, the valve leaflets are abnormally thickened, but obstruction to outflow is minimal.

Aphthous Stomatitis (Canker Sores)

WHITE LESIONS

- Leukoedema: filmy opalescent-appearing mucosa, which can be reverted to normal appearance by stretching. This condition is benign.
- Candidiasis
- White sponge nevus: thick, white corrugated folds involving the buccal mucosa; appears in childhood as an autosomal dominant trait; benign condition
- Darier's disease (keratosis follicularis): white papules on the gingivae, alveolar mucosa, and dorsal tongue; skin lesions also present (erythematous papules); inherited as an autosomal dominant trait
- Chemical injury: white sloughing mucosa
- Nicotine stomatitis: whitened palate with red papules
- Lichen planus: linear, reticular, slightly raised striae on buccal mucosa; skin is involved by pruritic violaceous papules on forearms and inner thighs
- Discoid lupus erythematosus: lesion resembles lichen planus
- Leukoplakia: white lesions that cannot be scraped off; 20% are premalignant epithelial dysplasia or squamous cell carcinoma
- Hairy leukoplakia: shaggy white surface that cannot be wiped off; seen in HIV infection, caused by Epstein-Barr virus

RED LESIONS

- Candidiasis may present with red instead of the more frequent white lesion (see White Lesions). Median rhomboid glossitis is a chronic variant.
- Benign migratory glossitis (geographic tongue): area of atrophic depapillated mucosa surrounded by a keratotic border
- Hemangiomas
- Histoplasmosis: ill-defined irregular patch with a granulomatous surface, sometimes ulcerated
- Allergy
- Anemia: atrophic reddened glossal mucosa seen with pernicious anemia

- Erythroplakia: red patch usually caused by epithelial dysplasia or squamous cell carcinoma
- Burning tongue (glossopyrosis): normal examination; sometimes associated with denture trauma, anemia, diabetes, vitamin B_{12} deficiency, psychogenic problems

DARK LESIONS (BROWN, BLUE, BLACK)
- Coated tongue: accumulation of keratin; harmless condition that can be treated by scraping
- Melanotic lesions: freckles, lentigines, lentigo, melanoma, Peutz-Jeghers syndrome, Addison's disease
- Varices
- Kaposi's sarcoma: red or purple macules that enlarge to form tumors; seen in patients with AIDS

RAISED LESIONS
- Papilloma
- Verruca vulgaris
- Condyloma acuminatum
- Fibroma
- Epulis
- Pyogenic granuloma
- Mucocele
- Retention cyst

BLISTERS
- Primary herpetic gingivostomatitis
- Pemphigus and pemphigoid
- Hand-foot-mouth disease: caused by coxsackievirus group A
- Erythema multiforme
- Herpangina: caused by echovirus
- Traumatic ulcer
- Primary syphilis
- Perlèche (angular cheilitis)
- Recurrent aphthous stomatitis (canker sores)
- Behçet's syndrome (aphthous ulcers, uveitis, genital ulcerations, arthritis, and aseptic meningitis)
- Reiter's syndrome (conjunctivitis, urethritis, and arthritis with occasional oral ulcerations)

Appendicitis

- Intestinal: regional cecal enteritis, incarcerated hernia, cecal diverticulitis, intestinal obstruction, perforated ulcer, perforated cecum, Meckel's diverticulitis
- Reproductive: ectopic pregnancy, ovarian cyst, torsion of ovarian cyst, salpingitis, tubo-ovarian abscess, mittelschmerz, endometriosis, seminal vesiculitis
- Renal: renal and ureteral calculi, neoplasms, pyelonephritis
- Vascular: leaking aortic aneurysm
- Psoas abscess
- Trauma
- Cholecystitis
- Mesenteric adenitis

Appetite Loss in Infants and Children[20]

ORGANIC DISEASE
- Infectious (acute or chronic)
- Neurologic: congenital degenerative disease
- Hypothalamic lesion: increased intracranial pressure (including a brain tumor), swallowing disorders (neuromuscular)
- Gastrointestinal: oral lesions (e.g., thrush or herpes simplex), gastroesophageal reflux, obstruction (especially with gastric or intestinal distention), inflammatory bowel disease (IBD), celiac disease, constipation
- Cardiac: congestive heart failure (CHF) (especially associated with cyanotic lesions)
- Metabolic: renal failure or renal tubular acidosis, liver failure, congenital metabolic disease, lead poisoning
- Nutritional: marasmus, iron deficiency, zinc deficiency
- Fever
- Rheumatoid arthritis (RA)
- Rheumatic fever
- Drugs: morphine, digitalis, antimetabolites, methylphenidate, amphetamines
- Miscellaneous: prolonged restriction of oral feedings, beginning in the neonatal period; systemic lupus erythematosus (SLE); tumor

PSYCHOLOGICAL FACTORS

- Anxiety, fear, depression, mania (limbic influence on the hypothalamus)
- Avoidance of symptoms associated with meals (abdominal pain, diarrhea, bloating, urgency, dumping syndrome)
- Anorexia nervosa
- Excessive weight loss and food aversion in athletes, simulating anorexia nervosa

Arterial Occlusion[15]

- Thromboembolism (post–myocardial infarction, mitral stenosis, rheumatic valve disease, atrial fibrillation, atrial myxoma, marantic endocarditis, bacterial endocarditis, Libman-Sacks endocarditis)
- Atheroembolism (microemboli composed of cholesterol, calcium, and platelets from proximal atherosclerotic plaques)
- Arterial thrombosis (endothelial injury, altered arterial blood flow, trauma, severe atherosclerosis, acute vasculitis)
- Vasospasm
- Trauma
- Hypercoagulable states
- Miscellaneous (irradiation, drugs, infections, necrotizing)

Arthritis and Abdominal Pain

- Viral syndrome
- Inflammatory bowel disease (IBD)
- Celiac disease
- Vasculitis
- Systemic lupus erythematosus (SLE)
- Rheumatoid arthritis (RA)
- Scleroderma
- Amyloidosis
- Chronic hepatitis C
- Whipple's disease
- Polyarteritis nodosa
- Behçet's disease
- Familial Mediterranean fever
- Blind loop syndrome

Arthritis and Diarrhea

- Viral syndrome
- Inflammatory bowel disease (IBD)
- Celiac disease
- Whipple's disease
- Enterogenic (bacterial) reactive arthritis
- Collagenous colitis
- Behçet's disease
- Hyperthyroidism
- Spondyloarthropathy
- Blind loop syndrome

Arthritis and Eye Lesions[5]

- Systemic lupus erythematosus (SLE)
- Sjögren's syndrome
- Behçet's syndrome
- Sarcoidosis
- Subacute bacterial endocarditis (SBE)
- Lyme disease
- Wegener's granulomatosis
- Giant cell arteritis
- Takayasu's arteritis
- Rheumatoid arthritis (RA), juvenile rheumatoid arthritis (JRA)
- Scleroderma
- Inflammatory bowel disease (IBD)
- Whipple's disease
- Ankylosing spondylitis
- Reactive arthritis
- Psoriatic arthritis

Arthritis and Heart Murmur[5]

- Subacute bacterial endocarditis (SBE)
- Cardiac myxoma
- Ankylosing spondylitis
- Reactive arthritis
- Acute rheumatic fever
- Rheumatoid arthritis (RA)

- Systemic lupus erythematosus (SLE) with Libman-Sacks endocarditis
- Relapsing polychondritis

Arthritis and Muscle Weakness[9]

- Rheumatoid arthritis (RA)
- Ankylosing spondylitis
- Polymyositis
- Dermatomyositis
- Systemic lupus erythematosus (SLE), scleroderma, mixed connective tissue disease
- Sarcoidosis
- HIV infection–associated arthritis
- Whipple's disease

Arthritis and Rash[5]

- Chronic urticaria
- Vasculitic urticaria
- Systemic lupus erythematosus (SLE)
- Dermatomyositis
- Polymyositis
- Psoriatic arthritis
- Reactive arthritis
- Chronic sarcoidosis
- Serum sickness
- Sweet's syndrome
- Leprosy

Arthritis and Subcutaneous Nodules[5]

- Rheumatoid arthritis (RA)
- Gout
- Pseudogout (rare)
- Sarcoidosis
- Light-chain amyloidosis (LA) (primary, multiple myeloma)
- Acute rheumatic fever (ARF)
- Hemochromatosis

- Whipple's disease
- Multicentric reticulohistiocytosis

Arthritis and Weight Loss[5]

- Severe rheumatoid arthritis (RA)
- RA with vasculitis
- Reactive arthritis
- RA or psoriatic arthritis or ankylosing spondylitis with amyloidosis
- Cancer
- Enteropathic arthritis (Crohn's disease, ulcerative colitis)
- HIV infection
- Whipple's disease
- Blind loop syndrome
- Scleroderma with intestinal bacterial overgrowth

Arthritis, Axial Skeleton

- Rheumatoid arthritis (RA)
- Psoriatic arthritis
- Reiter's syndrome
- Ankylosing spondylitis
- Juvenile RA
- Degenerative disease of the nucleus pulposus
- Spondylosis deformans
- Diffuse idiopathic skeletal hyperostosis (DISH)
- Alkaptonuria
- Infection

Arthritis, Fever, and Rash[5]

- Rubella, parvovirus B19
- Gonococcemia, meningococcemia
- Secondary syphilis, Lyme borreliosis
- Adult acute rheumatic fever, adult Still's disease, adult Kawasaki's disease
- Vasculitic urticaria
- Acute sarcoidosis

- Familial Mediterranean fever (FMF)
- Hyperimmunoglobulinemia D and periodic fever syndrome

Arthritis, Granulomatous

- Sarcoidosis
- Fungal arthritis
- Metastatic cancer
- Primary or metastatic synovial tumors

Arthritis, Juvenile, Rheumatoid

- Infectious causes of fever
- Systemic lupus erythematosus (SLE)
- Rheumatic fever
- Drug reaction
- Serum sickness
- "Viral arthritis"
- Lyme arthritis

Arthritis, Monarticular and Oligoarticular[2]

- Septic arthritis (*Staphylococcus aureus*, *Neisseria gonorrhoeae*, meningococci, streptococci, *Streptococcus pneumoniae*, enteric gram-negative bacilli)
- Crystalline-induced arthritis (gout, pseudogout; calcium oxalate, hydroxyapatite, and other basic calcium/phosphate crystals)
- Traumatic joint injury
- Hemarthrosis
- Monarticular or oligoarticular flare of an inflammatory polyarticular rheumatic disease (rheumatoid arthritis [RA], psoriatic arthritis, Reiter's syndrome, systemic lupus erythematosus [SLE])

Arthritis, Pediatric Age[20]

RHEUMATIC DISEASES OF CHILDHOOD
- Acute rheumatic fever
- Systemic lupus erythematosus (SLE)

- Juvenile ankylosing spondylitis
- Polymyositis and dermatomyositis
- Vasculitis
- Scleroderma
- Psoriatic arthritis
- Mixed connective tissue disease and overlap syndromes
- Kawasaki's disease
- Behçet's syndrome
- Familial Mediterranean fever
- Reiter's syndrome
- Reflex sympathetic dystrophy
- Fibromyalgia (fibrositis)

INFECTIOUS DISEASES
- Bacterial arthritis
- Viral or postviral arthritis
- Fungal arthritis
- Osteomyelitis
- Reactive arthritis

NEOPLASTIC DISEASES
- Leukemia
- Lymphoma
- Neuroblastoma
- Primary bone tumors

NONINFLAMMATORY DISORDERS
- Trauma
- Avascular necrosis syndromes
- Osteochondroses
- Slipped capital femoral epiphysis
- Diskitis
- Patellofemoral dysfunction (chondromalacia patellae)
- Toxic synovitis of the hip
- Overuse syndromes
- Genetic or congenital syndromes

HEMATOLOGIC DISORDERS
- Sickle cell disease
- Hemophilia
- Inflammatory bowel disease (IBD)

MISCELLANEOUS
- Growing pains
- Psychogenic arthralgias (conversion reactions)
- Hypermobility syndrome
- Villonodular synovitis
- Foreign body arthritis

Arthritis, Polyarticular

- Rheumatoid arthritis (RA), juvenile (rheumatoid) polyarthritis
- Systemic lupus erythematosus (SLE), other connective tissue diseases, erythema nodosum, palindromic rheumatism, relapsing polychondritis
- Psoriatic arthritis, ankylosing spondylitis
- Sarcoidosis
- Lyme arthritis, bacterial endocarditis, *N. gonorrhoeae* infection, rheumatic fever, Reiter's disease
- Crystal deposition disease
- Hypersensitivity to serum or drugs
- Hepatitis B, HIV infection, rubella, mumps
- Other: serum sickness, leukemias, lymphomas, enteropathic arthropathy, Whipple's disease, Behçet's syndrome, Henoch-Schönlein purpura, familial Mediterranean fever, hypertrophic pulmonary osteoarthropathy

Arthritis, Psoriatic

- Rheumatoid arthritis (RA)
- Erosive osteoarthritis
- Gouty arthritis
- Ankylosing spondylitis

Arthritis, Rheumatoid

- Systemic lupus erythematosus (SLE)
- Seronegative spondyloarthropathies
- Polymyalgia rheumatica
- Acute rheumatic fever
- Scleroderma
- Osteoarthritis

Arthritis, Septic

- Gout
- Pseudogout
- Trauma
- Hemarthrosis
- Rheumatic fever
- Adult or juvenile rheumatoid arthritis
- Spondyloarthropathies such as Reiter's syndrome
- Osteomyelitis
- Viral arthritides
- Septic bursitis

Asbestosis

- Silicosis
- Siderosis, other pneumoconioses
- Lung cancer
- Atelectasis

Ascites

- Hypoalbuminemia: nephrotic syndrome, protein-losing gastroenteropathy, starvation
- Cirrhosis
- Hepatic congestion: congestive heart failure (CHF), constrictive pericarditis, tricuspid insufficiency, hepatic vein obstruction (Budd-Chiari syndrome), inferior vena cava or portal vein obstruction
- Peritoneal infections: TB and other bacterial infections, fungal diseases, parasites
- Neoplasms: primary hepatic neoplasms, metastases to liver or peritoneum, lymphomas, leukemias, myeloid metaplasia
- Lymphatic obstruction: mediastinal tumors, trauma to the thoracic duct, filariasis
- Ovarian disease: Meigs' syndrome, struma ovarii
- Chronic pancreatitis or pseudocyst: pancreatic ascites
- Leakage of bile: bile ascites
- Urinary obstruction or trauma: urine ascites

- Myxedema
- Chylous ascites

Aspergillosis

- Tuberculosis
- Cystic fibrosis
- Carcinoma of the lung
- Eosinophilic pneumonia
- Bronchiectasis
- Sarcoidosis
- Lung abscess

Asthenia

- Depression
- Chronic fatigue syndrome
- Sleep disorders
- Anemia
- Hypothyroidism
- Sedentary lifestyle
- Medications (e.g., narcotics, sedatives)
- Infections
- Dehydration/electrolyte disorders
- COPD and other pulmonary disorders
- Renal failure
- Congestive heart failure (CHF)
- Diabetes
- Addison's disease
- Paraneoplastic syndrome

Asthma

- Congestive heart failure (CHF)
- Chronic obstructive pulmonary disease (COPD)
- Pulmonary embolism (in adult and elderly patients)
- Foreign body aspiration (most frequent in younger patients)
- Pneumonia and other upper respiratory infections
- Rhinitis with postnasal drip
- TB

- Hypersensitivity pneumonitis
- Anxiety disorder
- Wegener's granulomatosis
- Diffuse interstitial lung disease

Asthma, Childhood[4]

INFECTIONS
- Bronchiolitis (RSV)
- Pneumonia
- Croup
- Tuberculosis, histoplasmosis
- Bronchiectasis
- Bronchiolitis obliterans
- Bronchitis
- Sinusitis

ANATOMIC, CONGENITAL
- Cystic fibrosis
- Vascular rings
- Ciliary dyskinesia
- B lymphocyte immune defect
- Congestive heart failure (CHF)
- Laryngotracheomalacia
- Tumor, lymphoma
- H-type tracheoesophageal fistula
- Repaired tracheoesophageal fistula
- Gastroesophageal reflux

VASCULITIS, HYPERSENSITIVITY
- Allergic bronchopulmonary aspergillosis
- Allergic alveolitis, hypersensitivity pneumonitis
- Churg-Strauss syndrome
- Periarteritis nodosa

OTHER
- Foreign body aspiration
- Pulmonary thromboembolism
- Psychogenic cough
- Sarcoidosis

- Bronchopulmonary dysplasia
- Vocal cord dysfunction

Ataxia

- Vertebral-basilar artery ischemia
- Diabetic neuropathy
- Tabes dorsalis
- Vitamin B_{12} deficiency
- Multiple sclerosis and other demyelinating diseases
- Meningomyelopathy
- Cerebellar neoplasms, hemorrhage, abscess, infarct
- Nutritional (Wernicke's encephalopathy)
- Paraneoplastic syndromes
- Parainfectious: Guillain-Barré syndrome, acute ataxia of childhood and young adults
- Toxins: phenytoin, alcohol, sedatives, organophosphates
- Wilson's disease (hepatolenticular degeneration)
- Hypothyroidism
- Myopathy
- Cerebellar and spinocerebellar degeneration: ataxia-telangiectasia, Friedreich's ataxia
- Frontal lobe lesions: tumors, thrombosis of anterior cerebral artery, hydrocephalus
- Labyrinthine destruction: neoplasm, injury, inflammation, compression
- Hysteria
- AIDS

Ataxia, Acute or Recurrent[11]

- Drug ingestion (e.g., phenytoin, carbamazepine, sedatives, hypnotics, and phencyclidine) or intoxication (e.g., alcohol, ethylene glycol, hydrocarbon fumes, lead, mercury, or thallium)
- Postinfectious (cerebellitis [e.g., varicella], acute disseminated encephalomyelitis)
- Head trauma
- Basilar migraine
- Benign paroxysmal vertigo (migraine equivalent)

- Brain tumor or neuroblastoma (if accompanied by opsoclonus or myoclonus [i.e., "dancing eyes, dancing feet"])
- Hydrocephalus
- Infection (e.g., labyrinthitis, abscess)
- Seizure (ictal or postictal)
- Vascular events (e.g., cerebellar hemorrhage or stroke)
- Miller-Fisher variant of Guillain-Barré syndrome (ataxia, ophthalmoplegia, and areflexia). WARNING: If bulbar signs are present, disease is likely progressive; patient may lose ability to protect airway or ability to breathe.
- Inherited ataxias
- Inborn errors of metabolism (e.g., mitochondrial disorders, aminoacidopathies, urea cycle defects)
- Conversion reaction
- Multiple sclerosis

Ataxia, Chronic or Progressive[11]

- Hydrocephalus
- Hypothyroidism
- Tumor or paraneoplastic syndrome
- Low vitamin E levels (e.g., cystic fibrosis)
- Wilson's disease
- Inborn errors of metabolism
- Inherited ataxias (e.g., ataxia-telangiectasia, Friedreich's ataxia)

Ataxia-Telangiectasia

- Friedreich's ataxia
- Abetalipoproteinemia (Bassen-Kornzweig syndrome)
- Acquired vitamin E deficiency
- Early-onset cerebellar ataxia with retained reflexes (EOCA)
- Ataxia associated with biochemical abnormalities: associated with ceroid lipofuscinosis, xeroderma pigmentosa, Cockayne's syndrome, adrenoleukodystrophy, metachromatic leukodystrophy, mitochondrial disease, sialidosis, Niemann-Pick disease

Atelectasis

- Infection (pneumonia, TB, fungal, histoplasmosis)
- Lung neoplasm (primary or metastatic)

- Postoperative (lower lobes)
- Sarcoidosis
- Mucoid impaction
- Foreign body
- Postinflammatory (middle lobe syndrome)
- Pneumothorax
- Pleural effusion
- Pneumoconiosis
- Interstitial fibrosis
- Bulla
- Mediastinal or adjacent mass

Atrial Fibrillation

- Multifocal atrial tachycardia
- Atrial flutter
- Frequent atrial premature beats
- Baseline ECG artifact

Atrial Flutter

- Atrial fibrillation
- Paroxysmal atrial tachycardia
- ECG baseline artifact
- Atrial ectopy

Atrial Myxoma

- Mitral stenosis
- Mitral regurgitation
- Tricuspid stenosis
- Tricuspid regurgitation
- Pulmonary hypertension
- Endocarditis
- Vasculitis
- Left atrial thrombus
- Pulmonary embolism
- Cerebrovascular accidents
- Collagen-vascular disease

- Carcinoid heart disease
- Ebstein's anomaly

Atrial Septal Defect (ASD)

- Primary pulmonary hypertension
- Pulmonary stenosis
- Rheumatic heart disease
- Mitral valve prolapse
- Cor pulmonale

Atrioventricular Nodal Block[15]

- Idiopathic fibrosis (Lenègre's disease)
- Sclerodegenerative processes (e.g., Lev's disease with calcification of the mitral and aortic annuli)
- AV node radiofrequency ablation procedure
- Medications (e.g., digoxin, β-blockers, calcium channel blockers, class III antiarrhythmics)
- Acute inferior wall myocardial infarction (MI)
- Myocarditis
- Infections (endocarditis, Lyme disease)
- Infiltrative diseases (e.g., hemochromatosis, sarcoidosis, amyloidosis)
- Trauma (including cardiac surgical procedures)
- Collagen-vascular diseases
- Aortic root diseases (e.g., spondylitis)
- Electrolyte abnormalities (e.g., hyperkalemia)

Atrium Enlargement, Right Atrium

- Right ventricular failure
- Atrial septal defect
- Tricuspid regurgitation
- Tricuspid stenosis
- Pulmonary hypertension
- Restrictive cardiomyopathy
- Right atrial myxoma
- Ebstein's anomaly
- Anomalous pulmonary venous drainage to the right atrium

- Endomyocardial fibrosis
- Sinus of Valsalva fistula
- Arrhythmogenic right ventricular dysplasia

Attention-Deficit/Hyperactivity Disorder (ADHD)

- In early childhood, may be difficult to distinguish from normal active children
- ADHD may overlap symptoms in children with disruptive behavior, such as conduct disorder or oppositional defiant disorders
- School and behavioral problems are associated with a learning disability (these disorders often coexist)
- Bipolar disorder may be confused with ADHD, but it can be distinguished by the episodic nature of bipolar illness and the pervasive presence of ADHD

Atypical Mole

- Melanoma
- Lentigo maligna
- Compound nevus
- Flat wart
- Seborrheic keratosis

Autistic Spectrum Disorder

- Rett's syndrome: occurs in females; exhibits head growth deceleration, loss of previously acquired motor skills, and incoordination
- Childhood disintegration disorder: development normal until the age of 2 years, followed by regression
- Childhood-onset schizophrenia: follows period of normal development
- Asperger's syndrome: lacks the language developmental abnormalities of autism
- Isolated symptoms of autism: when occurring in isolation, defined as disorders (i.e., selective mutism, expressive language disorder,

mixed receptive-expressive language disorder, or stereotypic movement disorder)

AV Nodal Block[15]

- Idiopathic fibrosis (Lenègre's disease)
- Sclerodegenerative processes (e.g., Lev's disease with calcification of the mitral and aortic annuli)
- AV node radiofrequency ablation procedure
- Medications (e.g., digoxin, β-blockers, calcium channel blockers, class III antiarrhythmics)
- Acute inferior wall MI
- Myocarditis
- Infections (endocarditis, Lyme disease)
- Infiltrative diseases (e.g., hemochromatosis, sarcoidosis, amyloidosis)
- Trauma (including cardiac surgical procedures)
- Collagen-vascular diseases
- Aortic root diseases (e.g., spondylitis)
- Electrolyte abnormalities (e.g., hyperkalemia)

Babesiosis

- Amebiasis
- Ehrlichiosis
- Hepatic abscess
- Leptospirosis
- Malaria
- Salmonellosis, including typhoid fever
- Acute viral hepatitis
- Hemorrhagic fever

Bacillary Angiomatosis

- Pyogenic granuloma
- Angiokeratoma
- Kaposi's sarcoma
- Hemangioma
- Melanoma
- Abscess

Back Pain

- Trauma: injury to bone, joint, or ligament
- Mechanical: pregnancy, obesity, fatigue, scoliosis
- Degenerative: osteoarthritis
- Infections: osteomyelitis, subarachnoid or spinal abscess, TB, meningitis, basilar pneumonia
- Metabolic: osteoporosis, osteomalacia
- Vascular: leaking aortic aneurysm, subarachnoid or spinal hemorrhage/infarction
- Neoplastic: myeloma; Hodgkin's disease; carcinoma of pancreas; metastatic neoplasm from breast, prostate, lung
- GI: penetrating ulcer, pancreatitis, cholelithiasis, inflammatory bowel disease (IBD)
- Renal: hydronephrosis, calculus, neoplasm, renal infarction, pyelonephritis
- Hematologic: sickle cell crisis, acute hemolysis
- Gynecologic: neoplasm of uterus or ovary, dysmenorrhea, salpingitis, uterine prolapse
- Inflammatory: ankylosing spondylitis, psoriatic arthritis, Reiter's syndrome
- Lumbosacral strain
- Psychogenic: malingering, hysteria, anxiety
- Endocrine: adrenal hemorrhage or infarction

Back Pain, Children and Adolescents

- Trauma (muscle strain, vertebral fracture)
- Idiopathic scoliosis, kyphosis
- Psychological problem
- Infection (pyelonephritis, osteomyelitis)
- Inflammatory spondyloarthropathy
- Tumor
- Herniated disk
- Spondylolysis, spondylolisthesis
- Sickle cell crisis
- Syrinx

Back Pain, Viscerogenic Origin

- Urolithiasis
- Aortic aneurysm
- Colorectal carcinoma
- Endometriosis
- Tubal pregnancy
- Prostatitis
- Peptic ulcer
- Pancreatitis
- Diverticular spasm
- Metastatic neoplasm (e.g., bladder, uterus, ovary, kidney)

Baker's Cyst

- Deep venous thrombosis (DVT)
- Popliteal aneurysms
- Abscess
- Tumors
- Lymphadenopathy
- Varicosities
- Ganglion

Balanitis

- Leukoplakia
- Reiter's syndrome
- Lichen planus
- Balanitis xerotica obliterans
- Psoriasis
- Carcinoma of the penis
- Erythroplasia of Queyrat

Ballism*

- Cerebral infarction or hemorrhage
- Medications (e.g., dopamine agonists, phenytoin)

---

*Violent, flinging, non-patterned rapid movements.

- CNS neoplasm (primary or metastatic)
- Nonketotic hyperosmolar state

Barrett's Esophagus

- Gastroesophageal reflux disease (GERD), uncomplicated
- Erosive esophagitis
- Gastritis
- Hiatal hernia
- Peptic ulcer disease
- Angina
- Malignant neoplasm
- Stricture or Schatzki's ring

Bartter's Syndrome

- Diuretic abuse
- Surreptitious vomiting
- Gitelman's syndrome
- Autosomal dominant hypocalcemia
- Hyperprostaglandin E syndrome

Basal Cell Carcinoma

- Keratoacanthoma
- Squamous cell carcinoma
- Wart
- Seborrheic keratosis
- Melanoma (pigmented basal cell carcinoma)
- Xeroderma pigmentosum
- Basal cell nevus syndrome
- Molluscum contagiosum
- Sebaceous hyperplasia
- Psoriasis

Basophilia

- Inflammatory processes
- Leukemia
- Polycythemia vera

- Hodgkin's lymphoma
- Hemolytic anemia
- Post splenectomy
- Myeloid metaplasia
- Myxedema

Becker's Nevus

- Melanoma
- Congenital melanocytic nevus
- Postinflammatory pigmentation
- Nevus spilus
- Café au lait macule

Behçet's Syndrome

- Ulcerative colitis
- Crohn's disease
- Lichen planus
- Pemphigoid
- Herpes simplex infection
- Benign aphthous stomatitis
- Systemic lupus erythematosus (SLE)
- Reiter's syndrome
- Ankylosing spondylitis
- AIDS
- Hypereosinophilic syndrome
- Sweet's syndrome

Bell's Palsy

- Neoplasms affecting the base of the skull or the parotid gland
- Bacterial infectious process (meningitis, otitis media, osteomyelitis of the base of the skull)
- Brainstem stroke
- Multiple sclerosis
- Sarcoidosis
- Head trauma with fracture of temporal bone
- Other: Guillain-Barré syndrome, carcinomatous or leukemic meningitis, leprosy, Melkersson-Rosenthal syndrome

Bile Duct, Dilated[39]

- Normal variant
- Post cholecystectomy
- Unsuspected bile duct stone
- Sphincter of Oddi stenosis
- Occult bile duct stricture
- Previous bile duct injury
- Early carcinoma of the pancreas, carcinoma of the bile duct or carcinoma of the ampulla
- Extrinsic compression of the bile duct by a primary or secondary neoplasm

Bipolar Disorder

- Secondary manias caused by medical disorder (e.g., renal disease, AIDS, stroke, digoxin toxicity) are frequent.
- Onset of mania after the age of 40 years is suggestive of secondary mania.
- Less severe, and probably distinct, conditions of bipolar type II and cyclothymia are possible.
- Cross-sectional examination of acutely manic patient can be confused with schizophreniform or paranoid psychosis.

Bites and Stings, Arachnids

- Cellulitis
- Urticaria
- Other tick-borne illnesses
  - Babesiosis
  - Tick-borne relapsing fever
  - Tularemia
  - Rocky Mountain spotted fever
  - Ehrlichiosis
  - Colorado tick fever
  - Tick paralysis
- Community-acquired cutaneous methicillin-resistant *Staphylococcus aureus* infection

Bites and Stings, Insect

- Stings: cellulitis, bites
- Bites: stings, cellulitis

Bites, Snake

- Harmless snakebite
- Scorpion bite
- Insect bite
- Cellulitis
- Laceration or puncture wound

NOTE: Harmless snakebites are usually characterized by four rows of small scratches (teeth in upper jaw) separated from two rows of scratches (teeth in lower jaw). This is in distinction to venomous snakebites, which should have puncture wounds produced by the snake's fangs, whether other teeth marks are noted.

Bite Wounds

- Bite from a rabid animal (often the attack is unprovoked)
- Factitious injury

Bladder Cancer

- Urinary tract infection
- Frequency-urgency syndrome
- Interstitial cystitis
- Stone disease
- Endometriosis
- Neurogenic bladder

Blastomycosis

PULMONARY INFECTION
- Tuberculosis
- Bronchogenic carcinoma
- Histoplasmosis
- Bacterial pneumonia

CUTANEOUS INFECTION

- Bromoderma
- Pyoderma gangrenosum
- *Mycobacterium marinum* infection
- Squamous cell carcinoma
- Giant keratoacanthoma

Bleeding, Lower GI

(ORIGINATING BELOW THE LIGAMENT OF TREITZ)

Small Intestine

- Ischemic bowel disease (mesenteric thrombosis, embolism, vasculitis, trauma)
- Small bowel neoplasm: leiomyomas, carcinoids
- Hereditary hemorrhagic telangiectasia (Rendu-Osler-Weber syndrome)
- Meckel's diverticulum and other small intestine diverticula
- Aortoenteric fistula
- Intestinal hemangiomas: blue rubber bleb nevi, intestinal hemangiomas, cutaneous vascular nevi
- Hamartomatous polyps: Peutz-Jeghers syndrome (intestinal polyps, mucocutaneous pigmentation)
- Infections of small bowel: tuberculous enteritis, enteritis necroticans
- Volvulus
- Intussusception
- Lymphoma of small bowel, sarcoma, Kaposi's sarcoma
- Irradiation ileitis
- AV malformation of small intestine
- Inflammatory bowel disease (IBD)
- Polyarteritis nodosa
- Other: pancreaticoenteric fistulas, Henoch-Schönlein purpura, Ehlers-Danlos syndrome, systemic lupus erythematosus (SLE), amyloidosis, metastatic melanoma

Colon

- Carcinoma (particularly left colon)
- Diverticular disease
- Inflammatory bowel disease (IBD)
- Ischemic colitis

- Ischemic colitis
- Infective colitis

Bleeding Time Elevation

- Thrombocytopenia
- Capillary wall abnormalities
- Platelet abnormalities (Bernard-Soulier disease, Glanzmann's disease)
- Drugs (aspirin, warfarin, anti-inflammatory medications, streptokinase, urokinase, dextran, β-lactam antibiotics, moxalactam)
- Disseminated intravascular coagulation (DIC)
- Cirrhosis
- Uremia
- Myeloproliferative disorders
- von Willebrand disease

Bleeding, Upper GI

(ORIGINATING ABOVE THE LIGAMENT OF TREITZ)
- Oral or pharyngeal lesions: swallowed blood from nose or oropharynx
- Swallowed hemoptysis
- Esophageal: varices, ulceration, esophagitis, Mallory-Weiss tear, carcinoma, trauma
- Gastric: peptic ulcer (including Cushing's and Curling's ulcers), gastritis, angiodysplasia, gastric neoplasms, hiatal hernia, gastric diverticulum, pseudoxanthoma elasticum, Rendu-Osler-Weber syndrome
- Duodenal: peptic ulcer, duodenitis, angiodysplasia, aortoduodenal fistula, duodenal diverticulum, duodenal tumors, carcinoma of ampulla of Vater, parasites (e.g., hookworm), Crohn's disease
- Biliary: hematobilia (e.g., penetrating injury to liver, hepatobiliary malignant neoplasm, endoscopic papillotomy)

Bleeding, Upper GI, Pediatric[2]

<3 MONTHS
- Swallowed maternal blood
- Gastritis
- Ulcer, stress
- Bleeding diathesis
- Foreign body (nasogastric [NG] tube)
- Vascular malformation
- Duplication

<2 YEARS
- Esophagitis
- Gastritis
- Ulcer
- Pyloric stenosis
- Mallory-Weiss syndrome
- Vascular malformation
- Duplication

<5 YEARS
- Esophagitis
- Gastritis
- Ulcer
- Esophageal varices
- Foreign body
- Mallory-Weiss syndrome
- Hemophilia
- Vascular malformations

5–18 YEARS
- Esophagitis
- Gastritis
- Ulcer
- Esophageal varices
- Mallory-Weiss syndrome
- Inflammatory bowel disease (IBD)
- Hemophilia
- Vascular malformation

Blepharitis

- Keratoconjunctivitis sicca
- Eyelid malignant neoplasms
- Herpes simplex blepharitis
- Molluscum contagiosum
- Phthiriasis palpebrarum
- *Phthirus pubis* (pubic lice)
- *Demodex folliculorum* (transparent mites)
- Allergic blepharitis

Blindness, Geriatric Age

- Cataracts
- Glaucoma
- Diabetic retinopathy
- Macular degeneration
- Trauma
- Cerebrovascular accident (CVA)
- Corneal scarring

Blindness, Monocular, Transient

- Migraine (vasospasm)
- Embolic cerebrovascular disease
- Intermittent angle-closure glaucoma
- Partial retinal vein occlusion
- Hyphema
- Optic disc edema
- Giant cell arteritis
- Psychogenic
- Hypotension
- Hypercoagulopathy disorders
- Multiple sclerosis

Blindness, Pediatric Age[24]

CONGENITAL
- Optic nerve hypoplasia or aplasia
- Optic coloboma

- Congenital hydrocephalus
- Hydranencephaly
- Porencephaly
- Microencephaly
- Encephalocele, particularly occipital type
- Morning glory disc
- Aniridia
- Anterior microphthalmia
- Peters' anomaly
- Persistent pupillary membrane
- Glaucoma
- Cataracts
- Persistent hyperplastic primary vitreous

PHAKOMATOSES

- Tuberous sclerosis
- Neurofibromatosis (special association with optic glioma)
- Sturge-Weber syndrome
- von Hippel–Lindau disease

TUMORS

- Retinoblastoma
- Optic glioma
- Perioptic meningioma
- Craniopharyngioma
- Cerebral glioma
- Posterior and intraventricular tumors when complicated by hydrocephalus
- Pseudotumor cerebri

NEURODEGENERATIVE DISEASES

- Cerebral storage disease
- Gangliosidoses, particularly Tay-Sachs disease (infantile amaurotic familial idiocy), Sandhoff's variant, generalized gangliosidosis
- Other lipidoses and ceroid lipofuscinoses, particularly the late-onset amaurotic familial idiocies, such as those of Jansky-Bielschowsky disease and of Batten-Mayou disease and Spielmeyer-Vogt disease
- Mucopolysaccharidoses, particularly Hurler's syndrome and Hunter's syndrome

- Leukodystrophies (dysmyelination disorders), particularly metachromatic leukodystrophy and Canavan's disease
- Demyelinating sclerosis (myelinoclastic diseases), especially Schilder's disease and Devic's neuromyelitis optica
- Special types: Dawson's disease, Leigh disease, Bassen-Kornzweig syndrome, Refsum's disease
- Retinal degenerations: retinitis pigmentosa and its variants, Leber's congenital type
- Optic atrophies: congenital autosomal recessive type, infantile and congenital autosomal dominant types, Leber's disease, and atrophies associated with hereditary ataxias—the types of Behr, of Marie, and of Sanger Brown

INFECTIOUS PROCESSES
- Encephalitis, especially in the prenatal infection syndromes caused by *Toxoplasma gondii*, cytomegalovirus, rubella virus, *Treponema pallidum*, herpes simplex
- Meningitis, arachnoiditis
- Chorioretinitis
- Endophthalmitis
- Keratitis

HEMATOLOGIC DISORDERS
- Leukemia with CNS involvement

VASCULAR AND CIRCULATORY DISORDERS
- Collagen-vascular diseases
- Arteriovenous malformations—intracerebral hemorrhage, subarachnoid hemorrhage
- Central retinal occlusion

TRAUMA
- Contusion or avulsion of optic nerves, chiasm, globe, cornea
- Cerebral contusion or laceration
- Intracerebral, subarachnoid, or subdural hemorrhage

DRUGS/TOXINS
OTHER
- Retinopathy of prematurity
- Sclerocornea
- Conversion reaction

- Optic neuritis
- Osteopetrosis

Blisters, Subepidermal

- Burns
- Porphyria cutanea tarda
- Bullous pemphigoid
- Bullous drug reaction
- Arthropod bite reaction
- Toxic epidermal necrosis
- Dermatitis herpetiformis
- Polymorphous light eruption
- Variegate porphyria
- Lupus erythematosus
- Epidermolysis bullosa
- Pseudoporphyria
- Acute graft-versus-host reaction
- Linear IgA disease
- Leukocytoclastic vasculitis
- Pressure necrosis
- Urticaria pigmentosa
- Amyloidosis

Body Dysmorphic Disorder

- Anorexia nervosa
- Obsessive-compulsive disorder
- Anxiety disorder
- Social phobia
- Hypochondriasis
- Personality disorder

Bone Lesions, Preferential Site of Origin[36]

EPIPHYSIS
- Chondroblastoma
- Giant cell tumor—after fusion of growth plate
- Langerhans cell histiocytosis

- Clear cell chondrosarcoma
- Osteosarcoma

METAPHYSIS
- Parosteal sarcoma
- Chondrosarcoma
- Fibrosarcoma
- Nonossifying fibroma
- Giant cell tumor—before fusion of growth plate
- Unicameral bone cyst
- Aneurysmal bone cyst

DIAPHYSIS
- Myeloma
- Ewing's tumor
- Reticulum cell sarcoma

METADIAPHYSEAL
- Fibrosarcoma
- Fibrous dysplasia
- Enchondroma
- Osteoid osteoma
- Chondromyofibroma

Bone Marrow Failure Syndromes, Inherited[21]

BILINEAGE AND TRILINEAGE CYTOPENIAS
- Fanconi's anemia
- Shwachman-Diamond syndrome
- Dyskeratosis congenita
- Amegakaryocytic thrombocytopenia
- Other inherited thrombocytopenia disorders
- Other genetic syndromes
- Down syndrome
- Dubowitz syndrome
- Seckel's syndrome
- Reticular dysgenesis
- Schimke immuno-osseous dysplasia
- Noonan's syndrome
- Cartilage-hair hypoplasia
- Familial marrow failure (non-Fanconi)

UNILINEAGE CYTOPENIA
- Diamond-Blackfan anemia
- Kostmann's syndrome/congenital neutropenia
- *ELA2* mutations
- *HAX1* mutations
- GFII mutations
- WASP mutations
- Constitutive cell surface G-CSF-R mutations
- Other inherited neutropenia syndromes
- Barth syndrome
- Glycogen storage disease Ib
- Miscellaneous
- Thrombocytopenia with absent radii
- Congenital dyserythropoietic anemias (CDAs)
  - Types I, II, III, IV
  - Variants
  - Nonclassifiable CDAs
  - Groups IV, V, VI, VII

Bone Marrow Fibrosis[14]

- Myeloid disorders
- Myelofibrosis with myeloid metaplasia
- Metastatic cancer
- Chronic myeloid leukemia
- Myelodysplastic syndrome
- Atypical myeloid disorder
- Acute megakaryocytic leukemia
- Other acute myeloid leukemias
- Gray platelet syndrome
- Lymphoid disorders
- Hairy cell leukemia
- Multiple myeloma
- Lymphoma
- Nonhematologic disorders
- Connective tissue disorder
- Infections (tuberculosis, kala-azar)
- Vitamin D–deficiency rickets
- Renal osteodystrophy

Bone Mineral Density, Increased

- Paget's disease of bone
- Skeletal metastases
- DISH
- Osteonecrosis
- Sarcoidosis
- Hypoparathyroidism, pseudohypoparathyroidism
- Milk-alkali syndrome
- Osteopetrosis
- Hypervitaminosis A or D
- Dysplasias (craniodiaphyseal, craniometaphyseal, frontometaphyseal)
- Endosteal hyperostosis
- Fluorosis
- Heavy metal poisoning
- Ionizing radiation
- Other: lymphoma, leukemia, mastocytosis, multiple myeloma, polycythemia vera

Bone Pain

- Trauma
- Neoplasm (primary or metastatic)
- Osteoporosis with compression fracture
- Paget's disease of bone
- Infection (osteomyelitis, septic arthritis)
- Osteomalacia
- Viral syndrome
- Sickle cell disease
- Anxiety

Bone Resorption[36]

DISTAL CLAVICLE
- Hyperparathyroidism
- Rheumatoid arthritis (RA)
- Scleroderma
- Post-traumatic osteolysis

- Progeria
- Pycnodysostosis
- Cleidocranial dysplasia

INFERIOR ASPECT OF RIBS

- Vascular impression, associated with but not limited to coarctation of the aorta
- Hyperparathyroidism
- Neurofibromatosis

TERMINAL PHALANGEAL TUFTS

- Scleroderma
- Raynaud's phenomenon
- Vascular disease
- Frostbite, electrical burns
- Psoriasis
- Tabes dorsalis
- Hyperparathyroidism

GENERALIZED RESORPTION

- Paraplegia
- Myositis ossificans
- Osteoporosis

Bone Tumor, Primary Malignant

- Osteomyelitis
- Metastatic bone disease
- Bone cyst
- Benign bone neoplasm

Borderline Personality Disorder

- Histrionic and narcissistic personality disorders share some common features.
- Dysthymia and other depressive disorders: require a stability of affective symptoms not seen in BPD.
- Bipolar disorder: mood changes in BPD are often triggered by stressors and are less sustained than in bipolar disorder.
- Substance abuse or dependence: often induces impulsive, emotionally labile behavior.

- Post-traumatic stress disorder (PTSD): individuals with BPD often have history of trauma but do not avoid the feared stimulus or reexperience the trauma, as do individuals with PTSD.
- Mild cases of schizophrenia may superficially resemble BPD.

Botulism

- Myasthenia gravis
- Guillain-Barré syndrome
- Tick paralysis
- Cerebrovascular accident (CVA)

Bowen's Disease

- Psoriasis
- Basal cell carcinoma
- Lupus
- Actinic keratosis
- Seborrheic keratosis
- Paget's disease

Bradycardia, Sinus[15]

- Idiopathic
- Degenerative processes (e.g., Lev's disease, Lenègre's disease): medications, β-blockers, some calcium channel blockers (diltiazem, verapamil), digoxin (when vagal tone is high)
- Class I antiarrhythmic agents (e.g., procainamide), class III antiarrhythmic agents (amiodarone, sotalol), clonidine, lithium carbonate
- Acute myocardial ischemia and infarction
- Right or left circumflex coronary artery occlusion or spasm
- High vagal tone (e.g., athletes)

Brain Neoplasm

- Stroke
- Abscess/parasitic cyst
- Demyelinating disease: multiple sclerosis, postinfectious encephalomyelitis

- Metastatic tumors
- Primary central nervous system lymphoma
- Brain abscess

Breast Cancer

- Fibrocystic changes
- Fibroadenoma
- Hamartoma
- Fat necrosis
- Hematoma
- Duct ectasia
- Mammary adenosis

Breast Inflammatory Lesion[12]

- Mastitis (*Staphylococcus aureus*, beta-hemolytic streptococcus)
- Trauma
- Foreign body (sutures, breast implants)
- Granuloma (TB, fungal)
- Fat necrosis post biopsy
- Necrosis or infarction (anticoagulant therapy, pregnancy)
- Breast malignant neoplasm

Breast Mass

- Fibrocystic breasts
- Benign tumors (fibroadenoma, papilloma)
- Mastitis (acute bacterial mastitis, chronic mastitis)
- Malignant neoplasm
- Fat necrosis
- Hematoma
- Duct ectasia
- Mammary adenosis
- Breast abscess

Breath Odor[35]

- Sweet, fruity: diabetic ketoacidosis (DKA), starvation ketosis
- Fishy, stale: uremia (trimethylamines)

- Ammonia-like: uremia (ammonia)
- Musty fish, clover: fetor hepaticus (hepatic failure)
- Foul, feculent: intestinal obstruction/diverticulum
- Foul, putrid: nasal/sinus pathology (infection, foreign body, cancer), respiratory infections (empyema, lung abscess, bronchiectasis)
- Achalasia
- Halitosis: tonsillitis, gingivitis, respiratory infections, Vincent's angina, gastroesophageal reflux, *Helicobacter pylori* infection, Zenker's diverticulum
- Cinnamon: pulmonary TB

Breathing, Noisy[35]

- Infection: upper respiratory infection, peritonsillar abscess, retropharyngeal abscess, epiglottitis, laryngitis, tracheitis, bronchitis, bronchiolitis
- Irritants and allergens: hyperactive airway, asthma (reactive airway disease), rhinitis, angioneurotic edema
- Compression from outside of the airway: esophageal cysts or foreign body, neoplasms, lymphadenopathy
- Congenital malformation and abnormality: vascular rings, laryngeal webs, laryngomalacia, tracheomalacia, hemangiomas within the upper airway, stenoses within the upper airway, cystic fibrosis
- Acquired abnormality (at every level of the airway): nasal polyps, hypertrophied adenoids or tonsils, foreign body, intraluminal tumors, bronchiectasis
- Neurogenic disorder: vocal cord paralysis

Bronchiectasis

- TB
- Asthma
- Chronic bronchitis or chronic sinusitis
- Interstitial fibrosis
- Chronic lung abscess
- Foreign body aspiration
- Cystic fibrosis
- Lung carcinoma

Bronchitis, Acute

- Pneumonia
- Asthma
- Sinusitis
- Bronchiolitis
- Aspiration
- Cystic fibrosis
- Pharyngitis
- Cough secondary to medications
- Neoplasm (elderly patients)
- Influenza
- Allergic aspergillosis
- Gastroesophageal reflux disease (GERD)
- Congestive heart failure (CHF) (in elderly patients)
- Bronchogenic neoplasm

Brown Urine

- Bile pigments
- Myoglobin
- Concentrated urine
- Use of multivitamin supplements
- Medications (antimalarials, metronidazole, nitrofurantoin, levodopa, methyldopa, phenazopyridine)
- Diet rich in fava beans
- Urinary tract infection

Bruising

- Medication induced (warfarin, aspirin, NSAIDs, prednisone)
- Alcohol abuse
- Senile purpura
- Purpura simplex
- Physical abuse
- Vasculitis
- Platelet disorders
- Coagulation factor deficiencies
- Cushing's disease

- Vitamin C deficiency
- Marfan syndrome
- Ehlers-Danlos syndrome
- Disseminated intravascular coagulation
- Leukemia
- Hereditary hemorrhagic telangiectasia

Bruxism

- Anxiety disorder
- Dental compression syndrome
- Temporomandibular joint disorders
- Chronic orofacial pain disorders
- Oral motor disorders
- Malocclusion

Budd-Chiari Syndrome

- Shock liver/ischemic hepatitis
- Viral hepatitis
- Toxic hepatitis
- Hepatic veno-occlusive disease
- Alcoholic hepatitis
- Pancreatitis
- Cholecystitis
- Perforated viscus
- Peptic ulcer disease
- Cardiac cirrhosis (i.e., chronic right-sided heart failure)
- Alcoholic cirrhosis
- Cirrhosis of other etiologies: Wilson's disease, hemochromatosis, α_1-antitrypsin deficiency, autoimmune

Bulimia

- Schizophrenia
- GI disorders
- Neurologic disorders (seizures, Kleine-Levin syndrome, Klüver-Bucy syndrome)
- Brain neoplasms
- Psychogenic vomiting

Bullous Diseases

- Bullous pemphigoid
- Pemphigus vulgaris
- Pemphigus foliaceus
- Paraneoplastic pemphigus
- Cicatricial pemphigoid
- Erythema multiforme
- Dermatitis herpetiformis
- Herpes gestationis
- Impetigo
- Erosive lichen planus
- Linear IgA bullous dermatosis
- Epidermolysis bullosa acquisita

Bullous Pemphigoid

- Cicatricial pemphigoid
- Herpes gestationis
- Epidermolysis bullosa acquisita
- Systemic lupus erythematosus (SLE)
- Erythema multiforme
- Pemphigus
- Drug eruptions
- Pemphigoid nodularis

Burning Mouth Syndrome

- Mucosal disease such as lichen planus or candidiasis
- Nutritional deficiency in zinc, iron, or folate or vitamins B_1, B_2, B_6, B_9, B_{12}
- Dry mouth from Sjögren's syndrome or after chemotherapy or radiation therapy
- Cranial nerve injury
- Medication effect

Burns

- Cellulitis/abscess
- Insect bite (spider bite)

- Bullous erysipelas
- Carbuncle/furuncle
- Anthrax

Bursitis

- Degenerative joint disease
- Tendinitis (sometimes occurs in conjunction with bursitis)
- Cellulitis (if bursitis is septic)
- Infectious arthritis

Café au Lait Macule

- Seborrheic keratosis
- Multiple lentigines syndrome
- Lentigo
- Nevi

Calcification on Chest Radiograph

- Lung neoplasm (primary or metastatic)
- Silicosis
- Idiopathic pulmonary fibrosis
- Tuberculosis
- Histoplasmosis
- Disseminated varicella infection
- Mitral stenosis (end stage)
- Secondary hyperparathyroidism

Calcifications, Cutaneous

- Calcification, Raynaud's phenomenon, esophageal dysmotility, sclerodactyly, and telangiectasia (CREST) syndrome
- Trauma
- Pancreatitis or pancreatic cancer
- Chronic renal failure
- Sarcoidosis
- Hyperparathyroidism
- Milk-alkali syndrome
- Hypervitaminosis D

- Panniculitis
- Idiopathic
- Iatrogenic (e.g., application of calcium alginate dressing to skin)
- Multiple myeloma
- Dermatomyositis
- Parasitic infections
- Leukemia
- Lymphoma

Calcium Stones

- Medications (e.g., antacids, loop diuretics, vitamin D, acetazolamide, glucocorticoids)
- Primary hyperparathyroidism
- Hypercalcemia from malignant disease
- Sarcoidosis
- Prolonged immobilization
- Hyperoxaluria (e.g., Crohn's disease, celiac disease, chronic pancreatitis)
- Hyperuricosuria (e.g., hyperuricemia, excessive dietary purine, allopurinol, probenecid)
- Renal tubular acidosis
- Milk-alkali syndrome
- Thyrotoxicosis
- Hypocitraturia (e.g., metabolic acidosis, hypomagnesemia, hypokalemia)

Candidiasis

- Tinea
- Eczema
- Seborrheic dermatitis
- Psoriasis
- Cellulitis

Candidiasis, Vulvovaginal

- Bacterial vaginosis
- Trichomoniasis

Carbon Monoxide Poisoning

- Viral syndromes
- Cyanide
- Hydrogen sulfide
- Methemoglobinemia
- Amphetamines and derivatives
- Cocaine
- Cyclic antidepressants
- PCP
- Phenothiazines
- Theophylline toxicity

Carcinoid Syndrome

- Idiopathic flushing
- Anxiety
- Menopause
- Hyperthyroidism
- Medications (e.g., niacin)

Cardiac Arrest, Nontraumatic[27]

- Cardiac (coronary artery disease, cardiomyopathies, structural abnormalities, valve dysfunction, arrhythmias)
- Respiratory (upper airway obstruction, hypoventilation, pulmonary embolism, asthma, COPD exacerbation, pulmonary edema)
- Circulatory (tension pneumothorax, pericardial tamponade, pulmonary embolism [PE], hemorrhage, sepsis)
- Electrolyte abnormalities (hypokalemia or hyperkalemia, hypomagnesemia or hypermagnesemia, hypocalcemia)
- Medications (tricyclic antidepressants, digoxin, theophylline, calcium channel blockers)
- Drug abuse (cocaine, heroin, amphetamines)
- Toxins (carbon monoxide, cyanide)
- Environmental (drowning/near-drowning, electrocution, lightning, hypothermia or hyperthermia, venomous snakes)

Cardiac Death, Sudden[1]

NONCARDIAC
- CNS hemorrhage
- Massive pulmonary embolus
- Drug overdose
- Hypoxia secondary to lung disease
- Aortic dissection or rupture

CARDIAC
- Ventricular tachycardia
- Bradyarrhythmia, sick sinus syndrome
- Aortic stenosis
- Tetralogy of Fallot
- Pericardial tamponade
- Cardiac tumors
- Complications of infective endocarditis
- Hypertrophic cardiomyopathy (arrhythmia or obstruction)
- Myocardial ischemia
- Atherosclerosis
- Prinzmetal's angina
- Kawasaki's arteritis

Cardiac Enlargement[15]

CARDIAC CHAMBER ENLARGEMENT
- Chronic volume overload: mitral or aortic regurgitation, left-to-right shunt (patent ductus arteriosus [PDA], ventricular septal defect [VSD], arteriovenous [AV] fistula)
- Cardiomyopathy: ischemic, nonischemic
- Decompensated pressure overload: aortic stenosis, hypertension
- High-output states: severe anemia, thyrotoxicosis
- Bradycardia: severe sinus bradycardia, complete heart block

LEFT ATRIUM
- Left ventricular (LV) failure of any cause
- Mitral valve disease
- Myxoma

RIGHT VENTRICLE
- Chronic LV failure of any cause
- Chronic volume overload: tricuspid or pulmonic regurgitation, left-to-right shunt (atrial septal defect [ASD])
- Decompensated pressure overload: pulmonic stenosis, pulmonary veno-occlusive disease, pulmonary artery hypertension: primary, secondary (pulmonary embolism [PE], chronic obstructive pulmonary disease [COPD])

RIGHT ATRIUM
- Right ventricular (RV) failure of any cause
- Tricuspid valve disease
- Myxoma
- Ebstein's anomaly

MULTICHAMBER ENLARGEMENT
- Hypertrophic cardiomyopathy
- Acromegaly
- Severe obesity

PERICARDIAL DISEASE
- Pericardial effusion with or without tamponade
- Effusive constrictive disease
- Pericardial cyst, loculated effusion

PSEUDOCARDIOMEGALY
- Epicardial fat
- Chest wall deformity (pectus excavatum, straight back syndrome)
- Low lung volumes
- Anteroposterior (AP) chest radiograph
- Mediastinal tumor, cyst

Cardiac Murmurs

SYSTOLIC
- Mitral regurgitation (MR)
- Tricuspid regurgitation (TR)
- Ventricular septal defect (VSD)
- Aortic stenosis (AS)
- Hypertrophic obstructive cardiomyopathy
- Pulmonic stenosis (PS)

- Innocent murmur of childhood
- Coarctation of aorta
- Mitral valve prolapse (MVP)

DIASTOLIC
- Aortic regurgitation (AR)
- Atrial myxoma
- Mitral stenosis (MS)
- Pulmonary artery branch stenosis
- Tricuspid stenosis (TS)
- Graham Steell murmur (diastolic decrescendo murmur heard in severe pulmonary hypertension)
- Pulmonic regurgitation (PR)
- Severe MR
- Austin Flint murmur (diastolic rumble heard in severe AR)
- Severe VSD and patent ductus arteriosus

CONTINUOUS
- Patent ductus arteriosus
- Pulmonary arteriovenous (AV) fistula

Cardiac Tamponade

- Chronic obstructive pulmonary disease (COPD)
- Constrictive pericardial disease
- Restrictive cardiomyopathy
- Right ventricular infarction
- Pulmonary embolism

Cardioembolism

- Acute MI
- Atrial fibrillation
- Left ventricular aneurysm
- Valvular heart disease (e.g., rheumatic mitral valve disease, mitral valve prolapse)
- Dilated cardiomyopathy
- Atrial septal defect
- Patent foramen ovale
- Cardioversion for atrial fibrillation

- Infective endocarditis
- Atrial septal aneurysm
- Sick sinus syndrome and cardiac arrhythmias
- Nonbacterial thrombotic endocarditis
- Prosthetic heart valves
- Atrial myxoma and other intracardiac tumors
- Cyanotic heart disease
- Balloon angioplasty
- Coronary artery bypass grafting
- Aneurysms of sinus of Valsalva
- Other: VVI pacing, ventricular support devices, heart transplantation, intracardiac defects with paradoxical embolism

Cardiogenic Shock

- Myocardial infarction
- Arrhythmias
- Pericardial effusion/tamponade
- Chest trauma
- Valvular heart disease
- Myocarditis
- Cardiomyopathy
- Congestive heart failure (CHF), end stage

Cardiomyopathy, Congestive

- Frank pulmonary disease
- Valvular dysfunction
- Pericardial abnormalities
- Coronary atherosclerosis
- Psychogenic dyspnea

Cardiomyopathy, Dilated

- Frank pulmonary disease
- Valvular dysfunction
- Pericardial abnormalities
- Coronary atherosclerosis
- Psychogenic dyspnea

Cardiomyopathy, Hypertrophic

- Coronary atherosclerosis
- Valvular dysfunction
- Pericardial abnormalities
- Chronic pulmonary disease
- Psychogenic dyspnea

Cardiomyopathy, Restrictive

- Coronary atherosclerosis
- Valvular dysfunction
- Pericardial abnormalities
- Chronic lung disease
- Psychogenic dyspnea

Carpal Tunnel

- Cervical radiculopathy
- Chronic tendinitis
- Vascular occlusion
- Reflex sympathetic dystrophy
- Osteoarthritis
- Other arthritides
- Other entrapment neuropathies

Cataracts

- Corneal lesions
- Retinal lesions, detached retina, tumors
- Vitreous disease, chronic inflammation

Cat-Scratch Disease

- TB
- Sarcoidosis
- Sporotrichosis
- Toxoplasmosis
- Lymphogranuloma venereum
- Fungal diseases

- Benign and malignant tumors
- Tularemia

Cavernous Sinus Thrombosis

- Orbital cellulitis
- Internal carotid artery aneurysm
- Cerebrovascular accident (CVA)
- Migraine headache
- Allergic blepharitis
- Thyroid exophthalmos
- Brain tumor
- Meningitis
- Mucormycosis
- Trauma

Cavitary Lesion on Chest Radiograph[17]

NECROTIZING INFECTIONS

- Bacteria: anaerobes, *Staphylococcus aureus*, enteric gram-negative bacteria, *Pseudomonas aeruginosa*, *Legionella* species, *Haemophilus influenzae*, *Streptococcus pyogenes*, *Streptococcus pneumoniae*, *Rhodococcus*, *Actinomyces*
- Mycobacteria: *Mycobacterium tuberculosis*, *Mycobacterium kansasii*, *Mycobacterium avium-intracellulare* (MAI)
- Bacteria-like: *Nocardia* species
- Fungi: *Coccidioides immitis*, *Histoplasma capsulatum*, *Blastomyces hominis*, *Aspergillus* species, *Mucor* species
- Parasitic: *Entamoeba histolytica*, *Echinococcus*, *Paragonimus westermani*

CAVITARY INFARCTION

- Bland infarction (with or without superimposed infection)
- Lung contusion

SEPTIC EMBOLISM

- *S. aureus*, anaerobes, others

VASCULITIS

- Wegener's granulomatosis, periarteritis

NEOPLASMS
- Bronchogenic carcinoma, metastatic carcinoma, lymphoma

MISCELLANEOUS LESIONS
- Cysts, blebs, bullae, or pneumatocele with or without fluid collections
- Sequestration
- Empyema with air-fluid level
- Bronchiectasis

Celiac Disease

- Inflammatory bowel disease (IBD)
- Laxative abuse
- Intestinal parasitic infestations
- Other: irritable bowel syndrome, tropical sprue, chronic pancreatitis, Zollinger-Ellison syndrome, cystic fibrosis (children), lymphoma, eosinophilic gastroenteritis, short bowel syndrome, Whipple's disease

Cellulitis

- Erythrasma
- Septic arthritis
- DVT
- Peripheral vascular insufficiency
- Paget's disease of the breast
- Thrombophlebitis
- Acute gout
- Psoriasis
- *Candida* intertrigo
- Pseudogout
- Osteomyelitis
- Insect bite
- Lymphedema

Cerebral Infarction Secondary to Inherited Disorders

- Homocystinuria
- Marfan syndrome

- Ehlers-Danlos syndrome
- Rendu-Osler-Weber syndrome
- Pseudoxanthoma elasticum
- Fabry's disease

Cerebrovascular Disease, Ischemic[40]

VASCULAR DISORDERS
- Large-vessel atherothrombotic disease
- Lacunar disease
- Arterial-to-arterial embolization
- Carotid or vertebral artery dissection
- Fibromuscular dysplasia
- Migraine
- Venous thrombosis
- Radiation
- Complications of arteriography
- Multiple, progressive intracranial arterial occlusions

INFLAMMATORY DISORDERS
- Giant cell arteritis
- Polyarteritis nodosa
- Systemic lupus erythematosus (SLE)
- Granulomatous angiitis
- Takayasu's disease
- Arteritis associated with amphetamine, cocaine, or phenylpropanolamine
- Syphilis, mucormycosis
- Sjögren's syndrome
- Behçet's syndrome

CARDIAC DISORDERS
- Rheumatic heart disease
- Mural thrombus
- Arrhythmias
- Mitral valve prolapse
- Prosthetic heart valve
- Endocarditis
- Myxoma
- Paradoxical embolus

HEMATOLOGIC DISORDERS
- Thrombotic thrombocytopenic purpura
- Sickle cell disease
- Hypercoagulable states
- Polycythemia
- Thrombocytosis
- Leukocytosis
- Lupus anticoagulant

Cervical Cancer

- Cervical polyp
- Prolapsed uterine fibroid
- Preinvasive cervical lesions
- Neoplasia metastatic from a separate primary

Cervical Disk Disease

- Rotator cuff tendinitis
- Carpal tunnel syndrome
- Thoracic outlet syndrome
- Brachial neuritis

Cervical Dysplasia

- Metaplasia
- Hyperkeratosis
- Condyloma
- Microinvasive carcinoma
- Glandular epithelial abnormalities
- Adenocarcinoma in situ
- Metastatic tumor involvement of the cervix

Cervical Polyp

- Endometrial polyp
- Prolapsed myoma
- Retained products of conception
- Squamous papilloma

- Sarcoma
- Cervical malignant neoplasm

Cervicitis

- Carcinoma of the cervix
- Cervical erosion
- Cervical metaplasia

Chagas' Disease

- Acute disease: early African trypanosomiasis, New World cutaneous and mucocutaneous leishmaniasis
- Chronic disease: idiopathic cardiomyopathy, idiopathic achalasia, congenital or acquired megacolon

Chancroid

- Syphilis
- Herpes simplex
- Lymphogranuloma venereum
- Granuloma inguinale
- Traumatic ulceration
- Behçet's disease
- Crohn's disease

Charcot's Joint

- Osteomyelitis, cellulitis, abscess
- Infectious arthritis
- Osteoarthritis
- Rheumatoid and other inflammatory arthritides

Chest Pain, Children[4]

MUSCULOSKELETAL (COMMON)
- Trauma (accidental, abuse)
- Exercise, overuse injury (strain, bursitis)
- Costochondritis (Tietze's syndrome)

- Herpes zoster (cutaneous)
- Pleurodynia
- Fibrositis
- Slipping rib
- Sickle cell anemia vaso-occlusive crisis
- Osteomyelitis (rare)
- Primary or metastatic tumor (rare)

PULMONARY (COMMON)
- Pneumonia
- Pleurisy
- Asthma
- Chronic cough
- Pneumothorax
- Infarction (sickle cell anemia)
- Foreign body
- Embolism (rare)
- Pulmonary hypertension (rare)
- Tumor (rare)

GASTROINTESTINAL (LESS COMMON)
- Esophagitis (gastroesophageal reflux)
- Esophageal foreign body
- Esophageal spasm
- Cholecystitis
- Subdiaphragmatic abscess
- Perihepatitis (Fitz-Hugh–Curtis syndrome)
- Peptic ulcer disease

CARDIAC (LESS COMMON)
- Pericarditis
- Postpericardiotomy syndrome
- Endocarditis
- Mitral valve prolapse
- Aortic or subaortic stenosis
- Arrhythmias
- Marfan syndrome (dissecting aortic aneurysm)
- Anomalous coronary artery
- Kawasaki's disease
- Cocaine, sympathomimetic ingestion
- Angina (familial hypercholesterolemia)

IDIOPATHIC (COMMON)
- Anxiety, hyperventilation
- Panic disorder

OTHER (LESS COMMON)
- Spinal cord or nerve root compression
- Breast-related pathologic condition
- Castleman's disease (lymph node neoplasm)

Chest Pain, Nonpleuritic[9]

- Cardiac: myocardial ischemia/infarction, myocarditis
- Esophageal: spasm, esophagitis, ulceration, neoplasm, achalasia, diverticula, foreign body
- Referred pain from subdiaphragmatic GI structures
- Gastric and duodenal: hiatal hernia, neoplasm, peptic ulcer disease (PUD)
- Gallbladder and biliary: cholecystitis, cholelithiasis, impacted stone, neoplasm
- Pancreatic: pancreatitis, neoplasm
- Dissecting aortic aneurysm
- Pain originating from skin, breasts, and musculoskeletal structures: herpes zoster, mastitis, cervical spondylosis
- Mediastinal tumors: lymphoma, thymoma
- Pulmonary: neoplasm, pneumonia, pulmonary embolism/infarction
- Psychoneurosis
- Chest pain associated with mitral valve prolapse

Chest Pain, Pleuritic

- Cardiac: pericarditis, postpericardiotomy/Dressler's syndrome
- Pulmonary: pneumothorax, hemothorax, embolism/infarction, pneumonia, empyema, neoplasm, bronchiectasis, pneumomediastinum, TB, carcinomatous effusion
- GI: liver abscess, pancreatitis, esophageal rupture, Whipple's disease with associated pericarditis or pleuritis
- Subdiaphragmatic abscess
- Pain originating from skin and musculoskeletal tissues: costochondritis, chest wall trauma, fractured rib, interstitial

fibrositis, myositis, strain of pectoralis muscle, herpes zoster, soft tissue and bone tumors
- Collagen-vascular diseases with pleuritis
- Psychoneurosis
- Familial Mediterranean fever

Chickenpox (Varicella)

- Other viral infection
- Impetigo
- Scabies
- Drug rash
- Urticaria
- Dermatitis herpetiformis
- Smallpox

Cholangitis

- Biliary colic
- Acute cholecystitis
- Liver abscess
- Peptic ulcer disease (PUD)
- Pancreatitis
- Intestinal obstruction
- Right kidney stone
- Hepatitis
- Pyelonephritis

Cholecystitis

- Hepatic: hepatitis, abscess, hepatic congestion, neoplasm, trauma
- Biliary: neoplasm, stricture
- Gastric: peptic ulcer disease (PUD), neoplasm, alcoholic gastritis, hiatal hernia
- Pancreatic: pancreatitis, neoplasm, stone in the pancreatic duct or ampulla
- Renal: calculi, infection, inflammation, neoplasm, ruptured kidney
- Pulmonary: pneumonia, pulmonary infarction, right-sided pleurisy

- Intestinal: retrocecal appendicitis, intestinal obstruction, high fecal impaction
- Cardiac: myocardial ischemia (particularly involving the inferior wall), pericarditis
- Cutaneous: herpes zoster
- Trauma
- Fitz-Hugh–Curtis syndrome (perihepatitis)
- Subphrenic abscess
- Dissecting aneurysm
- Nerve root irritation caused by osteoarthritis of the spine

Cholelithiasis

- Peptic ulcer disease (PUD)
- Gastroesophageal reflux disease (GERD)
- Inflammatory bowel disease (IBD)
- Pancreatitis
- Neoplasms
- Nonulcer dyspepsia
- Irritable bowel syndrome

Cholestasis[14]

- Extrahepatic
- Choledocholithiasis
- Bile duct stricture
- Cholangiocarcinoma
- Pancreatic carcinoma
- Chronic pancreatitis
- Papillary stenosis
- Ampullary cancer
- Primary sclerosing cholangitis
- Choledochal cysts
- Parasites (e.g., *Ascaris*, *Clonorchis sinensis*)
- AIDS
- Cholangiography
- Biliary atresia
- Portal lymphadenopathy
- Mirizzi's syndrome
- Intrahepatic

- Viral hepatitis
- Alcoholic hepatitis
- Drug induced
- Ductopenia syndromes
- Primary biliary cirrhosis
- Benign recurrent intrahepatic cholestasis
- Byler's disease
- Primary sclerosing cholangitis
- Alagille's syndrome
- Sarcoid
- Lymphoma
- Postoperative
- Total parenteral nutrition
- α_1-Antitrypsin deficiency

Chorea

- Medications (e.g., neuroleptics, tricyclics, antiparkinsonian drugs)
- Cerebral palsy
- Huntington's disease
- Benign hereditary chorea
- Thyroid disorder (hyperthyroidism, hypothyroidism)
- Friedreich's ataxia
- Ataxia-telangiectasia
- Hypoglycemia, hyperglycemia
- Electrolyte abnormalities (hyponatremia, hypocalcemia, hypomagnesemia, hypernatremia)
- Vitamin B_{12} deficiency
- Systemic lupus erythematosus (SLE)
- Wilson's disease
- Alcohol
- Cocaine
- Carbon monoxide poisoning
- Mercury poisoning

Choreoathetosis[29]

SYSTEMIC DISEASES
- Systemic lupus erythematosus (SLE)
- Polycythemia

- Thyrotoxicosis
- Rheumatic fever
- Cirrhosis of the liver (acquired hepatocerebral degeneration)
- Diabetes mellitus (DM)
- Wilson's disease

PRIMARY DEGENERATIVE BRAIN DISEASES
- Huntington's chorea
- Olivopontocerebellar atrophies
- Neuroacanthocytosis

FOCAL BRAIN DISEASES
- Hemichorea
- Stroke
- Tumor
- Arteriovenous malformation

DRUG-INDUCED CHOREOATHETOSIS
- Parkinson's disease drugs: levodopa
- Epilepsy drugs: phenytoin, carbamazepine, phenobarbital, gabapentin, valproate
- Psychostimulant drugs: cocaine, amphetamine, methamphetamine, dextroamphetamine, methylphenidate, pemoline, psychotropic drugs, lithium, tricyclic antidepressant drugs
- Oral contraceptive drugs: cimetidine

Chronic Fatigue Syndrome

- Psychosocial depression, dysthymia, anxiety-related disorders, and other psychiatric diseases
- Infectious diseases (subacute bacterial endocarditis [SBE], Lyme disease, fungal diseases, mononucleosis, HIV infection, chronic hepatitis B or C, TB, chronic parasitic infections)
- Autoimmune diseases: systemic lupus erythematosus (SLE), myasthenia gravis, multiple sclerosis, thyroiditis, rheumatoid arthritis (RA)
- Endocrine abnormalities: hypothyroidism, hypopituitarism, adrenal insufficiency, Cushing's syndrome, diabetes mellitus (DM), hyperparathyroidism, pregnancy, reactive hypoglycemia
- Occult malignant disease

- Substance abuse
- Systemic disorders: chronic renal failure, chronic obstructive pulmonary disease (COPD), cardiovascular disease, anemia, electrolyte abnormalities, liver disease
- Other: inadequate rest, sleep apnea, narcolepsy, fibromyalgia, sarcoidosis, medications, toxic agent exposure, Wegener's granulomatosis

Chronic Inflammatory Demyelinating Polyneuropathy (CIDP)

- Guillain-Barré syndrome (GBS), the difference being that GBS evolves during a maximum of 4 weeks and CIDP usually progresses during at least 8 weeks.
- Diabetic neuropathy: the distinction can often be made with electrodiagnostic studies, which typically show axonal physiology in diabetic neuropathy.
- Mononeuritis multiplex
- Monoclonal gammopathy of undetermined significance, plasma cell dyscrasia, osteosclerotic myeloma, and HIV infection are not so much part of the differential diagnosis but may coexist and so should always be sought.

Chronic Obstructive Pulmonary Disease (COPD)

- Congestive heart failure (CHF)
- Asthma
- Respiratory infections
- Bronchiectasis
- Cystic fibrosis
- Neoplasm
- Pulmonary embolism
- Sleep apnea, obstructive
- Hypothyroidism

Churg-Strauss Syndrome

- Polyarteritis nodosa
- Wegener's granulomatosis

* Sarcoidosis
* Loeffler's syndrome
* Henoch-Schönlein purpura
* Allergic bronchopulmonary aspergillosis
* Rheumatoid arthritis (RA)
* Leukocytoclastic vasculitis

Chylothorax

* Post lymph node dissection of neck or chest
* Subclavian venous catheterization
* Thoracic aneurysm repair
* Trauma to chest and neck
* Mediastinal tumor resection
* Esophagectomy, pneumonectomy
* Lymphangitis, mediastinitis
* Neoplasms (lymphoma; carcinoma of esophagus, lung; mediastinal malignant neoplasms)
* Sympathectomy
* Venous thrombosis
* Congenital

Cicatricial Pemphigoid

* Bullous pemphigoid
* Erythema multiforme
* Dermatitis herpetiformis
* Linear IgA dermatosis
* Pemphigus
* Stevens-Johnson's syndrome
* Herpes simplex, herpes zoster

Cirrhosis, Primary Biliary

* Drug-induced cholestasis
* Other etiologies of chronic liver disease and cirrhosis: alcoholic cirrhosis, viral hepatitis (chronic), primary sclerosing cholangitis, autoimmune chronic active hepatitis, chemical/toxin-induced cirrhosis, other hereditary or familial disorders (e.g., cystic fibrosis, α_1-antitrypsin deficiency)

Claudication

- Spinal stenosis (neurogenic claudication)
- Muscle cramps
- Degenerative osteoarthritic joint disease, particularly of the lumbar spine and hips
- Compartment syndrome

Cloudy Urine

- Concentrated urine
- Use of multivitamin supplements
- Diet high in purine-rich foods
- Pyuria
- Phosphaturia
- Urinary tract infection
- Lipiduria
- Chyluria
- Hyperoxaluria

Clubbing

- Pulmonary neoplasm (lung, pleura)
- Other neoplasm (GI, liver, Hodgkin's disease, thymus, osteogenic sarcoma)
- Pulmonary infectious process (empyema, abscess, bronchiectasis, TB, chronic pneumonitis)
- Extrapulmonary infectious process (subacute bacterial endocarditis, intestinal TB, bacterial or amebic dysentery, arterial graft sepsis)
- Pneumoconiosis
- Cystic fibrosis
- Sarcoidosis
- Cyanotic congenital heart disease
- Endocrine (Graves' disease, hyperparathyroidism)
- Inflammatory bowel disease (IBD)
- Celiac disease
- Chronic liver disease, cirrhosis (particularly biliary and juvenile)
- Pulmonary arteriovenous (AV) malformations
- Idiopathic

- Thyroid acropachy
- Hereditary (pachydermoperiostitis)
- Chronic trauma (jackhammer operators, machine workers)

Cobalamin Deficiency[21]

NUTRITIONAL COBALAMIN DEFICIENCY (I.E., INSUFFICIENT COBALAMIN INTAKE)

- Vegetarians, poverty-imposed near-vegetarians, breast-fed infants of mothers with pernicious anemia

ABNORMAL INTRAGASTRIC EVENTS (I.E., INADEQUATE PROTEOLYSIS OF FOOD COBALAMIN)

- Atrophic gastritis, partial gastrectomy with hypochlorhydria, proton pump inhibitors, H_2 blockers

LOSS OR ATROPHY OF GASTRIC OXYNTIC MUCOSA (I.E., DEFICIENT INTRINSIC FACTOR [IF] MOLECULES)

- Total or partial gastrectomy, pernicious anemia, caustic destruction (lye)

ABNORMAL EVENTS IN SMALL BOWEL LUMEN

- Inadequate pancreatic protease (e.g., R-cobalamin not degraded, cobalamin not transferred to IF)
- Insufficient pancreatic protease (i.e., pancreatic insufficiency)
- Inactivation of pancreatic protease (i.e., Zollinger-Ellison syndrome)
- Usurping of luminal cobalamin (i.e., inadequate cobalamin binding to IF)
  - By bacteria; during stasis syndromes (e.g., blind loops, pouches of diverticulosis, strictures, fistulas, anastomosis); impaired bowel motility (e.g., scleroderma); hypogammaglobulinemia
  - By *Diphyllobothrium latum* (fish tapeworm)

DISORDERS OF ILEAL MUCOSA/IF-COBALAMIN RECEPTORS (I.E., IF-COBALAMIN NOT BOUND TO IF-COBALAMIN RECEPTORS)

- Diminished or absent IF-cobalamin receptors (e.g., ileal bypass, resection, fistula)

- Abnormal mucosal architecture/function (e.g., tropical or nontropical sprue, Crohn's disease, tuberculous ileitis, infiltration by lymphomas, amyloidosis)
- IF/post IF–cobalamin receptor defects (e.g., Imerslund-Graesbeck syndrome, transcobalamin II [TC II] deficiency)
- Drug effects (e.g., Slow-K, metformin, cholestyramine, colchicine, neomycin)

DISORDERS OF PLASMA COBALAMIN TRANSPORT (I.E., TC II–COBALAMIN NOT DELIVERED TO TC II RECEPTORS)

- Congenital TC II deficiency, defective binding of TC II–cobalamin to TC II receptors (rare)

METABOLIC DISORDERS (I.E., COBALAMIN NOT USED BY CELLS)

- Inborn enzyme errors (rare)
- Acquired disorders (e.g., cobalamin functionally inactivated by irreversible oxidation, N_2O inhalation)

Cocaine Overdose

- Methamphetamine ("speed") abuse
- Methylenedioxyamphetamine ("ecstasy") abuse
- Cathinone ("khat") abuse
- Lysergic acid diethylamide (LSD) abuse
- Hyperthyroidism, panic disorder, pheochromocytoma

Coccidioidomycosis

- Acute pulmonary coccidioidomycoses: community-acquired pneumonias caused by *Mycoplasma* and *Chlamydia*; granulomatous diseases, such as *Mycobacterium tuberculosis* and sarcoidosis; other fungal diseases, such as *Blastomyces dermatitidis* and *Histoplasma capsulatum*
- Coccidioidomas: true neoplasms

Colic, Acute Abdominal[39]

- Acute gastroenteritis
- Food poisoning
- Nonspecific causes, anxiety disorder

- Constipation
- Gastric outlet obstruction
  - Chronic peptic ulceration
  - Gastric cancer

SMALL BOWEL OBSTRUCTION
Adhesions
- Postsurgical
- Inflammatory (e.g., diverticular)
- Radiation
- Meckel's diverticulum
- Metastatic

Stricture
- Ischemic
- Radiation
- Inflammatory (e.g., Crohn's disease)

Volvulus

Intussusception
- Tumor (e.g., Peutz-Jeghers syndrome)

Superior Mesenteric Artery Syndrome

Intraluminal Bolus
- Gallstone
- Bezoar

Hernia
- Abdominal wall
- Internal

Neoplasm
- Benign (e.g., leiomyoma)
- Malignant (e.g., carcinoid tumor, adenocarcinoma)
- Large bowel obstruction
- Colon cancer
- Diverticular disease
- Volvulus
- Uterine
- Missed abortion
- Parturition
- Period pain

Color Changes, Cutaneous[35]

BROWN
- Generalized: pituitary, adrenal, liver disease; adrenocorticotropic hormone (ACTH)–producing tumor (e.g., oat cell lung carcinoma)
- Localized: nevi, neurofibromatosis

WHITE
- Generalized: albinism
- Localized: vitiligo, Raynaud's syndrome

RED (ERYTHEMA)
- Generalized: fever, polycythemia, urticaria, viral exanthems
- Localized: inflammation, infection, Raynaud's syndrome

YELLOW
- Generalized: liver disease, chronic renal disease, anemia
- Generalized (except sclera): hypothyroidism, increased intake of vegetables containing carotene
- Localized: resolving hematoma, infection, peripheral vascular insufficiency

BLUE
- Lips, mouth, nail beds: cardiovascular and pulmonary diseases, Raynaud's syndrome

Colorado Tick Fever

- Rocky Mountain spotted fever
- Influenza
- Leptospirosis
- Infectious mononucleosis
- Cytomegalovirus (CMV) infection
- Pneumonia
- Hepatitis
- Meningitis
- Endocarditis
- Scarlet fever
- Measles
- Rubella

- Typhus
- Lyme disease
- Idiopathic thrombocytopenic purpura (ITP)
- Thrombotic thrombocytopenic purpura (TTP)
- Kawasaki's disease
- Toxic shock syndrome
- Vasculitis

Colorectal Cancer

- Diverticular disease
- Strictures
- Inflammatory bowel disease (IBD)
- Infectious or inflammatory lesions
- Adhesions
- Arteriovenous malformations
- Metastatic carcinoma (prostate, sarcoma)
- Extrinsic masses (cysts, abscesses)

Coma

- Vascular: hemorrhage, thrombosis, embolism
- CNS infections: meningitis, encephalitis, cerebral abscess
- Cerebral neoplasms with herniation
- Head injury: subdural hematoma, cerebral concussion, cerebral contusion
- Drugs: narcotics, sedatives, hypnotics
- Ingestion or inhalation of toxins: carbon monoxide (CO), alcohol, lead
- Metabolic disturbances
- Hypoxia
- Acid-base disorders
- Hypoglycemia, hyperglycemia
- Hepatic failure
- Electrolyte disorders
- Uremia
- Hypothyroidism
- Hypothermia, hyperthermia
- Hypotension, malignant hypertension
- Postictal

Coma, Normal Computed Tomography[1]

MENINGEAL DISORDERS

- Subarachnoid hemorrhage (uncommon)
- Bacterial meningitis
- Encephalitis
- Subdural empyema

EXOGENOUS TOXINS

- Sedative drugs and barbiturates
- Anesthetics and γ-hydroxybutyrate*
- Alcohols
- Stimulants
- Phencyclidine[†]
- Cocaine and amphetamine[††]
- Psychotropic drugs
- Cyclic antidepressants
- Phenothiazines
- Lithium
- Anticonvulsants
- Opioids
- Clonidine[§]
- Penicillins
- Salicylates
- Anticholinergics
- Carbon monoxide (CO), cyanide, and methemoglobinemia

ENDOGENOUS TOXINS, DEFICIENCIES, OR DERANGEMENTS

- Hypoxia and ischemia
- Hypoglycemia

---

*General anesthetic, similar to γ-aminobutyric acid; recreational drug and bodybuilding aid. Rapid onset, rapid recovery often with myoclonic jerking and confusion. Deep coma (2–3 hr; Glasgow Coma Scale score = 3) with maintenance of vital signs.

[†]Coma associated with cholinergic signs: lacrimation, salivation, bronchorrhea, and hyperthermia.

[††]Coma after seizures or status (i.e., a prolonged postictal state).

[§]An antihypertensive agent active through the opiate receptor system; frequent overdose when it is used to treat narcotic withdrawal.

- Hypercalcemia
- Osmolar
- Hyperglycemia
- Hyponatremia
- Hypernatremia
- Organ system failure
- Hepatic encephalopathy
- Uremic encephalopathy
- Pulmonary insufficiency (carbon dioxide narcosis)

SEIZURES
- Prolonged postictal state
- Spike-wave stupor

HYPOTHERMIA OR HYPERTHERMIA
- Brainstem ischemia
- Basilar artery stroke
- Brainstem or cerebellar hemorrhage
- Conversion or malingering

Coma, Pediatric Population[32]

ANOXIA
- Birth asphyxia
- Carbon monoxide (CO) poisoning
- Croup/epiglottitis
- Meconium aspiration

INFECTION
- Hemolysis
- Blood loss
- Hydrops fetalis
- Meningoencephalitis
- Sepsis
- Postimmunization encephalitis

INCREASED INTRACRANIAL PRESSURE
- Anoxia
- Inborn metabolic errors
- Toxic encephalopathy

- Reye's syndrome
- Head trauma/intracranial bleed
- Hydrocephalus
- Posterior fossa tumors

HYPERTENSIVE ENCEPHALOPATHY
- Coarctation of aorta
- Nephritis
- Vasculitis
- Pheochromocytoma

ISCHEMIA
- Hypoplastic left side of heart
- Shunting lesions
- Aortic stenosis
- Cardiovascular collapse (any cause)

PURPURIC CAUSES
- Disseminated intravascular coagulation
- Hemolytic-uremic syndrome
- Leukemia
- Thrombotic purpura

HYPERCAPNIA
- Cystic fibrosis
- Bronchopulmonary dysplasia
- Congenital lung anomalies

NEOPLASM
- Medulloblastoma
- Glioma of brainstem
- Posterior fossa tumors

DRUGS/TOXINS
- Maternal sedation
- Alcohol
- Any drug
- Lead
- Salicylism
- Arsenic
- Pesticides

ELECTROLYTE ABNORMALITIES
- Hypernatremia (diarrhea, dehydration, salt poisoning)
- Hyponatremia (syndrome of inappropriate antidiuretic hormone [SIADH], androgenital syndrome, gastroenteritis)
- Hyperkalemia (renal failure, salicylism, androgenitalism)
- Hypokalemia (diarrhea, hyperaldosteronism, salicylism, diabetic ketoacidosis [DKA])
- Hypocalcemia (vitamin D deficiency, hyperparathyroidism)
- Severe acidosis (sepsis, cold injury, salicylism, DKA)

HYPOGLYCEMIA
- Birth injury or stress
- Diabetes
- Alcohol
- Salicylism
- Hyperinsulinemia
- Iatrogenic

POSTSEIZURE
- Renal causes: nephritis, hypoplastic kidneys
- Hepatic causes: acute hepatitis, fulminant hepatic failure, inborn metabolic errors, bile duct atresia

Condyloma Acuminatum

- Abnormal anatomic variants or skin tags around labia minora and introitus, pearly penile papules
- Dysplastic warts
- Seborrheic keratosis
- Erythroplasia of Queyrat
- Lichen planus
- Verrucous carcinoma
- Bowenoid papulosis
- Syphilis

Congenital Adrenal Hyperplasia

- Precocious puberty
- Polycystic ovary syndrome
- Androgen resistance syndromes

- Pseudohermaphroditism
- Mixed gonadal dysgenesis
- Testicular carcinoma
- Leydig cell tumors
- Adrenocortical carcinoma
- Addison's disease
- Pituitary adenoma

Congestive Heart Failure

- Cirrhosis
- Nephrotic syndrome
- Venous occlusive disease
- Chronic obstructive pulmonary disease (COPD), asthma
- Pulmonary embolism
- Acute respiratory distress syndrome (ARDS)
- Heroin overdose
- Pneumonia
- Hypothyroidism

Conjunctival Neoplasm

MALIGNANT
- Squamous cell carcinoma
- Melanoma
- Sebaceous carcinoma
- Kaposi's sarcoma
- Metastatic neoplasms

BENIGN
- Melanocytic nevus
- Squamous papilloma
- Hemangioma
- Lymphangioma
- Myxoma

Conjunctivitis

- Corneal lesions
- Acute iritis

- Episcleritis
- Scleritis
- Uveitis
- Canalicular obstruction
- Acute glaucoma

Constipation

- Intestinal obstruction
- Fecal impaction
- Diverticular disease
- GI neoplasm
- Strangulated femoral hernia
- Gallstone ileus
- Tuberculous stricture
- Adhesions
- Ameboma
- Volvulus
- Intussusception
- Inflammatory bowel disease (IBD)
- Hematoma of bowel wall, secondary to trauma or anticoagulants
- Poor dietary habits: insufficient bulk in diet, inadequate fluid intake
- Change from daily routine: travel, hospital admission, physical inactivity
- Acute abdominal conditions: renal colic, salpingitis, biliary colic, appendicitis, ischemia
- Hypercalcemia or hypokalemia, uremia
- Irritable bowel syndrome, pregnancy, anorexia nervosa, depression
- Painful anal conditions: hemorrhoids, fissure, stricture
- Decreased intestinal peristalsis: old age, spinal cord injuries, myxedema, diabetes, multiple sclerosis, parkinsonism and other neurologic diseases
- Drugs: codeine, morphine, antacids with aluminum, verapamil, anticonvulsants, anticholinergics, disopyramide, cholestyramine, alosetron, iron supplements
- Hirschsprung's disease, meconium ileus, congenital atresia in infants

Constipation, Adult Patient[39]

NO GROSS STRUCTURAL ABNORMALITY

- Inadequate fiber intake
- Irritable bowel syndrome (associated with abdominal pain) or functional constipation
- Idiopathic slow-transit constipation
- "Obstructed defecation": pelvic floor dysfunction (or dyssynergia)

STRUCTURAL DISORDERS

- Anal fissure, infection, or stenosis
- Colon cancer or stricture
- Aganglionosis or abnormal myenteric plexus
  - Hirschsprung's disease
  - Chagas' disease
  - Neuropathic pseudo-obstruction
- Abnormal colonic muscle
  - Myopathy
  - Dystrophia myotonica
  - Systemic sclerosis
  - Idiopathic megarectum or megacolon
  - Proximal megacolon

NEUROLOGIC CAUSES

- Diabetic autonomic neuropathy
- Damage to the sacral parasympathetic outflow
- Spinal cord damage or disease (e.g., multiple sclerosis)
- Parkinson's disease
- Blunting of consciousness, mental retardation, psychosis
- Pain induced by straining (e.g., sciatic nerve compression)

ENDOCRINE OR METABOLIC CAUSES

- Hypothyroidism
- Hypercalcemia
- Porphyria
- Pregnancy

PSYCHOLOGICAL DISORDERS

- Depression
- Anorexia nervosa
- Denied bowel habit

DRUG SIDE EFFECTS

Contact Dermatitis (Contact Eczema)

- Impetigo
- Lichen simplex chronicus
- Atopic dermatitis
- Nummular eczema
- Seborrheic dermatitis
- Psoriasis
- Scabies
- Insect bites
- Sunburn
- Candidiasis

Conversion Disorder

- Malingering: dysfunction is consciously created for the purpose of secondary gain or avoidance of noxious duties.
- Factitious disorder (e.g., Munchausen's syndrome): dysfunction is consciously created for the purpose of assuming the patient role.
- Somatization: a related disorder in which psychological difficulties are manifested with a wide range of somatic complaints that affect several organ systems.

Corneal Abrasion

- Herpes ulcers and other corneal ulcers
- Foreign body in the cornea (be certain it is not a keratitis)
- Acute angle glaucoma

Corneal Sensation, Decreased

- Herpes (simplex, zoster)
- Contact lens wear
- Topical agents (NSAIDs, anesthetics, β-blockers)
- Diabetes
- Eye trauma
- Post surgery

Corneal Ulceration

- *Pseudomonas* and pneumococcus infection—virulent
- *Moraxella*, *Staphylococcus*, alpha-streptococcus infection—less virulent
- Herpes simplex infection or disease caused by other viruses

Cor Pulmonale

- Pulmonary thromboembolic disease
- Chronic obstructive pulmonary disease (COPD)
- Interstitial lung disease
- Neuromuscular diseases causing hypoventilation (e.g., antilymphocyte serum [ALS])
- Collagen-vascular disease (e.g., systemic lupus erythematosus [SLE]; calcinosis cutis, Raynaud's phenomenon, esophageal dysfunction, sclerodactyly, telangiectasia [CREST]; systemic sclerosis)
- Pulmonary venous disease
- Primary pulmonary hypertension

Costochondritis

- Tietze's syndrome
- Cardiovascular disease
- GI disease
- Pulmonary disease
- Osteoarthritis
- Cervical disk syndrome

Cough

- Infectious process (viral, bacterial)
- Postinfectious
- "Smoker's cough"
- Rhinitis (allergic, vasomotor, postinfectious)
- Asthma
- Exposure to irritants (noxious fumes, smoke, cold air)
- Drug induced (especially angiotensin-converting enzyme [ACE] inhibitors, β-blockers)

- Gastroesophageal reflux disease (GERD)
- Interstitial lung disease
- Lung neoplasms
- Lymphomas, mediastinal neoplasms
- Bronchiectasis
- Cardiac (congestive heart failure, pulmonary edema, mitral stenosis, pericardial inflammation)
- Recurrent aspiration
- Inflammation of larynx, pleura, diaphragm, mediastinum
- Cystic fibrosis
- Anxiety
- Other: pulmonary embolism, foreign body inhalation, aortic aneurysm, Zenker's diverticulum, osteophytes, substernal thyroid, thyroiditis, polymyalgia rheumatica (PMR)

Craniopharyngioma

- Pituitary adenoma
- Empty sella syndrome
- Pituitary failure of any cause
- Primary brain tumors (e.g., meningiomas, astrocytomas)
- Metastatic brain tumors
- Other brain tumors
- Cerebral aneurysm

Creutzfeldt-Jakob Disease

- Alzheimer's disease
- Frontotemporal dementia
- Lewy body disease
- Vascular dementia
- Others (hydrocephalus, infectious, vitamin deficiency, endocrine)

Crohn's Disease

- Ulcerative colitis
- Infectious diseases (TB, *Yersinia*, *Salmonella*, *Shigella*, *Campylobacter*)
- Parasitic infections (amebic infection)
- Pseudomembranous colitis

- Ischemic colitis in elderly patients
- Lymphoma
- Colon carcinoma
- Diverticulitis
- Irradiation enteritis
- Collagenous colitis
- Fungal infections (*Histoplasma*, *Actinomyces*)
- Gay bowel syndrome (in homosexual patient)
- Carcinoid tumors
- Celiac sprue
- Mesenteric adenitis

Cryoglobulinemia

- Serum sickness
- Antiphospholipid antibody syndrome
- Sarcoidosis
- Waldenström's hyperglobulinemia
- Septic vasculitis
- Polyarteritis nodosa

Cryptococcosis

- Acute or subacute meningitis (caused by *Neisseria meningitidis*, *Streptococcus pneumoniae*, *Haemophilus influenzae*, *Listeria monocytogenes*, *Mycobacterium tuberculosis*, *Histoplasma capsulatum*, viruses)
- Intracranial mass lesion (neoplasms, toxoplasmosis, TB)
- Pulmonary involvement confused with *Pneumocystis jiroveci* pneumonia when diffuse or confused with TB or bacterial pneumonia when focal or involving the pleura
- Skin lesions confused with bacterial cellulitis or molluscum contagiosum

Cryptorchidism

- Retractile testis
- Ascended testis
- Dislocated testis
- Anorchia

Cryptosporidiosis

- *Campylobacter*
- *Clostridium difficile*
- *Entamoeba histolytica*
- *Giardia lamblia*
- *Salmonella*
- *Shigella*
- Microsporida
- Cytomegalovirus
- *Mycobacterium avium*

Cubital Tunnel Syndrome

- Medial epicondylitis
- Medial elbow instability
- Carpal tunnel syndrome
- Cervical disk syndrome with radicular arm symptoms
- Ulnar nerve compression at wrist (Guyon's canal)

Cushing's Syndrome

- Alcoholic pseudo-Cushing's syndrome (endogenous cortisol overproduction)
- Obesity associated with diabetes mellitus (DM)
- Adrenogenital syndrome

Cutaneous Infections, Athletes

- Tinea pedis
- Tinea cruris
- Molluscum contagiosum
- Herpes simplex
- Verruca vulgaris
- Folliculitis
- Impetigo
- Furuncles
- Otitis externa
- Erythrasma

Cutaneous Larva Migrans

- Superficial thrombophlebitis
- Mondor's disease
- Lichen striatus
- Phytophotodermatitis
- Herpes zoster
- Migratory myiasis
- Scabies
- Loiasis
- Dracunculiasis
- Cercarial dermatitis
- Onchocerciasis
- Dirofilariasis
- Contact dermatitis
- Creeping hair
- Jellyfish stings
- Fascioliasis
- Bacterial folliculitis
- Tinea pedis/corporis
- Impetigo
- Erythema chronicum migrans of Lyme disease
- Ground itch
- Toxocariasis

Cutis Laxa

- Anetoderma (localized area of lax skin often with herniation of underlying tissues)
- Morphea
- Atrophoderma (disorders characterized by a depression in the skin surface)
- Pseudoxanthoma elasticum
- Ehlers-Danlos syndrome
- Marfan syndrome

Cyanosis

- Congenital heart disease with right-to-left shunt
- Pulmonary embolism

- Hypoxia
- Pulmonary edema
- Pulmonary disease (oxygen diffusion and alveolar ventilation abnormalities)
- Hemoglobinopathies
- Decreased cardiac output
- Vasospasm
- Arterial obstruction
- Pulmonary atrioventricular (AV) fistulas
- Elevated hemidiaphragm
- Neoplasm (bronchogenic carcinoma, mediastinal neoplasm, intrahepatic lesion)
- Substernal thyroid
- Infectious process (pneumonia, empyema, TB, subphrenic abscess, hepatic abscess)
- Atelectasis
- Idiopathic
- Eventration
- Phrenic nerve dysfunction (myelitis, myotonia, herpes zoster)
- Trauma to phrenic nerve or diaphragm (e.g., surgery)
- Aortic aneurysm
- Intra-abdominal mass
- Pulmonary infarction
- Pleurisy
- Radiation therapy
- Rib fracture
- Superior vena cava syndrome

Cylindroma

- Basal cell carcinoma
- Pilar cyst
- Pilomatricoma
- Follicular neoplasm
- Eccrine spiradenoma

Cysticercosis

- Idiopathic epilepsy
- Migraine

- Vasculitides
- Primary neoplasia of CNS
- Toxoplasmosis
- Brain abscess
- Granulomatous disease such as sarcoidosis

Cystic Fibrosis

- Immunodeficiency states
- Celiac disease
- Asthma
- Recurrent pneumonia
- Chronic aspiration

Cytomegalovirus Infection

- Congenital: acute viral, bacterial, parasitic infections including other congenitally transmitted agents (toxoplasmosis, rubella, syphilis, pertussis, croup, bronchitis)
- Acquired: Epstein-Barr virus (EBV) mononucleosis; viral hepatitis: A, B, C; cryptosporidiosis; toxoplasmosis; *Mycobacterium avium* infections; human herpesvirus 6; drug reaction; acute HIV infection

Daytime Sleepiness

- Sleep deprivation
- Medication induced (e.g., benzodiazepines, β-blockers, narcotics, sedative antidepressants, gabapentin)
- Depression
- Obstructive sleep apnea

- Medical illness (e.g., severe anemia, hypothyroidism, COPD, hepatic failure, renal insufficiency, CHF, electrolyte disturbances)
- Circadian rhythm abnormalities (e.g., jet lag, shift work sleep disorder)
- Restless legs syndrome
- Post trauma
- Narcolepsy
- Neurologic disorders (e.g., neurodegenerative disorders; parkinsonism; multiple sclerosis; lesions affecting thalamus, hypothalamus, or brainstem)

Decubitus Ulcer

- Stasis ulcer
- Burns
- Contact dermatitis
- Pyoderma gangrenosum
- Squamous cell carcinoma
- Bullous pemphigoid
- Traumatic ulcer

Delirium[27]

PHARMACOLOGIC AGENTS
- Anxiolytics (benzodiazepines)
- Antidepressants (e.g., amitriptyline, doxepin, imipramine)
- Cardiovascular agents (e.g., methyldopa, digitalis, reserpine, propranolol, procainamide, captopril, disopyramide)
- Antihistamines
- Cimetidine
- Corticosteroids
- Antineoplastics

- Drugs of abuse (alcohol, cannabis, amphetamines, cocaine, hallucinogens, opioids, sedative-hypnotics, phencyclidine [PCP])

METABOLIC DISORDERS
- Hypercalcemia
- Hypercapnia
- Hypoglycemia
- Hyponatremia
- Hypoxia

INFLAMMATORY DISORDERS
- Sarcoidosis
- Systemic lupus erythematosus (SLE)
- Giant cell arteritis

ORGAN FAILURE
- Hepatic encephalopathy
- Uremia

NEUROLOGIC DISORDERS
- Alzheimer's disease
- Cerebrovascular accident (CVA)
- Encephalitis (including HIV infection)
- Encephalopathies
- Epilepsy
- Huntington's disease
- Multiple sclerosis (MS)
- Neoplasms
- Normal-pressure hydrocephalus (NPH)
- Parkinson's disease
- Pick's disease
- Wilson's disease

ENDOCRINE DISORDERS
- Addison's disease
- Cushing's disease
- Panhypopituitarism
- Parathyroid disease
- Postpartum psychosis
- Recurrent menstrual psychosis
- Sydenham's chorea
- Thyroid disease

DEFICIENCY STATES
- Niacin
- Thiamine, vitamin B_{12}, and folate

Delirium, Dialysis Patient[27]

STRUCTURAL
- Cerebrovascular accident (CVA) (particularly hemorrhage)
- Subdural hematoma
- Intracerebral abscess
- Brain tumor

METABOLIC
- Disequilibrium syndrome
- Uremia
- Drug effects
- Meningitis
- Hypertensive encephalopathy
- Hypotension
- Postictal state
- Hypernatremia or hyponatremia
- Hypercalcemia
- Hypermagnesemia
- Hypoglycemia
- Severe hyperglycemia
- Hypoxemia
- Dialysis dementia

Dementia with Lewy Bodies

- Parkinson's disease dementia (PDD): differentiated from DLB, in which dementia usually precedes parkinsonism. A somewhat arbitrary "1-year" rule is sometimes used to differentiate DLB from PDD in that if dementia presents within the first year after the parkinsonism, DLB can still be diagnosed.
- Alzheimer's disease (AD): differs from DLB, in which visual hallucinations and parkinsonism are prominent.
- Atypical parkinsonian syndromes (multiple systems atrophy, progressive supranuclear palsy, corticobasal degeneration): these

syndromes have other features, such as cerebellar degeneration, supranuclear gaze palsy, and asymmetric limb apraxia, that are not seen in DLB.

- Vascular dementia: differs from DLB in that despite the fluctuations in performance seen in DLB, there is no clear history of multiple strokes.
- Frontotemporal dementia (FTD, also known as Pick's disease)
- Creutzfeldt-Jakob disease (CJD): differs from DLB in that it is usually more rapidly progressive, can have cerebellar signs and symptoms, and often has distinctive EEG abnormalities.
- Toxic-, metabolic-, or pharmacologic-related delirium

Demyelinating Diseases[40]

MULTIPLE SCLEROSIS (MS)
- Relapsing and chronic progressive forms
- Acute MS
- Neuromyelitis optica (Devic's disease)

DIFFUSE CEREBRAL SCLEROSIS
- Schilder's encephalitis periaxialis diffusa
- Baló's concentric sclerosis

ACUTE DISSEMINATED ENCEPHALOMYELITIS
- After measles, chickenpox, rubella, influenza, mumps
- After rabies or smallpox vaccination

NECROTIZING HEMORRHAGIC ENCEPHALITIS
- Hemorrhagic leukoencephalitis

LEUKODYSTROPHIES
- Krabbe's globoid leukodystrophy
- Metachromatic leukodystrophy
- Adrenoleukodystrophy
- Adrenomyeloneuropathy
- Pelizaeus-Merzbacher leukodystrophy
- Canavan's disease
- Alexander's disease

Dependent Personality

- Dependency and personality changes arising as a consequence of an Axis I disorder, such as mood disorders, social anxiety, panic disorder, and agoraphobia
- Dependency arising as a consequence of a general medical condition
- Most common comorbid Axis I conditions are major depressive and other mood disorders, anxiety disorders, including social phobia, and adjustment disorder.
- Most common comorbid personality disorders are histrionic, avoidant, and borderline. Each of these disorders is characterized by dependent features. Dependent personality disorder (DPD) is distinguished by its predominantly submissive, reactive, and clinging behavior.
- Borderline: also fears abandonment but reacts to abandonment with rage rather than urgent efforts to replace the relationship. Also unstable relationships in borderline.
- Histrionic: also strong need for reassurance with associated clinging, but behavior is flamboyant with active demands for attention rather than docile and self-effacing.
- Avoidant: also experiences strong feelings of inadequacy but avoids contact until certain of acceptance rather than active seeking of connection.

Depression

- Hypothyroidism
- Major organ system disease (e.g., cardiovascular, liver, renal, neuronal diseases) with depressive symptoms
- Elderly patients: frequently coexists with dementia
- Bipolar patients will frequently present with depression, but routine treatment with antidepressant medications may be detrimental in this group.
- Neurosyphilis

de Quervain's Tenosynovitis

- Carpal tunnel syndrome
- Ostearthritis

- Gout
- Infiltrative tenosynovitis
- Radiculopathy
- Compression neuropathy (e.g., superficial branch of the radial nerve "bracelet syndrome")
- Infection (e.g., TB, bacterial)

Dermatitis, Atopic

- Scabies
- Psoriasis
- Dermatitis herpetiformis
- Contact dermatitis
- Photosensitivity
- Seborrheic dermatitis
- Candidiasis
- Lichen simplex chronicus
- Other: Wiskott-Aldrich syndrome, phenylketonuria (PKU), mycosis fungoides, ichthyosis, HIV dermatitis, non-nummular eczema, histiocytosis X

Dermatitis, Contact

- Impetigo
- Lichen simplex chronicus
- Atopic dermatitis
- Nummular eczema
- Seborrheic dermatitis
- Psoriasis
- Scabies

Dermatitis Herpetiformis

- Linear IgA bullous dermatosis (not associated with gluten-sensitive enteropathy)
- Herpes simplex infection
- Herpes zoster infection
- Erythema multiforme
- Bullous pemphigoid

Dermatofibroma

- Insect bite
- Foreign body reaction
- Angioma
- Melanoma
- Wart
- Prurigo nodularis
- Basal cell carcinoma
- Scar
- Keloid
- Nevus

Dermatographism

- Cholinergic urticaria
- Solar urticaria
- Heat urticaria
- Exercise-induced urticaria
- Cold urticaria
- Lupus
- Aquagenic urticaria
- Polymorphous light eruption

Dermatomyositis

- Polymyositis
- Inclusion body myositis
- Muscular dystrophies
- Amyotrophic lateral sclerosis
- Myasthenia gravis
- Eaton-Lambert syndrome
- Drug-induced myopathies
- Diabetic amyotrophy
- Guillain-Barré syndrome
- Hyperthyroidism or hypothyroidism
- Lichen planus
- Systemic lupus erythematosus (SLE)
- Contact dermatitis
- Atopic dermatitis

- Psoriasis
- Seborrheic dermatitis

Dermatosis by Morphology[16]

MACULES
Hypopigmented
- Halo nevus
- Leprosy
- Postinflammatory
- Sarcoidosis
- Tinea versicolor
- Tuberous sclerosis
- Vitiligo

Hyperpigmented
- Café au lait spot
- Drug eruption
- Ephelis (freckle)
- Lentigo
- Mastocytosis
- Melanoma
- Melasma
- Mongolian spot
- Nevus
- Ochronosis
- Postinflammatory
- Purpura
- Stasis dermatitis

Erythematous
- Drug eruption
- Rheumatic fever
- Secondary syphilis
- Viral exanthem

PAPULES
Isolated Papules
- Acrochordon
- Actinic keratosis
- Angiofibroma

- Angioma
- Appendageal tumors (benign or malignant)
- Bacillary angiomatosis
- Basal cell carcinoma
- Chondrodermatitis nodularis helicis
- Dermatofibroma
- Fungal infections, early
- Hemangioma
- Keratoacanthoma
- Melanoma
- Milia
- Molluscum contagiosum
- Neurofibroma
- Nevus
- Pyogenic granuloma
- Sebaceous hyperplasia
- Seborrheic keratosis
- Squamous cell carcinoma
- Wart

Papular Eruptions
- Acne rosacea
- Acne vulgaris
- Appendageal tumors (usually benign)
- Arthropod bite
- Bacillary angiomatosis
- Dermatomyositis
- Drug eruption
- Eczematous dermatitis
- Flat warts
- Folliculitis
- Granuloma annulare
- Keratosis pilaris
- Lichen nitidus
- Lichen planus
- Lichen sclerosus
- Lupus erythematosus
- Lymphoma
- Miliaria

- Molluscum contagiosum
- Neurofibromatosis
- Pediculosis corporis
- Perioral dermatitis
- Pityriasis rosea
- Polymorphous light eruption
- Pruritic urticarial papules, plaques of pregnancy
- Psoriasis
- Sarcoidosis
- Sarcoma (Kaposi's, other)
- Scabies
- Syphilis
- Urticaria
- Vasculitis
- Venous lake
- Viral exanthem
- Xanthoma

PUSTULES
- Acne rosacea/perioral dermatitis
- Acne vulgaris
- Arthropod bite (fire ants)
- Drug eruption
- Eosinophilic folliculitis
- Erythema toxicum neonatorum
- Folliculitis
- Fungal or yeast infections, especially tinea capitis and Majocchi's granuloma
- Furunculosis
- Gonorrhea, disseminated
- Herpes simplex/zoster
- Impetigo
- Keratosis pilaris
- Neonatal pustulosis
- Pseudofolliculitis barbae
- Pustular psoriasis
- Pyoderma gangrenosum
- Syphilis
- Varicella

PLAQUES

- Acanthosis nigricans
- Candidiasis
- Cellulitis
- Deep fungal infections
- Dermatomyositis
- Diaper dermatitis
- Eczematous dermatitis, including lichen simplex chronicus
- Erythrasma
- Fungal infections (e.g., tinea corporis, pedis, cruris, manus)
- Granuloma annulare
- Ichthyosis
- Lichen planus
- Lichen sclerosus
- Lupus erythematosus
- Lyme disease
- Lymphoma, cutaneous T-cell
- Morphea
- Myxedema
- Necrobiosis lipoidica diabeticorum
- Paget's disease, mammary/extramammary
- Pityriasis rosea
- Psoriasis
- Sarcoidosis
- Seborrheic dermatitis
- Sweet's syndrome
- Syphilis
- Tinea versicolor
- Vasculitis
- Xanthelasma

NODULES AND TUMORS

- Acrochordon
- Angioma
- Appendageal tumors
- Basal cell carcinoma
- Callus/clavus
- Chondrodermatitis nodularis helicis
- Erythema nodosum
- Hidradenitis suppurativa

- Histiocytosis
- Inclusion cyst
- Kaposi's sarcoma
- Keloid
- Lipoma
- Lymphoma, cutaneous
- Melanoma
- Metastatic carcinoma
- Neurofibroma
- Nevus
- Prurigo nodularis
- Pyogenic granuloma
- Seborrheic keratosis
- Squamous cell carcinoma
- Syphilis
- Tuberous sclerosis
- Venous lake
- Wart
- Xanthoma

VESICLES AND BULLAE
- Bullous disease in diabetes
- Bullous pemphigoid
- Burn
- Cellulitis
- Congenital syphilis
- Contact dermatitis
- Dermatitis herpetiformis
- Eczema, especially of the hand/foot
- Epidermolysis bullosa
- Erythema multiforme
- Fixed drug eruption
- Fungal infections, especially tinea pedis
- Herpes gestationis
- Herpes simplex
- Herpes zoster
- Id reaction
- Impetigo
- Insect bite reaction
- Lichen planus

- Lupus erythematosus, bullous
- Pemphigus vulgaris/foliaceus
- Porphyria cutanea tarda
- Scabies
- Staphylococcal scalded skin syndrome
- Streptococcal toxic shock–like syndrome
- Toxic epidermal necrolysis
- Varicella
- Vasculitis

EROSIONS AND ULCERS

Mouth

- Aphthae
- Avitaminosis
- Bullous pemphigoid
- Burn
- Candidiasis
- Epidermolysis bullosa
- Erythema multiforme
- Hand-foot-mouth disease
- Herpangina
- Herpes simplex
- Lichen planus
- Lupus erythematosus
- Pemphigus vulgaris
- Perlèche
- Toxic epidermal necrolysis

Genital

- Balanitis
- Candidiasis
- Chancroid
- Diaper dermatitis, severe
- Erythema multiforme
- Fixed drug eruption
- Fungal infections, tinea cruris
- Herpes simplex
- Intertrigo
- Lichen planus
- Lichen sclerosus
- Lymphogranuloma venereum

- Squamous cell carcinoma
- Syphilis

Other
- Basal cell carcinoma
- Bullous pemphigoid
- Ecthyma
- Erythema multiforme
- Ischemia
- Necrobiosis lipoidica
- Pemphigus vulgaris
- Porphyria cutanea tarda
- Pyoderma gangrenosum
- Spider bite
- Squamous cell carcinoma
- Stasis ulcer
- Toxic epidermal necrosis

DESQUAMATION
- Exfoliative dermatitis
- Kawasaki's syndrome
- Keratolysis exfoliativa (hands and feet)
- Scarlet fever
- Scarlatiniform eruption
- Staphylococcal scalded skin syndrome
- Toxic shock syndrome (late)

Dermatosis by Region[16]

SCALP
Papules/Plaques
- Actinic keratosis
- Appendageal tumor
- Cyst
- Hemangioma
- Lichen planopilaris
- Lupus erythematosus
- Melanoma
- Nevus
- Seborrheic keratosis

Nodules
- Actinic keratosis
- Appendageal tumor
- Basal cell carcinoma
- Cyst
- Hemangioma
- Kerion
- Metastatic carcinoma
- Nevus
- Prurigo nodularis
- Seborrheic keratosis

Eruptions
- Contact dermatitis
- Dissecting cellulitis
- Eczema
- Folliculitis
- Herpes zoster
- Pediculosis capitis
- Psoriasis
- Seborrheic dermatitis
- Tinea capitis

Alopecias
- Alopecia areata
- Anagen effluvium
- Androgenic alopecia
- Discoid lupus erythematosus
- Hypervitaminosis A
- Lichen planopilaris
- Syphilis
- Systemic disease
- Telogen effluvium
- Tinea capitis
- Traction/chemical alopecia
- Trichotillomania

FACE

Isolated Papules
- Acrochordon
- Actinic keratosis

- Angioma
- Appendageal tumors
- Basal cell carcinoma
- Cyst
- Dermatosis papulosa nigra
- Hemangioma
- Keratoacanthoma
- Lentigo maligna
- Milia
- Nevus
- Sebaceous hyperplasia
- Seborrheic keratosis
- Solar lentigo
- Squamous cell carcinoma
- Telangiectasia
- Venous lake
- Xanthelasma

Eruptions
- Acne rosacea
- Acne vulgaris
- Adenoma sebaceum
- Dermatomyositis
- Eczema, including contact dermatitis
- Erysipelas
- Favre-Racouchot (comedones in actinically damaged skin)
- Fifth disease
- Herpes simplex/zoster
- Impetigo
- Lupus erythematosus
- Lymphocytoma cutis
- Melasma
- Pemphigoid/pemphigus
- Perioral dermatitis
- Photodrug eruption
- Pityriasis alba
- Postinflammatory hypopigmentation
- Psoriasis
- Sarcoidosis
- Scleroderma

- Seborrheic dermatitis
- Steroid rosacea
- Syphilis
- Tinea corporis
- Urticaria, angioedema
- Warts, especially flat or molluscum

ORAL MUCOSA

See also Dermatosis by Morphology, Erosions, and Ulcers.

- Kaposi's sarcoma
- Leukoplakia
- Melanoma
- Mucous cysts
- Oral hairy leukoplakia
- Oral melanotic macule
- Pyogenic granuloma
- Verruca

AXILLA

- Acanthosis nigricans
- Acrochordon
- Axillary freckling in neurofibromatosis
- Bullous pemphigoid
- Contact dermatitis
- Epidermal inclusion cyst
- Erythrasma
- Fox-Fordyce disease
- Fungal or yeast infections
- Hailey-Hailey disease
- Hidradenitis suppurativa
- Intertrigo
- Pediculosis corporis
- Pseudoxanthoma elasticum
- Scabies
- Striae distensae
- Trichomycosis axillaris

HANDS AND FEET

Isolated Papules

- Actinic keratosis
- Arsenical keratosis

- Basal cell carcinoma
- Callus/clavus
- Felon
- Keratoacanthoma
- Melanoma
- Nevus
- Painful fat herniations
- Pyogenic granuloma
- Solar lentigo
- Squamous cell carcinoma
- Warts

Eruptions

- Acute or chronic paronychia
- Cutaneous larva migrans (feet)
- Dermatomyositis
- Drug eruption
- Eczema, including contact dermatitis
- Emboli
- Epidermolysis bullosa
- Erythema multiforme
- Granuloma annulare
- Hand-foot-mouth disease
- Herpetic whitlow
- Hyperhidrosis
- Juvenile plantar dermatosis
- Keratolysis exfoliativa
- Lichen planus (wrists, ankles)
- Lupus erythematosus
- Pitted keratolysis (feet)
- Pityriasis rubra pilaris
- Porphyria cutanea tarda
- Psoriasis
- Reiter's syndrome
- Rocky Mountain spotted fever
- Scabies
- Scleroderma
- Syphilis
- Tinea pedis, manus
- Viral exanthems
- Vitiligo

GENITALIA/INGUINAL

- Acrochordons
- Acrodermatitis enteropathica
- Angiokeratoma
- Balanitis
- Bowen's disease
- Candidiasis
- Chancroid
- Condylomata acuminata
- Contact dermatitis
- Diaper dermatitis
- Erythema multiforme
- Erythrasma
- Fixed drug eruption
- Folliculitis
- Furunculosis
- Herpes simplex/zoster
- Hidradenitis suppurativa
- Intertrigo
- Kawasaki's syndrome
- Lichen planus
- Lichen sclerosus
- Lichen simplex chronicus
- Lymphogranuloma venereum
- Molluscum contagiosum
- Paget's disease, extramammary
- Pearly penile papules
- Pediculosis pubis
- Perianal streptococcal cellulitis
- Pinworm
- Pityriasis rubra pilaris
- Psoriasis
- Reiter's syndrome
- Scabies
- Seborrheic dermatitis
- Squamous cell carcinoma
- Syphilis
- Tinea cruris

PHOTODISTRIBUTED
- Dermatomyositis
- Lupus erythematosus
- Pellagra
- Photodrug eruption
- Polymorphous light eruption
- Porphyria cutanea tarda

Dermoid Cyst

- Epidermoid cyst
- Nevus sebaceus
- Enlarged lymph node
- Pilomatricoma

Diabetes Insipidus

- Diabetes mellitus (DM), nephropathies
- Primary polydipsia, medications (e.g., chlorpromazine)
- Osmotic diuresis (glucose, mannitol, anticholinergics)
- Psychogenic polydipsia, electrolyte disturbances

Diabetes Mellitus

- Diabetes insipidus
- Stress hyperglycemia
- Diabetes secondary to hormonal excess, drugs, pancreatic disease
- Excessive use of diuretics

Diabetic Ketoacidosis

- Hyperosmolar nonketotic state
- Alcoholic ketoacidosis
- Uremic acidosis
- Metabolic acidosis secondary to methyl alcohol, ethylene glycol
- Salicylate poisoning

Diarrhea, Acute Watery and Bloody[39]

ACUTE WATERY DIARRHEA

- Gastrointestinal infections
- Protozoal (e.g., *Giardia*)
- Bacterial (e.g., enterotoxigenic *Escherichia coli*, cholera)
- Viral (e.g., rotavirus, Norwalk virus)
- Drugs
- Toxins
- Dietary constituents (e.g., lactose intolerance)
- Onset of chronic diarrheal illness

ACUTE BLOODY DIARRHEA

- Infectious colitis
- Confluent proctocolitis (e.g., *Shigella, Campylobacter, Salmonella, Entamoeba histolytica*)
- Segmental colitis (e.g., *Campylobacter, Salmonella*, enteroinvasive *E. coli, Aeromonas, E. histolytica*)
- Drug-induced colitis (e.g., nonsteroidal anti-inflammatory drugs [NSAIDs])
- Inflammatory bowel disease
- Ischemic colitis (usually elderly patient with underlying heart disease or arrhythmias)
- Antibiotic-associated colitis

Diarrhea, Tube-Fed Patient[14]

COMMON CAUSES UNRELATED TO TUBE FEEDING

- Elixir medications containing sorbitol
- Magnesium-containing antacids
- Antibiotic-induced sterile gut
- Pseudomembranous colitis

POSSIBLE CAUSES RELATED TO TUBE FEEDING

- Inadequate fiber to form stool bulk
- High fat content of formula (in the presence of fat malabsorption syndrome)
- Bacterial contamination of enteral products and delivery systems (causal association with diarrhea not documented)

- Rapid advancement in rate (after the GI tract is unused for prolonged periods)

UNLIKELY CAUSES RELATED TO TUBE FEEDING
- Formula hyperosmolality (proven not to be the cause of diarrhea)
- Lactose (absent from nearly all enteral feeding formulas)

Diffuse Interstitial Lung Disease

- Congestive heart failure (CHF)
- Chronic renal failure
- Lymphangitic carcinomatosis
- Sarcoidosis
- Allergic alveolitis

Digitalis Overdose

- Medications
  - β-Blockers
  - Calcium channel blockers
  - Clonidine
  - Cyclic antidepressants
  - Encainide and flecainide
  - Procainamide
  - Propoxyphene
  - Quinidine
- Plants producing digitalis-like glycosides
  - Foxglove
  - Oleander
  - Lily of the valley
- Cardiac conduction abnormalities
  - Sick sinus syndrome
  - AV node dysfunction
- Electrolyte abnormalities
  - Hyperkalemia

Diphtheria

- Streptococcal pharyngitis
- Viral pharyngitis
- Mononucleosis

Diplopia, Binocular

- Cranial nerve palsy (third, fourth, sixth)
- Thyroid eye disease
- Myasthenia gravis
- Decompensated strabismus
- Orbital trauma with blowout fracture
- Orbital pseudotumor
- Cavernous sinus thrombosis

Diplopia, Monocular

- Postoperative corrected long-standing tropia
- Defective contact lenses
- Poorly fitting bifocals
- Trauma to iris
- Corneal disorder (e.g., dry eye, astigmatism)
- Cataracts
- Lens subluxation
- Nystagmus
- Eyelid twitching
- Foreign body in aqueous or vitreous media
- Migraine
- Lesions of occipital cortex
- Psychogenic

Diplopia, Vertical

- Myasthenia
- Superior oblique palsy
- Myositis or pseudotumor with orbital involvement
- Lymphoma or metastases affecting the orbits
- Brainstem or cerebellar lesions
- Hydrocephalus
- Third nerve palsy
- Botulism
- Wernicke's encephalopathy
- Dysthyroid orbitopathy (muscle infiltration)

Discoid Lupus Erythematosus (DLE)

- Psoriasis
- Lichen planus
- Secondary syphilis
- Superficial fungal infections
- Photosensitivity eruption
- Sarcoidosis
- Subacute cutaneous lupus erythematosus
- Rosacea
- Keratoacanthoma
- Actinic keratosis
- Dermatomyositis

Disseminated Intravascular Coagulation (DIC)

- Hepatic necrosis: normal or elevated factor VIII concentrations
- Vitamin K deficiency: normal platelet count
- Hemolytic-uremic syndrome (HUS)
- Thrombocytopenic purpura
- Renal failure, systemic lupus erythematosus (SLE), sickle cell crisis, dysfibrinogenemias

Diverticular Disease

- Irritable bowel syndrome (IBS)
- Inflammatory bowel disease (IBD)
- Carcinoma of colon
- Endometriosis
- Ischemic colitis
- Infections (pseudomembranous colitis, appendicitis, pyelonephritis, pelvic inflammatory disease [PID])
- Lactose intolerance

Dizziness

- Viral syndrome
- Anxiety, hyperventilation
- Benign positional paroxysmal vertigo

- Medications (e.g., sedatives, antihypertensives, analgesics)
- Withdrawal from medications (e.g., benzodiazepines, SSRIs)
- Alcohol or drug abuse
- Postural hypotension
- Hypoglycemia, hyperglycemia
- Hematologic disorders (e.g., anemia, polycythemia, leukemia)
- Head trauma
- Meniere's disease
- Vertebrobasilar ischemia
- Cervical osteoarthritis
- Cardiac abnormalities (arrhythmias, cardiomyopathy, CHF, pericarditis)
- Multiple sclerosis
- Peripheral vestibulopathy
- Air or sea travel
- Electrolyte abnormalities
- Eye problems (cornea, lens, retina)
- Migraine
- Brainstem infarct
- Autonomic neuropathy
- Chronic otomastoiditis
- Complex partial seizures
- Ramsay Hunt syndrome
- Arteritis
- Syncope and presyncope
- Perilymph fistula
- Cerebellopontine tumor
- Hepatic or renal disease

Drug Eruption

- Scarlet fever
- Measles
- Rubella
- Viral exanthem such as enterovirus, echovirus, cytomegalovirus
- Kawasaki's disease
- Juvenile rheumatoid arthritis
- Secondary syphilis
- Primary HIV disease

Dry Eye

- Contacts
- Medications (antihistamines, clonidine, β-blockers, ibuprofen, scopolamine)
- Keratoconjunctivitis sicca
- Trauma
- Environmental causes (air-conditioning in patient with contacts)

Dumping Syndrome

- Pancreatic insufficiency
- Inflammatory bowel disease (IBD)
- Afferent loop syndromes
- Bile acid reflux after surgery
- Bowel obstruction
- Gastroenteric fistula

Dysfunctional Uterine Bleeding

- Pregnancy-related cause
- Anatomic uterine causes: leiomyomas, adenomyosis, polyps, endometrial hyperplasia, cancer, STDs, intrauterine contraceptive device (IUD)
- Anatomic nonuterine causes: cervical neoplasia, cervicitis; vaginal neoplasia, adhesions, trauma, foreign body, atrophic vaginitis, infections, condyloma; vulvar trauma, infections, neoplasia, condyloma, dystrophy, varices
- Urinary tract: urethral caruncle, diverticulum, hematuria
- GI tract: hemorrhoids, anal fissure, colorectal lesions
- Systemic diseases: exogenous hormone intake, renal disease
- Coagulopathies: von Willebrand disease, thrombocytopenia, hepatic failure
- Endocrinopathies: thyroid disorder, hypothyroidism and hyperthyroidism, diabetes mellitus (DM)

Dysmenorrhea

- Adenomyosis
- Adhesions

- Allen-Masters syndrome
- Cervical strictures or stenosis
- Congenital malformation of müllerian system
- Ectopic pregnancy
- Endometriosis, endometritis
- Imperforate hymen
- Intrauterine contraceptive device (IUD) use
- Leiomyomas
- Ovarian cysts
- Pelvic congestion syndrome, pelvic inflammatory disease (PID)
- Polyps
- Transverse vaginal septum

Dyspareunia[12]

INTROITAL
- Vaginismus
- Intact or rigid hymen
- Clitoral problems
- Vulvovaginitis
- Vaginal atrophy: hypoestrogen
- Vulvar dystrophy
- Bartholin's or Skene's gland infection
- Inadequate lubrication
- Operative scarring

MIDVAGINAL
- Urethritis
- Trigonitis
- Cystitis
- Short vagina
- Operative scarring
- Inadequate lubrication

DEEP
- Endometriosis
- Pelvic infection
- Uterine retroversion
- Ovarian pathology
- Gastrointestinal

- Orthopedic
- Abnormal penile size or shape

Dyspepsia, Nonulcerative

Other possible causes of dyspepsia:
- Peptic ulcer disease
- Gastroesophageal reflux
- Gastric, esophageal, and all abdominal cancers
- Biliary tract disease
- Gastroparesis
- Pancreatitis
- Medications (i.e., NSAIDs, erythromycin, steroids)
- Infiltrative diseases of the stomach (i.e., Crohn's disease or sarcoidosis)
- Metabolic disturbances (i.e., hypercalcemia or hyperkalemia)
- Ischemic bowel disease
- System disorders (i.e., diabetes, thyroid disorders, or connective tissue diseases)

Dysphagia

- Esophageal obstruction: neoplasm, foreign body, achalasia, stricture, spasm, esophageal web, diverticulum, Schatzki's ring
- Peptic esophagitis with stricture, Barrett's stricture
- External esophageal compression: neoplasms (thyroid neoplasm, lymphoma, mediastinal tumors), thyroid enlargement, aortic aneurysm, vertebral spurs, aberrant right subclavian artery (dysphagia lusoria)
- Hiatal hernia, gastroesophageal reflux disease (GERD)
- Oropharyngeal lesions: pharyngitis, glossitis, stomatitis, neoplasms
- Hysteria: globus hystericus
- Neurologic or neuromuscular disturbances: bulbar paralysis, myasthenia gravis, amyotrophic lateral sclerosis (ALS), multiple sclerosis (MS), parkinsonism, cerebrovascular accident (CVA), diabetic neuropathy
- Toxins: poisoning, botulism, tetanus, post-diphtheritic dysphagia
- Systemic diseases: scleroderma, amyloidosis, dermatomyositis
- *Candida* and herpes esophagitis
- Presbyesophagus

Dyspnea

- Upper airway obstruction: trauma, neoplasm, epiglottitis, laryngeal edema, tongue retraction, laryngospasm, abductor paralysis of vocal cords, aspiration of foreign body
- Lower airway obstruction: neoplasm, chronic obstructive pulmonary disease (COPD), asthma, aspiration of foreign body
- Pulmonary infection: pneumonia, abscess, empyema, TB, bronchiectasis
- Pulmonary hypertension
- Pulmonary embolism/infarction
- Parenchymal lung disease
- Pulmonary vascular congestion
- Cardiac disease: arteriosclerotic heart disease (ASHD), valvular lesions, cardiac dysrhythmias, cardiomyopathy, pericardial effusion, cardiac shunts
- Space-occupying lesions: neoplasm, large hiatal hernia, pleural effusions
- Disease of chest wall: severe kyphoscoliosis, fractured ribs, sternal compression, morbid obesity
- Neurologic dysfunction: Guillain-Barré syndrome, botulism, polio, spinal cord injury
- Interstitial pulmonary disease: sarcoidosis, collagen-vascular diseases, desquamative interstitial pneumonia (DIP), Hamman-Rich pneumonitis, others
- Pneumoconioses: silicosis, berylliosis, others
- Mesothelioma
- Pneumothorax, hemothorax, pleural effusion
- Inhalation of toxins
- Cholinergic drug intoxication
- Carcinoid syndrome
- Hematologic: anemia, polycythemia, hemoglobinopathies
- Thyrotoxicosis, myxedema
- Diaphragmatic compression caused by abdominal distention, subphrenic abscess, ascites
- Lung resection
- Metabolic abnormalities: uremia, hepatic coma, diabetic ketoacidosis (DKA)
- Sepsis
- Atelectasis

- Psychoneurosis
- Diaphragmatic paralysis
- Pregnancy

Dystonia

- Parkinson's disease
- Progressive supranuclear palsy
- Wilson's disease
- Huntington's disease
- Drug effects

Dysuria

- Urinary tract infection (UTI)
- Estrogen deficiency (in postmenopausal woman)
- Vaginitis
- Genital infection (e.g., herpes, condyloma)
- Interstitial cystitis
- Chemical irritation (e.g., deodorant aerosols, douches)
- Meatal stenosis or stricture
- Reiter's syndrome
- Bladder neoplasm
- GI (diverticulitis, Crohn's disease)
- Impaired bladder or sphincter action
- Urethral carbuncle
- Chronic fibrosis post trauma
- Radiation therapy
- Prostatitis
- Urethritis (gonococcal, chlamydial)
- Behçet's syndrome
- Stevens-Johnson syndrome

Earache[34]

- Otitis media
- Serous otitis media
- Eustachitis
- Otitis externa
- Otitic barotrauma

- Mastoiditis
- Foreign body
- Impacted cerumen
- Referred otalgia, as with temporomandibular joint (TMJ) dysfunction, dental problems, and tumors

Echinococcosis

- Cystic neoplasms
- Abscess (amebic or bacterial)
- Congenital polycystic disease

Eclampsia

- Preexisting seizure disorder
- Metabolic abnormalities (hypoglycemia, hyponatremia, hypocalcemia)
- Substance abuse
- Head trauma, infection (meningitis, encephalitis)
- Intracerebral bleeding or thrombosis
- Amniotic fluid embolism
- Space-occupying brain lesions or neoplasms
- Pseudoseizure

Ectopic Adrenocorticotropic Hormone (ACTH) Secretion[14]

- Small cell carcinoma of lung
- Endocrine tumors of foregut origin
- Thymic carcinoid
- Islet cell tumor
- Medullary carcinoid, thyroid
- Bronchial carcinoid
- Pheochromocytoma
- Ovarian tumor

Ectopic Pregnancy

- Corpus luteum cyst
- Rupture or torsion of ovarian cyst

- Threatened or incomplete abortion
- Pelvic inflammatory disease (PID)
- Appendicitis
- Gastroenteritis
- Dysfunctional uterine bleeding
- Degenerating uterine fibroids
- Endometriosis

Eczema Herpeticum

- Impetigo
- Contact dermatitis
- Pemphigus
- Dermatitis herpetiformis
- Bullous pemphigoid

Edema, Children[20]

CARDIOVASCULAR
- Congestive heart failure (CHF)
- Acute thrombi or emboli
- Vasculitis of many types

RENAL
- Nephrotic syndrome
- Glomerulonephritis of many types
- End-stage renal failure

ENDOCRINE OR METABOLIC
- Thyroid disease
- Starvation
- Hereditary angioedema

IATROGENIC
- Drugs (diuretics and steroids)
- Water or salt overload

HEMATOLOGIC
- Hemolytic disease of the newborn

- Gastritis, duodenitis
- Intussusception
- Incarcerated hernia: inguinal, internal secondary to old adhesions
- Cow's milk protein intolerance, food allergy, eosinophilic gastroenteritis
- Disaccharidase deficiency
- Celiac disease: presents after introduction of gluten in diet; inherited risk
- Adynamic ileus: the mediator for many nongastrointestinal causes
- Neonatal necrotizing enterocolitis
- Chronic granulomatous disease with gastric outlet obstruction

Non–Gastrointestinal Tract
- Infectious: otitis, urinary tract infection (UTI), pneumonia, upper respiratory tract infection, sepsis, meningitis
- Metabolic: aminoaciduria and organic aciduria, galactosemia, fructosemia, adrenogenital syndrome, renal tubular acidosis, diabetic ketoacidosis, Reye's syndrome
- CNS: trauma, tumor, infection, diencephalic syndrome, rumination, autonomic responses (pain, shock)
- Medications: anticholinergics, aspirin, alcohol, idiosyncratic reaction (e.g., codeine)

CHILDHOOD
Gastrointestinal Tract
- Peptic ulcer: vomiting is a common presentation in children younger than 6 years.
- Trauma: duodenal hematoma, traumatic pancreatitis, perforated bowel
- Pancreatitis: mumps, trauma, CF, hyperparathyroidism, hyperlipidemia, organic acidemias
- Crohn's disease
- Idiopathic intestinal pseudo-obstruction
- Superior mesenteric artery syndrome

Non–Gastrointestinal Tract
- CNS: cyclic vomiting, migraine, anorexia nervosa, bulimia

Empyema

- Uninfected parapneumonic effusion
- Congestive heart failure (CHF)
- Malignant neoplasm involving the pleura
- Tuberculous pleurisy
- Collagen-vascular disease (particularly rheumatoid lung and systemic lupus erythematosus [SLE])

Encephalitis, Viral

- Bacterial infections: brain abscess, toxic encephalopathies, TB
- Protozoal infections
- Behçet's syndrome
- Lupus encephalitis
- Sjögren's syndrome
- Multiple sclerosis (MS)
- Syphilis
- Cryptococcosis
- Toxoplasmosis
- Brucellosis
- Leukemic or lymphomatous meningitis
- Other metastatic tumors
- Lyme disease
- Cat-scratch disease
- Vogt-Koyanagi-Harada syndrome
- Mollaret's meningitis

Encephalomyelitis, Nonviral Causes[26]

- Subacute bacterial endocarditis
- Rocky Mountain spotted fever
- Typhus
- *Ehrlichia*
- Q fever
- *Chlamydia*
- *Mycoplasma*
- *Legionella*
- Brucellosis

- *Listeria*
- Whipple's disease
- Cat-scratch disease
- Syphilis (meningovascular)
- Relapsing fever
- Lyme disease
- Leptospirosis
- *Nocardia*
- Actinomycosis
- Tuberculosis
- *Cryptococcus*
- *Histoplasma*
- *Toxoplasma*
- *Plasmodium falciparum*
- Trypanosomiasis
- Behçet's disease
- Vasculitis
- Carcinoma
- Drug reactions

Encephalopathy

- Dementia: distinguished from encephalopathy by a history of slowly progressive cognitive decline over time (fluctuating cognitive function is rare except in diffuse Lewy body disease).
- Hypersomnia
- Aphasia: distinguished from encephalopathy by virtue of its representing a specific disorder of language rather than a global disturbance of cognitive function.
- Depression
- Psychosis: some overlap with encephalopathy because delusions and hallucinations may be common to both.
- Mania
- Vegetative state from cerebral injury; these patients appear awake (eyes are open), but there is no content to their consciousness.
- Akinetic mutism: these patients do not talk and do not move; there is little fluctuation in their state, and there is no asterixis.
- Locked-in syndrome: may be distinguished from encephalopathy by the presence of fixed neurologic deficits (e.g., paralysis of all four limbs).

Encephalopathy, Metabolic[37]

- Substrate deficiency: hypoxia/ischemia, carbon monoxide (CO) poisoning, hypoglycemia
- Cofactor deficiency: thiamine, vitamin B_{12}, pyridoxine (isoniazid [INH] administration)
- Electrolyte disorders: hyponatremia, hypercalcemia, carbon dioxide narcosis, dialysis, hypermagnesemia, disequilibrium syndrome
- Endocrinopathies: diabetic ketoacidosis (DKA), hyperosmolar coma, hypothyroidism, hyperadrenocorticism, hyperparathyroidism
- Endogenous toxins: liver disease, uremia, porphyria
- Exogenous toxins: drug overdose (sedative-hypnotics, ethanol, narcotics, salicylates, tricyclic antidepressants), drug withdrawal, toxicity of therapeutic medications, industrial toxins (e.g., organophosphates, heavy metals), sepsis
- Heat stroke
- Epilepsy (postictal)

Encopresis

- Hirschsprung's disease
- Cerebral palsy
- Myelomeningocele
- Pseudo-obstruction
- Anorectal lesions
- Malformations
- Trauma
- Rectal prolapse
- Hypothyroidism
- Medications

Endocarditis, Infective

- Brain abscess
- Fever of undetermined origin (FUO)
- Pericarditis
- Meningitis
- Rheumatic fever

- Osteomyelitis
- Salmonella
- TB
- Bacteremia
- Pericarditis
- Glomerulonephritis

Endometrial Cancer

- Atypical hyperplasia
- Other genital tract malignant disease
- Polyps
- Atrophic vaginitis
- Granuloma cell tumor
- Fibroid uterus

Endometriosis

- Ectopic pregnancy
- Acute appendicitis
- Chronic appendicitis
- Pelvic inflammatory disease (PID)
- Pelvic adhesions
- Hemorrhagic cyst
- Hernia
- Psychological disorder
- Irritable bowel syndrome (IBS)
- Uterine leiomyomas
- Adenomyosis
- Nerve entrapment syndrome
- Scoliosis
- Muscular/skeletal strain
- Interstitial cystitis

Enthesopathy

- Viremia or bacteremia
- Ankylosing spondylitis
- Psoriatic arthritis
- Drug induced (quinolones, etretinate)

- Reactive arthritis
- Disseminated idiopathic skeletal hyperostosis (DISH)
- Reiter's syndrome

Enuresis

- May be associated with encopresis and sleep disorders such as sleep terrors; much less likely to be a primary psychological disorder
- Organic causes of enuresis include diabetes mellitus, diabetes insipidus, bladder outlet obstruction, small bladder capacity, detrusor instability, urethral valves, meatal stenosis, cerebral palsy, spina bifida, pelvic mass, impacted stool, sedating medications, and nocturnal seizures.

Eosinophilic Fasciitis

- Systemic sclerosis
- Chemical-induced sclerosis
- Generalized lichen sclerosus et atrophicus
- Graft-versus-host disease
- Porphyria cutanea tarda
- Chronic Lyme borreliosis

Eosinophilic Pneumonia

- TB
- Brucellosis
- Fungal diseases
- Bronchogenic carcinoma
- Hodgkin's disease
- Immunoblastic lymphadenopathy
- Rheumatoid lung disease
- Sarcoidosis

Eosinophiluria

- Interstitial nephritis
- Tyrosinase-negative oculocutaneous albinism (ATN)
- Urinary tract infection (UTI)

- Kidney transplant rejection
- Hepatorenal syndrome

Ephelides (Freckles)

- Melanocytic nevus
- Lentigo
- Tinea versicolor
- Seborrheic keratosis
- Café au lait spots

Epicondylitis

- Cervical radiculopathy
- Intra-articular elbow pathology (osteoarthritis, osteochondritis dissecans, loose body)
- Radial nerve compression
- Ulnar neuropathy
- Medial collateral ligament instability

Epidermoid Cyst (Sebaceous Cyst, Epidermal Inclusion Cyst)

- Insect bite
- Cylindroma
- Trichilemmoma
- Pilar cyst
- Granuloma annulare
- Dermoid cyst
- Lipoma
- Milia

Epididymitis

- Orchitis
- Testicular torsion, trauma, or tumor
- Epididymal cyst
- Hydrocele
- Varicocele
- Spermatocele

Epiglottitis

- Croup
- Angioedema
- Peritonsillar abscess
- Retropharyngeal abscess
- Diphtheria
- Foreign body aspiration
- Lingual tonsillitis

Epilepsy

- Psychogenic spells
- Transient ischemic attack (TIA)
- Hypoglycemia
- Syncope
- Narcolepsy
- Migraine
- Paroxysmal vertigo
- Arrhythmias
- Drug reaction

Episcleritis

- Acute glaucoma
- Conjunctivitis
- Scleritis
- Subconjunctival hemorrhage
- Congenital or lymphoid masses

Epistaxis

- Trauma
- Medications (nasal sprays, nonsteroidal anti-inflammatory drugs [NSAIDs], anticoagulants, antiplatelets)
- Nasal polyps
- Cocaine use
- Coagulopathy (hemophilia, liver disease, disseminated intravascular coagulation [DIC], thrombocytopenia)

- Systemic disorders (hypertension, uremia)
- Infections
- Anatomic malformations
- Rhinitis
- Nasal polyps
- Local neoplasms (benign and malignant)
- Desiccation
- Foreign body

Epstein-Barr Infection

- Heterophil-negative infectious mononucleosis caused by cytomegalovirus (CMV)
- Although clinical presentation is similar, CMV more frequently follows transfusion.
- Bacterial and viral causes of pharyngitis
- Toxoplasmosis
- Acute retroviral syndrome of HIV
- Lymphoma

Erectile Dysfunction, Organic[32]

- Neurogenic abnormalities: somatic nerve neuropathy, CNS abnormalities
- Psychogenic causes: depression, performance anxiety, marital conflict
- Endocrine causes: hyperprolactinemia, hypogonadotropic hypogonadism, testicular failure, estrogen excess
- Trauma: pelvic fracture, prostate surgery, penile fracture
- Systemic disease: diabetes mellitus (DM), renal failure, hepatic cirrhosis
- Medications: β-blockers, diuretics, antidepressants, H_2 blockers, exogenous hormones, alcohol, α-blockers, nicotine abuse, finasteride, others
- Structural abnormalities: Peyronie's disease

Erosions, Genitalia

- Candidiasis
- Intraepithelial neoplasia

- Squamous cell carcinoma
- Lichen planus
- Pemphigus vulgaris
- Erythema multiforme
- Lichen sclerosus
- Bullous pemphigoid
- Extramammary Paget's disease
- Impetigo

Erysipelas

- Other types of cellulitis
- Necrotizing fasciitis
- Deep venous thrombosis (DVT)
- Contact dermatitis
- Erythema migrans (Lyme disease)
- Insect bite
- Herpes zoster
- Erysipeloid
- Acute gout
- Pseudogout

Erythema Multiforme

- Chronic urticaria
- Secondary syphilis
- Pityriasis rosea
- Contact dermatitis
- Pemphigus vulgaris
- Lichen planus
- Serum sickness
- Drug eruption
- Granuloma annulare
- Polymorphic light eruption
- Viral exanthem

Erythema Nodosum

- Insect bites
- Post-traumatic ecchymoses

- Vasculitis
- Weber-Christian disease
- Fat necrosis associated with pancreatitis
- Necrobiosis lipoidica
- Scleroderma
- Lupus panniculitis
- Subcutaneous granuloma
- α_1-Antitrypsin deficiency

Erythematous Annular Skin Lesions

- Tinea corporis
- Warfarin plaques
- Erythema multiforme
- Erythema annulare
- Cutaneous lupus
- Cutaneous sarcoidosis
- Trauma
- Acute febrile neutrophilic dermatosis (Sweet's syndrome)

Erythrasma

- Intertrigo
- Tinea
- Contact dermatitis
- Eczema
- Pityriasis rosea

Erythroderma

- Atopic eczema
- Seborrheic dermatitis
- Drug eruption (sulfonamides, allopurinol, anticonvulsants, penicillins)
- Cutaneous T-cell lymphoma
- Pityriasis rubra pilaris
- Norwegian (crusted) scabies
- Fungal infection
- Lichen planus

Esophageal Cancer

- Achalasia of the esophagus
- Scleroderma of the esophagus
- Diffuse esophageal spasm
- Esophageal rings and webs
- Gastroesophageal reflux disease (GERD)
- Barrett's esophagus

Esophageal Perforation[27]

- Trauma
- Caustic burns
- Iatrogenic
- Foreign bodies
- Spontaneous rupture (Boerhaave's syndrome)
- Postoperative breakdown of anastomosis

Esophagitis[26]

INFECTIOUS
- Candidiasis
- Cytomegalovirus
- Herpes simplex virus
- HIV infection, acute

NONINFECTIOUS
- Gastroesophageal reflux
- Mucositis from cancer chemotherapy
- Mucositis from radiation therapy
- Aphthous ulcers

Esotropia

- Congenital
- Accommodative esotropia
- Myasthenia gravis
- Abducens palsy
- Pseudo–sixth nerve palsy
- Medial rectus entrapment (e.g., blowout fracture)

- Posterior internuclear ophthalmoplegia
- Wernicke's encephalopathy
- Thyroid myopathy
- Chiari malformation

Essential Tremor

- Parkinson's disease: tremor is usually asymmetric, especially early in the disease, and it is predominantly a resting tremor. Patients with Parkinson's disease will also have increased tone, decreased facial expression, slowness of movement, and shuffling gait.
- Cerebellar tremor: an intention tremor that increases at the end of a goal-directed movement (such as finger to nose testing). Other associated neurologic abnormalities include ataxia, dysarthria, and difficulty with tandem gait.
- Drug induced: many drugs enhance normal, physiologic tremor. These include caffeine, nicotine, lithium, levothyroxine, β-adrenergic bronchodilators, valproate, and selective serotonin reuptake inhibitors (SSRIs).
- Wilson's disease: wing-beating tremor that is most pronounced with shoulders abducted, elbows flexed, and fingers pointing toward each other. There are usually other neurologic abnormalities, including dysarthria, dystonia, and Kayser-Fleischer rings on ophthalmologic examination.

Exanthems[29]

- Measles
- Rubella
- Erythema infectiosum (fifth disease)
- Roseola exanthema
- Varicella
- Enterovirus
- Adenovirus
- Epstein-Barr virus
- Kawasaki's disease
- Staphylococcal scalded skin
- Scarlet fever
- Meningococcemia
- Rocky Mountain spotted fever

Eyelid Neoplasm

MALIGNANT
- Melanoma
- Basal cell carcinoma
- Squamous cell carcinoma
- Bowen's disease
- Sebaceous cell carcinoma
- Metastatic lymphoma/leukemia

BENIGN
- Melanocytic nevus
- Pilar, eccrine, or apocrine tumor
- Neurofibroma
- Keratosis
- Squamous papilloma
- Keratoacanthoma

Eyelid Retraction

- Congenital
- Graves' ophthalmopathy
- Myasthenia gravis
- Postsurgical
- Guillain-Barré syndrome
- Cerebellar disease
- Horizontal gaze palsy
- Partial palsy of superior rectus muscle
- Encephalitis
- Closed head injury
- Disseminated sclerosis
- Eye trauma
- Contact lens wear
- Proptosis
- Eyelid neoplasm
- Atopic dermatitis
- Herpes zoster ophthalmicus
- Botulinum toxin injection
- Cyclic oculomotor paralysis
- Spheroid wing meningioma

Felty's Syndrome

- Drug reaction
- Myeloproliferative disorders
- Lymphoma/reticuloendothelial malignant neoplasms
- Hepatic cirrhosis with portal hypertension
- Sarcoidosis
- TB
- Amyloidosis
- Chronic infections

Femoral Neck Fracture

- Osteoarthritis of hip
- Pathologic fracture
- Lumbar disk syndrome with radicular pain
- Insufficiency fracture of pelvis

Fetal Alcohol Syndrome

- Other causes of symmetric growth retardation including intrauterine infection and aneuploidy
- Aneuploidy (T21, T18, T13)
- Syndromes with overlapping features of FAS
- Fetal anticonvulsant syndrome
- Maternal phenylketonuria
- Toluene embryopathy
- Velocardiofacial syndrome
- Williams syndrome
- Dubowitz syndrome
- Cornelia de Lange syndrome

Fever and Jaundice

- Cholecystitis
- Hepatic abscess (pyogenic, amebic)
- Ascending cholangitis
- Pancreatitis
- Malaria
- Neoplasm (hepatic, pancreatic, biliary tract, metastatic)

- Mononucleosis
- Viral hepatitis
- Sepsis
- Babesiosis
- HIV infection *(Cryptosporidium)*
- Biliary ascariasis
- Toxic shock syndrome
- *Yersinia* infection, leptospirosis, yellow fever, dengue fever, relapsing fever

Fever and Rash

- Drug hypersensitivity: penicillin, sulfonamides, thiazides, anticonvulsants, allopurinol
- Viral infection: measles, rubella, varicella, erythema infectiosum, roseola, enterovirus infection, viral hepatitis, infectious mononucleosis, acute HIV infection
- Other infections: meningococcemia, staphylococcemia, scarlet fever, typhoid fever, *Pseudomonas* bacteremia, Rocky Mountain spotted fever, Lyme disease, secondary syphilis, bacterial endocarditis, babesiosis, brucellosis, listeriosis
- Serum sickness
- Erythema multiforme
- Erythema marginatum
- Erythema nodosum
- Systemic lupus erythematosus (SLE)
- Dermatomyositis
- Allergic vasculitis
- Pityriasis rosea
- Herpes zoster

Fever in Returning Travelers and Immigrants[29]

Differential diagnosis of some selected systemic febrile illnesses to consider in returned travelers and immigrants*

---

*Diagnoses for which particular symptoms are indicative are in italics. Exposure to regions of the world that are most likely to be significant to the diagnosis are presented in (parentheses). Vectors, risk behaviors, and sources associated with acquisition are presented in [brackets]. Special clinical characteristics are listed within {braces}

COMMON

- *Acute respiratory tract infection* (worldwide)
- *Gastroenteritis* (worldwide) [food-borne, water-borne, fecal-oral]
- Enteric fever, including typhoid (worldwide) [food, water]
- *Urinary tract infection* (worldwide) [sexual contact]
- Drug reactions [antibiotics, prophylactic agents, other] {rash frequent}
- Malaria (tropics, limited areas of temperate zones) [mosquitoes]
- Arboviruses (Africa, tropics) [mosquitoes, ticks, mites]
- Dengue (Asia, Caribbean, Africa) [mosquitoes]
- Viral hepatitis (worldwide)
- Hepatitis A (worldwide) [food, fecal-oral]
- Hepatitis B (worldwide, especially Asia, sub-Saharan Africa) [sexual contact] {long incubation period}
- Hepatitis C (worldwide) [blood or sexual contact]
- Hepatitis E (Asia, North Africa, Mexico, others) [food, water]
- TB (worldwide) [airborne, milk] {long period to symptomatic infection}
- *STDs* (worldwide) [sexual contact]

LESS COMMON

- Filariasis (Asia, Africa, South America) [biting insects] {long incubation period, eosinophilia}
- *Measles* (developing world) [airborne] {in susceptible individual}
- Amebic abscess (worldwide) [food]
- Brucellosis (worldwide) [milk, cheese, food, animal contact]
- Listeriosis (worldwide) [food-borne] {meningitis}
- Leptospirosis (worldwide) [animal contact, open fresh water] {jaundice, meningitis}
- Strongyloidiasis (warm and tropical areas) [soil contact] {eosinophilia}
- Toxoplasmosis (worldwide) [undercooked meat]

RARE

- Relapsing fever (western Americas, Asia, northern Africa) [ticks, lice]
- *Hemorrhagic fevers* (worldwide) [arthropod and nonarthropod transmitted]
- Yellow fever (tropics) [mosquitoes] {hepatitis}
- Hemorrhagic fever with renal syndrome (Europe, Asia, North America) [rodent urine] {renal impairment}

- Hantavirus pulmonary syndrome (western North America, others) [rodent urine] {respiratory distress syndrome}
- Lassa fever (Africa) [rodent excreta, person to person] {high mortality rate}
- Other: chikungunya, Rift Valley, Ebola-Marburg, others (various) [insect bites, rodent excreta, aerosols, person to person] {often severe}
- *Rickettsial infections* {rashes and eschars}
- Leishmaniasis, visceral (Middle East, Mediterranean, Africa, Asia, South America) [biting flies] {long incubation period}
- Acute schistosomiasis (Africa, Asia, South America, Caribbean) [fresh water]
- Chagas' disease (South and Central America) [reduviid bug bites] {often asymptomatic}
- African trypanosomiasis (Africa) [tsetse fly bite] {neurologic syndromes, sleeping sickness}
- Bartonellosis (South America) [sandfly bite; cb] {skin nodules}
- HIV infection/AIDS (worldwide) [sexual and blood contact]
- Trichinosis (worldwide) [undercooked meat] {eosinophilia}
- *Plague* (temperate and tropical plains) [animal exposures and fleas]
- *Tularemia* (worldwide) [animal contact, fleas, aerosols] {ulcers, lymph nodes}
- *Anthrax* (worldwide) [animal, animal product contact] {ulcers}
- *Lyme disease* (North America, Europe) [tick bites] {arthritis, meningitis, cardiac abnormalities}

Fever of Undetermined Origin (FUO), Possible Causes

The most common causes are italicized.
- Infection (16%)
  - *Abscess: abdominal, pelvic*
  - Tuberculosis
  - *HIV infection*
  - *Nosocomial* (febrile for 3 days in hospital): urinary tract infection, pneumonia, line-related bacteremia, *Clostridium difficile* diarrhea, sinusitis
  - Bacterial endocarditis (especially caused by difficult-to-isolate organisms)

- Biliary tract infection
- Osteomyelitis, vertebral and mandibular
- Less common infections: Q fever, leptospirosis, psittacosis, tularemia, secondary syphilis, gonococcemia, chronic meningococcemia, Whipple's disease, yersiniosis, fungal infections
- Malignant neoplasia (7%)
  - *Lymphoma* and *leukemia*, renal cell carcinoma, hepatocellular carcinomas, other tumors metastatic to liver
- Noninfectious inflammatory disease (22%)
  - Juvenile rheumatoid arthritis (younger patients)
  - Temporal arteritis (elderly patients)
  - Other vasculitis: polyarteritis nodosa, Takayasu's arteritis, Wegener's granulomatosis, mixed cryoglobulinemia, adult Still's disease
- Other (4%)
  - Drug-induced fever
  - Inflammatory bowel disease
  - Sarcoidosis
  - Granulomatous hepatitis
  - Deep venous thrombosis
  - Alcoholic hepatitis

Fibrocystic Breast Disease

- If presenting as dominant mass or masses, exclude possible carcinoma
- Breast abscess
- If presenting with nipple discharge, differentiate from discharge of possible malignant origin
- Mastitis
- Mastodynia

Fibromyalgia

- Polymyalgia rheumatica
- Referred discogenic spine pain
- Rheumatoid arthritis (RA)
- Localized tendinitis
- Connective tissue disease

- Osteoarthritis
- Thyroid disease
- Spondyloarthropathies

Fifth Disease

- Juvenile rheumatoid arthritis (JRA) (Still's disease)
- Rubella, measles (rubeola), and other childhood viral exanthems
- Mononucleosis
- Lyme disease
- Acute HIV infection
- Drug eruption

Filariasis

- Chronic lymphedema
- Milroy's disease
- Postoperative scarring
- Lymphedema of malignant disease

Finger Lesions, Inflammatory

- Paronychia
- Herpes simplex type 1 (herpetic whitlow)
- Dyshidrotic eczema (pompholyx)
- Herpes zoster
- Bacterial endocarditis (Osler's nodes)
- Psoriatic arthritis

Flank Pain

- Urolithiasis
- Radicular/muscular
- Pyelonephritis
- Herpes zoster
- Renal abscess
- Renal vein thrombosis
- Renal infarction
- Abdominal aortic aneurysm (AAA)

Flatulence and Bloating[34]

- Ingestion of nonabsorbable carbohydrates
- Ingestion of carbonated beverages
- Malabsorption: pancreatic insufficiency, biliary disease, celiac disease, bacterial overgrowth in small intestine
- Lactase deficiency
- Irritable bowel syndrome (IBS)
- Anxiety disorders
- Food poisoning, giardiasis

Flushing[28]

- Physiologic flushing: menopause, ingestion of monosodium glutamate (Chinese restaurant syndrome), ingestion of hot drinks
- Drugs: alcohol (with or without disulfiram, metronidazole, or chlorpropamide), nicotinic acid, diltiazem, nifedipine, levodopa, bromocriptine, vancomycin, amyl nitrate
- Neoplastic disorders: carcinoid syndrome, VIPoma syndrome, medullary carcinoma of thyroid, systemic mastocytosis, basophilic chronic myelocytic leukemia, renal cell carcinoma
- Anxiety
- Agnogenic flushing

Folate Deficiency[21]

NUTRITIONAL CAUSES
- Decreased dietary intake
- Poverty and famine
- Institutionalized individuals (e.g., psychiatric, nursing homes), chronic debilitating disease
- Prolonged feeding of infants with goat's milk, special slimming diets or food fads (i.e., folate-rich foods not consumed), cultural or ethnic cooking techniques (i.e., food folate destroyed)
- Decreased diet and increased requirements
- Physiologic (e.g., pregnancy and lactation, prematurity, hyperemesis gravidarum, infancy)
- Pathologic (e.g., intrinsic hematologic diseases involving hemolysis with compensatory erythropoiesis, abnormal

hematopoiesis, or bone marrow infiltration with malignant disease and dermatologic disease such as psoriasis)

FOLATE MALABSORPTION

- With normal intestinal mucosa
  - Some drugs (controversial)
  - Congenital folate malabsorption (rare)
- With mucosal abnormalities (e.g., tropical and nontropical sprue, regional enteritis)

DEFECTIVE CELLULAR FOLATE UPTAKE

- Familial aplastic anemia (rare)
- Acute cerebral folate deficiency

INADEQUATE CELLULAR USE

- Folate antagonists (e.g., methotrexate)
- Hereditary enzyme deficiencies involving folate

DRUGS

- Multiple effects on folate metabolism (e.g., alcohol, sulfasalazine, triamterene, pyrimethamine, trimethoprim-sulfamethoxazole, diphenylhydantoin, barbiturates)

ACUTE FOLATE DEFICIENCY

- Intensive care unit setting
- Uncertain origin

Folliculitis

- Pseudofolliculitis barbae (ingrown hairs)
- Acne vulgaris
- Dermatophyte fungal infections
- Keratosis pilaris
- Cutaneous candidiasis
- Superficial fungal infections
- Miliaria

Food Poisoning, Bacterial

- Viral gastroenteritis (Norwalk or rotavirus)
- Parasitic gastroenteritis (*Entamoeba histolytica*, *Giardia lamblia*)
- Toxins (ciguatoxins, mushrooms, heavy metals)

Foot Dermatitis

- Tinea pedis
- Dyshidrotic eczema
- Tylosis (mechanically induced hyperkeratosis, fissuring, and dryness)
- Allergic contact dermatitis
- Psoriasis
- Peripheral vascular insufficiency
- Neuropathic foot ulcers (DM, poorly fitting shoes)
- Acquired plantar keratoderma
- Sézary's syndrome

Footdrop

- Peripheral neuropathy
- L5 radiculopathy
- Peroneal nerve compression
- Sciatic nerve palsy
- Scapuloperoneal syndromes
- Spasticity
- Myopathy
- Dystonia

Foot Lesion, Ulcerating

- Cellulitis
- Plantar wart
- Squamous cell carcinoma
- Actinomycosis (Madura foot)
- Plantar fibromatosis
- Pseudoepitheliomatous hyperplasia

Foot Pain

- Trauma (fractures, musculoskeletal and ligamentous strain)
- Inflammation (plantar fasciitis, Achilles tendinitis or bursitis, calcaneal apophysitis)

- Arterial insufficiency, Raynaud's phenomenon, thromboangiitis obliterans
- Gout, pseudogout
- Calcaneal spur
- Infection (cellulitis, abscess, lymphangitis, gangrene)
- Decubitus ulcer
- Paronychia, ingrown toenail
- Thrombophlebitis, postphlebitic syndrome

Forearm and Hand Pain

- Epicondylitis
- Tenosynovitis
- Osteoarthritis
- Cubital tunnel syndrome
- Carpal tunnel syndrome
- Trauma
- Herpes zoster
- Peripheral vascular insufficiency
- Infection (cellulitis, abscess)

Friedreich's Ataxia

- Charcot-Marie-Tooth disease type (in early cases)
- Abetalipoproteinemia (Bassen-Kornzweig syndrome)
- Severe vitamin E deficiency with malabsorption
- Early-onset cerebellar ataxia with retained reflexes
- Autosomal dominant cerebellar ataxia (spinocerebellar ataxia)

Frostbite

- Other induced cold injuries including:
  - Frostnip: transient tingling and numbness without associated permanent tissue damage
  - Pernio (chilblains): a self-limited, cold-induced vasculitis of dermal vessels associated with purple plaques or nodules, often affecting dorsum of hands and feet and seen with prolonged cold exposure to above-freezing temperatures

- Cold immersion (trench) foot: caused by ischemic injury resulting from sustained severe vasoconstriction in appendages exposed to wet cold at temperatures above freezing

Frozen Shoulder

- Secondary causes of shoulder stiffness (prolonged immobilization after trauma or surgery)
- Posterior shoulder dislocation
- Ruptured rotator cuff
- Glenohumeral osteoarthritis
- Rotator cuff inflammation
- Superior sulcus tumor
- Cervical disk disease
- Brachial neuritis

Furuncle

- Folliculitis
- Pseudofolliculitis
- Foreign body reaction
- Acne
- Hidradenitis suppurativa
- Epidermoid cyst

Gait Abnormalities

- Parkinsonism
- Degenerative joint disease (hips, back, knees)
- Multiple sclerosis (MS)
- Trauma, foot pain
- Cerebrovascular accident (CVA)
- Cerebellar lesions
- Infections (tabes, encephalitis, meningitis)
- Sensory ataxia
- Dystonia, cerebral palsy, neuromuscular disorders
- Metabolic abnormalities

Galactorrhea

- Intraductal papilloma
- Breast cancer
- Paget's disease of breast
- Breast abscess
- True galactorrhea
- Prolonged suckling
- Drugs (isonicotinic acid hydrazide [INH], phenothiazines, reserpine derivatives, amphetamines, spironolactone, tricyclic antidepressants)
- Major stressors (surgery, trauma)
- Hypothyroidism
- Pituitary tumors

Ganglia

- Lipoma
- Fibroma
- Epidermoid inclusion cyst
- Osteochondroma
- Hemangioma
- Infection (TB, fungi, secondary syphilis)
- Gout
- Rheumatoid nodule
- Radial artery aneurysm

Gardner's Syndrome

- Familial adenomatous polyposis (FAP)
- Turcot's syndrome
- Attenuated adenomatous polyposis coli
- Peutz-Jeghers syndrome
- Juvenile polyposis
- Hereditary nonpolyposis colorectal cancer
- Cowden syndrome

Gastric Cancer

- Gastric lymphoma (5% of gastric malignant neoplasms)
- Hypertrophic gastritis

- Peptic ulcer
- Reflux esophagitis
- Nonulcer dyspepsia

Gastric Emptying, Delayed[1]

MECHANICAL OBSTRUCTION
- Duodenal or pyloric channel ulcer
- Pyloric stricture
- Tumor of the distal stomach

FUNCTIONAL OBSTRUCTION (GASTROPARESIS)
- Drugs: anticholinergics, β-adrenergics, opiates
- Electrolyte imbalance: hypokalemia, hypocalcemia, hypomagnesemia
- Metabolic disorders: diabetes mellitus (DM), hypoparathyroidism, hypothyroidism, pregnancy
- Vagotomy
- Viral infections
- Neuromuscular disorders (myotonic dystrophy, autonomic neuropathy, scleroderma, polymyositis)
- Gastric pacemaker (i.e., tachygastria)
- Brainstem tumors
- Gastroesophageal reflux disease (GERD)
- Psychiatric disorders: anorexia nervosa, psychogenic vomiting
- Idiopathic

Gastric Emptying, Rapid

- Pancreatic insufficiency
- Dumping syndrome
- Peptic ulcer
- Celiac disease
- Promotility agents
- Zollinger-Ellison disease

Gastritis

- Gastroesophageal reflux disease (GERD)
- Nonulcer dyspepsia

- Gastric lymphoma or carcinoma
- Pancreatitis
- Gastroparesis

Gastroesophageal Reflux Disease

- Peptic ulcer disease
- Unstable angina
- Esophagitis (from infections such as herpes, *Candida*), medication induced (doxycycline, potassium chloride)
- Esophageal spasm (nutcracker esophagus)
- Cancer of esophagus

Genital Discharge, Female[12]

- Physiologic discharge: cervical mucus, vaginal transudation, bacteria, squamous epithelial cells
- Individual variation
- Pregnancy
- Sexual response
- Menstrual cycle variation
- Infection
- Foreign body: tampon, cervical cap, other
- Neoplasm
- Fistula
- Intrauterine contraceptive device (IUD)
- Cervical ectropion
- Spermicide
- Nongenital causes: urinary incontinence, urinary tract fistula, Crohn's disease, rectovaginal fistula

Genital Sores[1]

- Herpes genitalis
- Syphilis
- Chancroid
- Lymphogranuloma venereum
- Granuloma inguinale

- Condyloma acuminatum
- Neoplastic lesion
- Trauma

Giant Cell Arteritis

- Other vasculitic syndromes
- Nonarteritic anterior ischemic optic neuropathy (AION)
- Transient ischemic attack (TIA), stroke
- Infections
- Occult neoplasm, multiple myeloma
- Primary amyloidosis

Giardiasis

- Other agents of infective diarrhea (e.g., amebae, *Salmonella* sp., *Shigella* sp., *Staphylococcus aureus*, *Cryptosporidium*)
- Noninfectious causes of malabsorption

Gilbert's Disease

- Hemolytic anemia
- Liver disease (chronic hepatitis, cirrhosis)
- Crigler-Najjar syndrome

Gingivitis

- Gingival hyperplasia, which may be caused by long-term use of phenytoin or nifedipine
- Necrotizing ulcerative gingivitis (NUG)
- Acute herpetic gingivostomatitis
- Aphthous stomatitis
- Chronic periodontal disease
- Desquamative gingivitis
- Gonococcal and streptococcal gingivostomatitis
- Oral candidiasis
- Ludwig's angina
- HIV infection–associated idiopathic ulcerations

Glaucoma, Chronic Open-Angle

- Other optic neuropathies
- Secondary glaucoma from inflammation and steroid therapy
- Red eye differential
- Trauma
- Contact lens injury

Glaucoma, Primary Angle-Closure

- High pressure
- Optic nerve cupping
- Field loss
- Shallow chamber
- Open-angle glaucoma
- Conjunctivitis
- Corneal disease, keratitis
- Uveitis
- Scleritis
- Allergies
- Contact lens wearing with irritation

Glenohumeral Dislocation

- Rotator cuff rupture
- Frozen shoulder (posterior dislocation)
- Suprascapular nerve paralysis
- Anterior instability

Glomerulonephritis, Acute

- Cirrhosis with edema and ascites
- Congestive heart failure (CHF)
- Acute interstitial nephritis
- Severe hypertension
- Hemolytic-uremic syndrome (HUS)
- Systemic lupus erythematosus (SLE), diabetes mellitus (DM), amyloidosis, preeclampsia, sclerodermal renal crisis

Glomus Tumor

- Schwannoma (neurilemmoma)
- Eccrine spiradenoma
- Hemangioma
- Arteriovenous malformation (AVM)
- Blue nevus
- Melanoma
- Angiolipoma

Glossitis

- Infections
- Use of chemical irritants
- Neoplasms
- Skin disorders (e.g., Behçet's syndrome, erythema multiforme)

Glossodynia[39]

DENTURE RELATED
- Dentures (ill-fitting, monomer from denture base)
- Dental plaque
- Oral parafunction

INFECTIVE/DERMATOLOGIC
- Candidiasis
- Lichen planus

DEFICIENCY STATES
- Iron, B_{12}, folate, B_2 (riboflavin), B_6 (pyridoxine), zinc

ENDOCRINE
- Diabetes
- Myxedema*
- Hormonal changes occurring during menopause*

NEUROLOGICALLY MEDIATED
- Referred from tonsils, teeth
- Lingual nerve neuropathy

---

*Unproven associations.

- Glossopharyngeal neuralgia
- Esophageal reflux*

IATROGENIC

- Mouthwash xerostomia

PSYCHOGENIC

IDIOPATHIC

Glucocorticoid Deficiency[14]

- Adrenocorticotropic hormone (ACTH)–independent causes
  - TB
  - Autoimmune (idiopathic)
  - Other rare causes
  - Fungal infection
  - Adrenal hemorrhage
  - Metastases
  - Sarcoidosis
  - Amyloidosis
  - Adrenoleukodystrophy
  - Adrenomyeloneuropathy
  - HIV infection
  - Congenital adrenal hyperplasia
  - Medications (e.g., ketoconazole)
- ACTH-dependent causes
  - Hypothalamic-pituitary-adrenal suppression
  - Exogenous: glucocorticoid, ACTH
  - Endogenous: cure of Cushing's syndrome
  - Hypothalamic: pituitary lesions
  - Neoplasm: primary pituitary tumor, metastatic tumor
  - Craniopharyngioma
  - Infection: TB, actinomycosis, nocardiosis
  - Sarcoid
  - Head trauma
  - Isolated ACTH deficiency

Goiter

- Thyroiditis
- Toxic multinodular goiter

---

*Unproven associations.

- Graves' disease
- Medications (e.g., propylthiouracil [PTU], methimazole, sulfonamides, sulfonylureas, ethionamide, amiodarone, lithium)
- Iodine deficiency
- Sarcoidosis, amyloidosis
- Defective thyroid hormone synthesis
- Resistance to thyroid hormone

Gonorrhea

- Nongonococcal urethritis (NGU)
- Nongonococcal mucopurulent cervicitis
- *Chlamydia trachomatis*

Goodpasture's Syndrome

- Wegener's granulomatosis
- Systemic lupus erythematosus (SLE)
- Systemic necrotizing vasculitis
- Idiopathic rapidly progressive glomerulonephritis
- Drug-induced renal pulmonary disease (e.g., penicillamine)

Gout

- Pseudogout
- Rheumatoid arthritis
- Osteoarthritis
- Cellulitis
- Infectious arthritis

Granuloma Annulare

- Tinea corporis
- Lichen planus
- Necrobiosis lipoidica diabeticorum
- Sarcoidosis
- Rheumatoid nodules
- Late secondary or tertiary syphilis

- Arcuate and annular plaques of mycosis fungoides
- Papular granuloma annulare can simulate insect bites, secondary syphilis, xanthoma.
- Annular elastolytic giant cell granuloma

Granuloma Inguinale

- Carcinoma
- Secondary syphilis: condylomata lata
- Amebiasis: necrotic ulceration
- Concurrent infections
- Lymphogranuloma venereum
- Chancroid
- Genital herpes

Granulomatous Dermatitides

- Granuloma annulare
- Sarcoidosis
- Necrobiosis lipoidica diabeticorum
- Cutaneous Crohn's disease
- Rheumatoid nodules
- Annular elastolytic giant cell granuloma (actinic granuloma)
- Foreign body granuloma

Granulomatous Disorders[33]

INFECTIONS
Fungi
- *Histoplasma*
- *Coccidioides*
- *Blastomyces*
- *Sporothrix*
- *Aspergillus*
- *Cryptococcus*

Protozoa
- *Toxoplasma*
- *Leishmania*

Metazoa
- *Toxocara*
- *Schistosoma*

Spirochetes
- *Treponema pallidum*
- *Treponema pertenue*
- *Treponema carateum*

Mycobacteria
- *Mycobacterium tuberculosis*
- *Mycobacterium leprae*
- *Mycobacterium kansasii*
- *Mycobacterium marinum*
- *Mycobacterium avium*
- Bacille Calmette-Guérin (BCG) vaccine

Bacteria
- *Brucella*
- *Yersinia*

Other Infections
- Cat-scratch disease
- Lymphogranuloma

NEOPLASIA
- Carcinoma
- Reticulosis
- Pinealoma
- Dysgerminoma
- Seminoma
- Reticulum cell sarcoma
- Malignant nasal granuloma

CHEMICALS
- Beryllium
- Zirconium
- Silica
- Starch
- Immunologic aberrations
- Sarcoidosis
- Crohn's disease
- Primary biliary cirrhosis

- Wegener's granulomatosis
- Giant cell arteritis
- Peyronie's disease
- Hypogammaglobulinemia
- Systemic lupus erythematosus (SLE)
- Lymphomatoid granulomatosis
- Histiocytosis X
- Hepatic granulomatous disease
- Immune complex disease
- Rosenthal-Melkersson syndrome
- Churg-Strauss allergic granulomatosis

LEUKOCYTE OXIDASE DEFECT
- Chronic granulomatous disease of childhood

EXTRINSIC ALLERGIC ALVEOLITIS
- Farmer's lung
- Bird fancier's lung
- Mushroom worker's lung
- Suberosis (cork dust)
- Bagassosis
- Maple bark stripper's lung
- Paprika splitter's lung
- Coffee bean dust
- Spatlese lung

OTHER DISORDERS
- Whipple's disease
- Pyrexia of unknown origin
- Radiotherapy
- Cancer chemotherapy
- Panniculitis
- Chalazion
- Sebaceous cyst
- Dermoid
- Sea urchin spine injury

Granulomatous Liver Disease

- Sarcoidosis
- Wegener's granulomatosis

- Vasculitis
- Inflammatory bowel disease (IBD)
- Allergic granulomatosis
- Erythema nodosum
- Infections (fungal, viral, parasitic)
- Primary biliary cirrhosis
- Lymphoma
- Hodgkin's disease
- Drugs (e.g., allopurinol, hydralazine, sulfonamides, penicillins)
- Toxins (copper sulfate, beryllium)

Graves' Disease

- Anxiety disorder
- Premenopausal state
- Thyroiditis
- Other causes of hyperthyroidism (e.g., toxic multinodular goiter, toxic adenoma)
- Other: metastatic neoplasm, diabetes mellitus (DM), pheochromocytoma

Green or Blue Urine

- Pseudomonal urinary tract infection
- Medications: triamterene, amitriptyline, IV cimetidine, IV promethazine
- Biliverdin
- Dyes (methylene blue, indigo carmine)

Groin Lump[39]

COMMON CAUSES
- Inguinal hernia
- Femoral hernia
- Lymph node

OTHER CAUSES
- Saphena varix
- Femoral artery aneurysm/pseudoaneurysm
- Psoas abscess

- Lipoma of the cord
- Encysted hydrocele of the cord (male)
- Testicular maldescent (male)
- Hydrocele of canal of Nuck (female)

Groin Pain, Active Patient[38]

MUSCULOSKELETAL
- Avascular necrosis of the femoral head
- Avulsion fracture (lesser trochanter, anterior superior iliac spine, anterior inferior iliac spine)
- Bursitis (iliopectineal, trochanteric)
- Entrapment of the ilioinguinal or iliofemoral nerve
- Gracilis syndrome
- Muscle tear (adductors, iliopsoas, rectus abdominis, gracilis, sartorius, rectus femoris)
- Myositis ossificans of the hip muscles
- Osteitis pubis
- Osteoarthritis of the femoral head
- Slipped capital femoral epiphysis
- Stress fracture of the femoral head or neck and pubis
- Synovitis

HERNIA RELATED
- Avulsion of the internal oblique muscle in the conjoined tendon
- Defect at the insertion of the rectus abdominis muscle
- Direct inguinal hernia
- Femoral ring hernia
- Indirect inguinal hernia
- Inguinal canal weakness

UROLOGIC
- Epididymitis
- Fracture of the testis
- Hydrocele
- Kidney stone
- Posterior urethritis
- Prostatitis
- Testicular cancer
- Torsion of the testis

- Urinary tract infection (UTI)
- Varicocele

GYNECOLOGIC
- Ectopic pregnancy
- Ovarian cyst
- Pelvic inflammatory disease (PID)
- Torsion of the ovary
- Vaginitis

LYMPHATIC ENLARGEMENT IN GROIN

Guillain-Barré Syndrome

- Toxic peripheral neuropathies: heavy metal poisoning (lead, thallium, arsenic), medications (vincristine, disulfiram), organophosphate poisoning, hexacarbon (glue sniffer's neuropathy)
- Nontoxic peripheral neuropathies: acute intermittent porphyria, vasculitic polyneuropathy, infectious (poliomyelitis, diphtheria, Lyme disease), tick paralysis
- Neuromuscular junction disorders: myasthenia gravis, botulism, snake envenomations
- Myopathies such as polymyositis, acute necrotizing myopathies caused by drugs
- Metabolic derangements such as hypermagnesemia, hypokalemia, hypophosphatemia
- Acute CNS disorders such as basilar artery thrombosis with brainstem infarction, brainstem encephalomyelitis, transverse myelitis, or spinal cord compression
- Hysterical paralysis or malingering

Gynecomastia

- Physiologic (puberty, newborns, aging)
- Drugs (estrogen and estrogen precursors, digitalis, testosterone and exogenous androgens, clomiphene, cimetidine, spironolactone, ketoconazole, amiodarone, angiotensin-converting enzyme [ACE] inhibitors, isoniazid, phenytoin, methyldopa, metoclopramide, phenothiazine)

- Increased prolactin level (prolactinoma)
- Liver disease
- Adrenal disease
- Thyrotoxicosis
- Increased estrogen production (human chorionic gonadotropin [hCG]–producing tumor, testicular tumor, bronchogenic carcinoma)
- Secondary hypogonadism
- Primary gonadal failure (trauma, castration, viral orchitis, granulomatous disease)
- Defects in androgen synthesis
- Testosterone deficiency
- Klinefelter's syndrome

Hairy Tongue

- Oral hairy leukoplakia
- Candidiasis
- Lichen planus
- Stomatitis

Halitosis

- Tobacco use
- Alcohol use
- Dry mouth (mouth breathing, inadequate fluid intake)
- Foods (onion, garlic, meats, nuts)
- Disease of mouth or nose (infections, cancer, inflammation)
- Medications (antihistamines, antidepressants)
- Systemic disorders (diabetes, uremia)
- GI disorders (esophageal diverticula, hiatal hernia, gastroesophageal reflux disease [GERD], achalasia)
- Sinusitis
- Pulmonary disorders (bronchiectasis, pneumonia, neoplasms, TB)

Hand-Foot-Mouth Disease

- Aphthous stomatitis
- Herpes simplex infection
- Herpangina

- Erythema multiforme
- Pemphigus
- Gonorrhea
- Acute leukemia
- Lymphoma
- Allergic contact dermatitis

Hand Pain and Swelling[5]

- Trauma
- Gout
- Pseudogout
- Cellulitis
- Lymphangitis
- Deep venous thrombosis (DVT) of upper extremity
- Thrombophlebitis
- Rheumatoid arthritis (RA)
- Remitting seronegative symmetric synovitis with pitting edema
- Polymyalgia rheumatica
- Mixed connective tissue disease
- Scleroderma
- Rupture of the olecranon bursa
- Medsger's syndrome (neoplasia)
- The puffy hand of drug addiction
- Reflex sympathetic dystrophy
- Eosinophilic fasciitis
- Sickle cell (hand-foot syndrome)
- Leprosy
- Factitial (the rubber band syndrome)

Headache[13]

- Vascular: migraine, cluster headaches, temporal arteritis, hypertension, cavernous sinus thrombosis
- Musculoskeletal: neck and shoulder muscle contraction, strain of extraocular or intraocular muscles, cervical spondylosis, temporomandibular arthritis
- Infections: meningitis, encephalitis, brain abscess, sepsis, sinusitis, osteomyelitis, parotitis, mastoiditis

- Cerebral neoplasm
- Subdural hematoma
- Cerebral hemorrhage/infarct
- Pseudotumor cerebri
- Normal-pressure hydrocephalus (NPH)
- Post lumbar puncture
- Cerebral aneurysm, arteriovenous malformations
- Post trauma
- Dental problems: abscess, periodontitis, poorly fitting dentures
- Trigeminal neuralgia, glossopharyngeal neuralgia
- Otitis and other ear diseases
- Glaucoma and other eye diseases
- Metabolic: uremia, carbon monoxide inhalation, hypoxia
- Pheochromocytoma, hypoglycemia, hypothyroidism
- Effort induced: benign exertional headache, cough headache, coital cephalalgia
- Drugs: alcohol, nitrates, histamine antagonists
- Paget's disease of the skull
- Emotional, psychiatric

Headache, Acute[11]

DIFFERENTIAL DIAGNOSIS OF ACUTE HEADACHE
Evaluation of the first acute headache should exclude pathologic causes listed here before consideration of more common etiologies.
- Increased intracranial pressure (ICP): trauma, hemorrhage, tumor, hydrocephalus, pseudotumor cerebri, abscess, arachnoid cyst, cerebral edema
- Decreased ICP: after ventriculoperitoneal shunt, lumbar puncture, cerebrospinal fluid leak from basilar skull fracture
- Meningeal inflammation: meningitis, leukemia, subarachnoid or subdural hemorrhage
- Vascular: vasculitis, arteriovenous malformation, hypertension, cerebrovascular accident
- Bone, soft tissue: referred pain from scalp, eyes, ears, sinuses, nose, teeth, pharynx, cervical spine, temporomandibular joint
- Infection: systemic infection, encephalitis, sinusitis, others
- First migraine

Headache and Facial Pain[37]

VASCULAR HEADACHES

- Migraine
  - Migraine with headaches and inconspicuous neurologic features
    - Migraine without aura ("common migraine")
  - Migraine with headaches and conspicuous neurologic features
    - With transient neurologic symptoms: migraine with typical aura ("classic migraine"), sensory, basilar, and hemiplegic migraine
    - With prolonged or permanent neurologic features ("complicated migraine"): ophthalmoplegic migraine, migrainous infarction
  - Migraine without headaches but with conspicuous neurologic features ("migraine equivalents")
    - Abdominal migraine
    - Benign paroxysmal vertigo of childhood
  - Migraine aura without headache ("isolated auras," transient migrainous accompaniments)
- Cluster headaches
  - Episodic cluster headache ("cyclic cluster headaches")
  - Chronic cluster headaches
  - Chronic paroxysmal hemicrania
- Other vascular headaches
  - Headaches of reactive vasodilation (fever, drug induced, postictal, hypoglycemia, hypoxia, hypercapnia, hyperthyroidism)
  - Headaches associated with arterial hypertension
    - Chronic severe hypertension (diastolic >120 mm Hg)
    - Paroxysmal severe hypertension (pheochromocytoma, some coital headaches)
  - Headaches caused by cranial arteritis
    - Giant cell arteritis ("temporal arteritis")
    - Other vasculitides

HEADACHES ASSOCIATED WITH DEMONSTRABLE MUSCLE SPASM

- Headache caused by posturally induced or paralesional muscle spasm

- Headaches of sustained or impaired posture (e.g., prolonged close work, driving)
- Headaches associated with cervical spondylosis and other diseases of cervical spine
- Myofascial pain dysfunction syndrome (headache or facial pain associated with disorders of teeth, jaws, and related structures, or "temporomandibular joint [TMJ] syndrome")
- Headaches caused by psychophysiologic muscle contraction ("muscle contraction headaches," or tension type of headache associated with disorder of pericranial muscles)

HEADACHES AND FACIAL PAIN WITHOUT DEMONSTRABLE PHYSICAL SUBSTRATE

- Headaches of uncertain etiology: "tension headaches" (tension type of headache unassociated with disorder of pericranial muscles)
- Some forms of post-traumatic headache
- Psychogenic headaches (e.g., hypochondriacal, conversional, delusional, malingering)
- Facial pain of uncertain etiology ("atypical facial pain")

COMBINED TENSION-MIGRAINE HEADACHES

- Episodic migraine superimposed on chronic tension headaches
- Chronic daily headaches: associated with analgesic or ergotamine overuse ("rebound headaches")
- Not associated with drug overuse

HEADACHES AND HEAD PAINS CAUSED BY DISEASES OF EYES, EARS, NOSE, SINUSES, TEETH, OR SKULL

HEADACHES CAUSED BY MENINGEAL INFLAMMATION

- Subarachnoid hemorrhage
- Meningitis and meningoencephalitis
- Others (e.g., meningeal carcinomatosis)

HEADACHES ASSOCIATED WITH ALTERED INTRACRANIAL PRESSURE ("TRACTION HEADACHES")

Increased Intracranial Pressure

- Intracranial mass lesions (e.g., neoplasm, hematoma, abscess)
- Hydrocephalus
- Benign intracranial hypertension
- Venous sinus thrombosis

Decreased Intracranial Pressure
- Post–lumbar puncture headaches
- Spontaneous hypoliquorrheic headaches

HEADACHES AND HEAD PAINS CAUSED BY CRANIAL NEURALGIAS

Presumed Irritation of Superficial Nerves
- Occipital neuralgia
- Supraorbital neuralgia

Presumed Irritation of Intracranial Nerves
- Trigeminal neuralgia ("tic douloureux")
- Glossopharyngeal neuralgia

Headache, Cluster

- Migraine
- Trigeminal neuralgia
- Temporal arteritis
- Postherpetic neuralgia
- Pheochromocytoma
- Glaucoma

Headache, Migraine

- Subarachnoid hemorrhage
- Cluster headache
- Chronic daily headaches (including drug rebound headaches)
- Arteriovenous malformation
- Vasculitis
- Intracranial mass lesion

Headache, Tension Type

- Migraine (would expect associated symptoms; see Headache, Migraine)
- Cervical spine disease
- Intracranial mass (may present with focal neurologic signs, seizures, or headache awakening patient from sleep)

- Idiopathic intracranial hypertension (found more often in obese women of childbearing age; may have papilledema, visual loss, or diplopia)
- Rebound headache from overuse of analgesics
- Secondary headache (e.g., temporomandibular joint syndrome, thyrotoxicosis, polycythemia, drug side effects)
- Migraine and tension-type headache may often coexist and may be difficult to differentiate (suggest headache calendar).

Head and Neck, Soft Tissue Masses

- Lipoma
- Pilar cyst
- Epidermal inclusion cyst
- Dermoid cyst
- Bone cyst
- Hemangioma
- Eosinophilic granuloma
- Other: facial nerve neuroma, teratoma, rhabdomyoma, rhabdomyosarcoma, branchial cleft cyst

Hearing Loss, Acute[27]

- Infectious: mumps, measles, influenza, herpes simplex, herpes zoster, cytomegalovirus (CMV), mononucleosis, syphilis
- Vascular: macroglobulinemia, sickle cell disease, Berger's disease, leukemia, polycythemia, fat emboli, hypercoagulable states
- Metabolic: diabetes, pregnancy, hyperlipoproteinemia
- Conductive: cerumen impaction, foreign bodies, otitis media, otitis externa, barotrauma, trauma
- Medications: aminoglycosides, loop diuretics, antineoplastics, salicylates, vancomycin
- Neoplasm: acoustic neuroma, metastatic neoplasm

Heartburn and Indigestion[34]

- Reflux esophagitis
- Gastritis
- Nonulcer dyspepsia

- Functional GI disorder (anxiety disorder, social/environmental stresses)
- Excessive intestinal gas (ingestion of flatulogenic foods, GI stasis, constipation)
- Gas entrapment (hepatitis or splenic flexure syndrome)
- Neoplasm (adenocarcinoma of stomach or esophagus, lymphoma)
- Gallbladder disease

Heart Failure, Pregnancy

- Congenital valvular heart disease exacerbated by pregnancy
- Peripartum cardiomyopathy
- Untreated thyrotoxicosis
- Hypothyroidism
- Pulmonary hypertension
- Myocardial infarction

Heat Illness

- Infections (meningitis, encephalitis, sepsis)
- Head trauma
- Epilepsy
- Thyroid storm
- Acute cocaine intoxication
- Malignant hyperthermia
- Heat exhaustion can be differentiated from heat stroke by the following:
  - Essentially intact mental function and lack of significant fever in heat exhaustion
  - Mild or absent increases in creatine kinase (CK), aspartate transaminase (AST), lactate dehydrogenase (LDH), and alanine aminotransferase (ALT) in heat exhaustion

Heel Pain

- Achilles tendinitis/tendinopathy (insertional, noninsertional)
- Retrocalcaneal bursitis (superficial, deep)
- Plantar fasciopathy
- Neuropathy (tarsal tunnel, posterior tibial nerve [medial calcaneal branch], abductor digiti quinti)

- Calcaneal stress fracture
- Puncture wound, foreign body
- Cellulitis
- Spondyloarthropathy
- Fat pad atrophy
- Soft tissue tumor
- S1 radiculopathy
- Paget's disease of bone
- Haglund deformity
- Primary or metastatic bone tumor

Heel Pain, Plantar[25]

SKIN

- Keratoses
- Verruca
- Ulcer
- Fissure

FAT

- Atrophy
- Panniculitis

DENSE CONNECTIVE TISSUE

- Inflammatory fasciitis
- Fibromatosis
- Enthesopathy
- Bursitis

BONE (CALCANEUS)

- Stress fracture
- Paget's disease
- Benign bone cyst/tumor
- Malignant bone tumor
- Metabolic bone disease (osteopenia)

NERVE

- Tarsal tunnel
- Plantar nerve entrapment
- S1 nerve root radiculopathy
- Painful peripheral neuropathy

INFECTION
- Dermatomycoses
- Acute osteomyelitis
- Plantar abscess

MISCELLANEOUS
- Foreign body
- Nonunion calcaneus fracture
- Psychogenic
- Idiopathic

HELLP Syndrome

- Appendicitis
- Gallbladder disease
- Peptic ulcer
- Enteritis
- Hepatitis
- Pyelonephritis
- Systemic lupus erythematosus (SLE)
- Thrombotic thrombocytopenic purpura
- Hemolytic-uremic syndrome (HUS)
- Acute fatty liver of pregnancy

Hemarthrosis

- Trauma
- Anticoagulant therapy
- Thrombocytopenia, thrombocytosis
- Bleeding disorders (e.g., von Willebrand disease)
- Charcot's joint
- Idiopathic
- Other: pigmented villonodular synovitis, hemangioma, synovioma, arteriovenous (AV) fistula, ruptured aneurysm

Hematemesis[39]

Causes of hematemesis:
VERY COMMON
- Gastric or duodenal ulcer or erosions

COMMON
- Mallory-Weiss tear (a laceration at the gastroesophageal junction)
- Ulcerative esophagitis
- Esophageal varices

UNCOMMON
- Vascular malformations
- Ulcerated gastrointestinal stromal tumor
- Carcinoma of esophagus or stomach
- Aortoenteric fistula

Hematuria

Use the mnemonic TICS:
- T
  - Trauma: blow to kidney, insertion of Foley catheter or foreign body in urethra, prolonged and severe exercise, very rapid emptying of overdistended bladder
  - Tumor: hypernephroma, Wilms' tumor, papillary carcinoma of the bladder, prostatic and urethral neoplasms
  - Toxins: turpentine, phenols, sulfonamides and other antibiotics, cyclophosphamide, nonsteroidal anti-inflammatory drugs (NSAIDs)
- I
  - Infections: glomerulonephritis, TB, cystitis, prostatitis, urethritis, *Schistosoma haematobium*, yellow fever, blackwater fever
  - Inflammatory processes: Goodpasture's syndrome, periarteritis, post irradiation
- C
  - Calculi: renal, ureteral, bladder, urethra
  - Cysts: simple cysts, polycystic disease
  - Congenital anomalies: hemangiomas, aneurysms, arteriovenous malformation (AVM)
- S
  - Surgery: invasive procedures, prostatic resection, cystoscopy
  - Sickle cell disease and other hematologic disturbances: hemophilia, thrombocytopenia, anticoagulants
  - Somewhere else: bleeding genitals, factitious (drug addicts)

Hematuria, Cause by Age and Sex

0–20 YEARS
- Acute urinary tract infection (UTI)
- Acute glomerulonephritis
- Congenital urinary tract anomalies with obstruction
- Trauma to genitals

20–40 YEARS
- Acute UTI
- Trauma to genitals
- Urolithiasis
- Bladder cancer

40–60 YEARS (WOMEN)
- Acute UTI
- Bladder cancer
- Urolithiasis

40–60 YEARS (MEN)
- Acute UTI
- Bladder cancer
- Urolithiasis

60 YEARS AND OLDER (WOMEN)
- Acute UTI
- Bladder cancer
- Vaginal trauma or irritation
- Urolithiasis

60 YEARS AND OLDER (MEN)
- Acute UTI
- Benign prostatic hyperplasia
- Bladder cancer
- Urolithiasis
- Trauma

Hemiparesis/Hemiplegia

- Cerebrovascular accident (CVA)
- Transient ischemic attack (TIA)
- Cerebral neoplasm

- Multiple sclerosis (MS) or other demyelinating disorder
- CNS infection
- Migraine
- Hypoglycemia
- Subdural hematoma
- Vasculitis
- Todd's paralysis
- Epidural hematoma
- Metabolic (hyperosmolar state, electrolyte imbalance)
- Psychiatric disorders
- Congenital disorders
- Leukodystrophies
- Acute fatty liver of pregnancy

Hemochromatosis

- Hereditary anemias with defect of erythropoiesis
- Cirrhosis
- Repeated blood transfusions

Hemolysis and Hemoglobinuria

- Erythrocyte trauma (prosthetic cardiac valves, marching and severe trauma, extensive burns)
- Infections (malaria, *Bartonella*, *Clostridium welchii*)
- Brown recluse spider bite
- Incompatible blood transfusions
- Hemolytic-uremic syndrome (HUS)
- Thrombotic thrombocytopenic purpura (TTP)
- Paroxysmal nocturnal hemoglobinuria (PNH)
- Drugs (penicillins, quinidine, methyldopa, sulfonamides, nitrofurantoin)
- Erythrocyte enzyme deficiencies (e.g., exposure to fava beans in patients with glucose-6-phosphate dehydrogenase [G6PD] deficiency)

Hemolysis, Intravascular

- Infections
- Exertional hemolysis (e.g., prolonged march)

- Valve hemolysis
- Microangiopathic hemolytic anemia
- Osmotic and chemical agents
- Thermal injury
- Cold agglutinins
- Venoms (snakes, spiders)
- Paroxysmal nocturnal hemoglobinuria (PNH)

Hemolysis, Mechanical

- Prosthetic heart valves
- Aortic stenosis
- Malignant hypertension
- Metastatic adenocarcinoma
- Traumatic exercise
- Renal transplants
- Renal cortical necrosis
- Glomerulonephritis
- Thrombotic thrombocytopenic purpura (TTP), hemolytic-uremic syndrome (HUS)
- Renal vasculitis
- Scleroderma
- Diabetes

Hemolytic-Uremic Syndrome (HUS)

- The differential is vast, including all causes of bloody and nonbloody diarrhea, because the GI symptoms usually precede the triad of HUS.
- Thrombotic thrombocytopenic purpura
- Disseminated intravascular coagulation
- Prosthetic valve hemolysis
- Malignant hypertension
- Vasculitis

Hemoperitoneum

- Ruptured graafian follicle
- Ruptured spleen
- Ectopic pregnancy

- Traumatic laceration of liver
- Ruptured aneurysm
- Ruptured bladder
- Traumatic laceration of bowel, pancreas, uterus

Hemophilia

- Other clotting factor deficiencies
- Platelet function disorders
- Vitamin K deficiency
- Anticoagulant overdose

Hemoptysis

CARDIOVASCULAR
- Pulmonary embolism/infarction
- Left ventricular (LV) failure
- Mitral stenosis
- Arteriovenous (AV) fistula
- Severe hypertension
- Erosion of aortic aneurysm

PULMONARY
- Neoplasm (primary or metastatic)
- Infection
- Pneumonia: *Streptococcus pneumoniae, Klebsiella pneumoniae, Staphylococcus aureus, Legionella pneumophila*
- Bronchiectasis
- Abscess
- TB
- Bronchitis
- Fungal infections (aspergillosis, coccidioidomycosis)
- Parasitic infections (amebiasis, ascariasis, paragonimiasis)
- Vasculitis: Wegener's granulomatosis, Churg-Strauss syndrome, Henoch-Schönlein purpura
- Goodpasture's syndrome
- Trauma (needle biopsy, foreign body, right-sided heart catheterization, prolonged and severe cough)
- Cystic fibrosis (CF), bullous emphysema
- Pulmonary sequestration
- Pulmonary arteriovenous (AV) fistula

- Systemic lupus erythematosus (SLE)
- Idiopathic pulmonary hemosiderosis
- Drugs: aspirin, anticoagulants, penicillamine
- Pulmonary hypertension
- Mediastinal fibrosis

OTHER
- Epistaxis, trauma
- Laryngeal bleeding (laryngitis, laryngeal neoplasm)
- Hematologic disorders (clotting abnormalities, disseminated intravascular coagulation [DIC], thrombocytopenia)

Hemorrhoids

- Fissure
- Abscess
- Anal fistula
- Condylomata acuminata
- Hypertrophied anal papillae
- Rectal prolapse
- Rectal polyp
- Neoplasm

Hemosiderinuria

- Paroxysmal nocturnal hemoglobinuria (PNH)
- Chronic hemolytic anemia
- Hemochromatosis
- Blood transfusion
- Thalassemias

Henoch-Schönlein Purpura

- Polyarteritis nodosa
- Meningococcemia
- Thrombocytopenic purpura
- Viral syndrome

Hepatic Coma

- Delirium secondary to medications or illicit drugs
- Cerebrovascular accident (CVA), subdural hematoma

- Meningitis, encephalitis
- Hypoglycemia
- Uremia
- Cerebral anoxia
- Hypercalcemia
- Metastatic neoplasm to brain
- Alcohol withdrawal syndrome

Hepatic Cysts[37]

CONGENITAL HEPATIC CYSTS
- Parenchymal: solitary cyst, polycystic disease
- Ductal: localized dilatation, multiple cystic dilatations of intrahepatic ducts (Caroli's disease)

ACQUIRED HEPATIC CYSTS
- Inflammatory cysts: retention cysts, echinococcal cyst, amebic cyst
- Neoplastic cyst
- Peliosis hepatis

Hepatic Encephalopathy

- Delirium caused by medications or illicit drugs
- Cerebrovascular accident, subdural hematoma
- Meningitis, encephalitis
- Hypoglycemia
- Uremia
- Cerebral anoxia
- Hypercalcemia
- Metastatic neoplasm to brain
- Alcohol withdrawal syndrome

Hepatic Granulomas[1]

INFECTIONS
- Bacterial, spirochetal: TB and atypical mycobacterial infections, tularemia, brucellosis, leprosy, syphilis, Whipple's disease, listeriosis
- Viral: mononucleosis, cytomegalovirus (CMV)

- Rickettsial: Q fever
- Fungal: coccidioidomycosis, histoplasmosis, cryptococcal infections, actinomycosis, aspergillosis, nocardiosis
- Parasitic: schistosomiasis, clonorchiasis, toxocariasis, ascariasis, toxoplasmosis, amebiasis

HEPATOBILIARY DISORDERS

- Primary biliary cirrhosis, granulomatous hepatitis, jejunoileal bypass

SYSTEMIC DISORDERS

- Sarcoidosis, Wegener's granulomatosis, inflammatory bowel disease, Hodgkin's disease, lymphoma

DRUGS/TOXINS

- Beryllium, parenteral foreign material (e.g., starch, talc, methyldopa, procainamide, allopurinol, α-silicone), phenylbutazone, phenytoin, nitrofurantoin, hydralazine

Hepatitis, Acute[26]

INFECTIOUS

- Hepatitis A, B, C, D, G
- Epstein-Barr virus
- Cytomegalovirus
- Herpes simplex virus
- Yellow fever
- Leptospirosis
- Q fever
- HIV infection
- Brucellosis
- Lyme disease
- Syphilis

NONINFECTIOUS

- Drug induced
- Autoimmune
- Ischemic
- Acute fatty liver of pregnancy
- Acute Budd-Chiari syndrome
- Wilson's disease

Hepatitis, Autoimmune

- Acute viral hepatitis (A, B, C, D, E; cytomegalovirus [CMV], Epstein-Barr virus, herpes)
- Chronic viral hepatitis (B, C)
- Toxic hepatitis (alcohol, drugs)
- Primary biliary cirrhosis
- Primary sclerosing cholangitis
- Hemochromatosis
- Nonalcoholic steatohepatitis
- Systemic lupus erythematosus (SLE)
- Wilson's disease
- α_1-Antitrypsin deficiency

Hepatitis, Chronic[26]

- Chronic viral hepatitis
- Hepatitis B
- Hepatitis C
- Hepatitis D
- Autoimmune hepatitis and variant syndromes
- Hereditary hemochromatosis
- Wilson's disease
- α_1-Antitrypsin deficiency
- Fatty liver and nonalcoholic steatohepatitis
- Alcoholic liver disease
- Drug-induced liver disease
- Hepatic granulomas
- Infectious
- Drug induced
- Neoplastic
- Idiopathic

Hepatitis A

- Other hepatitis virus (B, C, D, E)
- Infectious mononucleosis
- Cytomegalovirus (CMV) infection
- Herpes simplex virus infection
- Leptospirosis

- Brucellosis
- Drug-induced liver disease
- Ischemic hepatitis
- Autoimmune hepatitis

Hepatitis B

- Other hepatitis virus (A, C, D, E)
- Infectious mononucleosis
- Cytomegalovirus (CMV) infection
- Herpes simplex virus infection
- Leptospirosis
- Brucellosis
- Drug-induced liver disease
- Ischemic hepatitis
- Autoimmune hepatitis

Hepatitis C

- Other hepatitis virus (A, B, D, E)
- Infectious mononucleosis
- Cytomegalovirus (CMV) infection
- Herpes simplex virus infection
- Leptospirosis
- Brucellosis
- Drug-induced liver disease
- Ischemic hepatitis
- Autoimmune hepatitis

Hepatitis D

- Other hepatitis virus (A, B, C, E)
- Infectious mononucleosis
- Cytomegalovirus (CMV) infection
- Herpes simplex virus infection
- Leptospirosis
- Brucellosis
- Drug-induced liver disease
- Ischemic hepatitis
- Autoimmune hepatitis

Hepatitis E

- Other hepatitis virus (A, B, C, D)
- Infectious mononucleosis
- Cytomegalovirus (CMV) infection
- Herpes simplex virus infection
- Leptospirosis
- Brucellosis
- Drug-induced liver disease
- Ischemic hepatitis
- Autoimmune hepatitis

Hepatocellular Carcinoma

- Metastatic neoplasm to liver
- Benign liver tumors (adenomas)
- Focal nodular hyperplasia
- Hemangiomas
- Focal fatty infiltration

Hepatomegaly

FREQUENT JAUNDICE
- Infectious hepatitis
- Toxic hepatitis
- Carcinoma: liver, pancreas, bile ducts, metastatic neoplasm to liver
- Cirrhosis
- Obstruction of common bile duct
- Alcoholic hepatitis
- Biliary cirrhosis
- Cholangitis
- Hemochromatosis with cirrhosis

INFREQUENT JAUNDICE
- Congestive heart failure (CHF)
- Amyloidosis
- Liver abscess
- Sarcoidosis
- Infectious mononucleosis

- Alcoholic fatty infiltration
- Nonalcoholic steatohepatitis
- Lymphoma
- Leukemia
- Budd-Chiari syndrome
- Myelofibrosis with myeloid metaplasia
- Familial hyperlipoproteinemia type I
- Other: amebiasis, hydatid disease of liver, schistosomiasis, kala-azar (*Leishmania donovani*), Hurler's syndrome, Gaucher's disease, kwashiorkor

Hepatomegaly, by Shape of Liver[39]

DIFFUSELY ENLARGED AND SMOOTH

Massive
- Metastatic disease
- Alcoholic liver disease with fatty infiltration
- Myeloproliferative diseases (e.g., polycythemia rubra vera, myelofibrosis)

Moderate
- The above causes
- Hemochromatosis
- Hematologic disease (e.g., chronic myeloid leukemia, lymphoma)
- Fatty liver (e.g., diabetes mellitus, obesity)
- Infiltrative disorders (e.g., amyloid)

Mild
- The above causes
- Hepatitis (viral, drugs)
- Cirrhosis
- Biliary obstruction
- Granulomatous disorders (e.g., sarcoid)
- HIV infection

DIFFUSELY ENLARGED AND IRREGULAR
- Metastatic disease
- Cirrhosis
- Hydatid disease
- Polycystic liver disease

LOCALIZED SWELLINGS
- Riedel's lobe (a normal variant; the lobe may be palpable in the right lumbar region)
- Metastasis
- Large simple hepatic cyst
- Hydatid cyst
- Hepatoma
- Liver abscess (e.g., amebic abscess)

Hepatorenal Syndrome

- Prerenal azotemia: response to sustained plasma expansion is good (prompt diuresis with volume expansion).
- Acute tubular necrosis: urinary sodium >30, FE_{Na} >1.5%, urinary/plasma creatinine ratio <30, urine/plasma osmolality ratio = 1, urine sediment reveals casts and cellular debris; there is no significant response to sustained plasma expansion.

Hermaphroditism[4]

FEMALE PSEUDOHERMAPHRODITISM
- Androgen exposure
  - Fetal source
    - 21-Hydroxylase (P450c21) deficiency
    - 11β-Hydroxylase (P450c11) deficiency
    - 3β-Hydroxysteroid dehydrogenase II (3) deficiency
    - Aromatase (P450arom) deficiency
  - Maternal source
    - Virilizing ovarian tumor
    - Virilizing adrenal tumor
    - Androgenic drugs
- Undetermined origin
- Associated with GU and GI tract defects

MALE PSEUDOHERMAPHRODITISM
- Defects in testicular differentiation
  - Denys-Drash syndrome (mutation in *WT1* gene)
  - WAGR syndrome (Wilms' tumor, aniridia, GU malformation, retardation)

- Deletion of 11p13
- Camptomelic syndrome (autosomal gene at 17q24.3-q25.1) and *SOX9* mutation
- XY pure gonadal dysgenesis (Swyer syndrome)
  - Mutation in *SRY* gene
  - Unknown cause
  - XY gonadal agenesis
- Deficiency of testicular hormones
  - Leydig cell aplasia
  - Mutation in luteinizing hormone (LH) receptor
  - Lipoid adrenal hyperplasia (P450scc) deficiency; mutation in StAR (steroidogenic acute regulatory protein)
  - 3β-Hydroxysteroid dehydrogenase II deficiency
  - 17-Hydroxylase/17,20-lyase (P450c17) deficiency
  - Persistent müllerian duct syndrome
  - Gene mutations, müllerian-inhibiting substance (MIS)
  - Receptor defects for MIS
- Defect in androgen action
  - 5α-Reductase 2 mutations
  - Androgen receptor defects
  - Complete androgen insensitivity syndrome
  - Partial androgen insensitivity syndrome
    - Reifenstein's and other syndromes
    - Smith-Lemli-Opitz syndrome
- Defect in conversion of 7-dehydrocholesterol to cholesterol

TRUE HERMAPHRODITISM
- XX
- XY
- XX/XY chimeras

Herpangina

- Herpes simplex
- Bacterial pharyngitis
- Tonsillitis
- Aphthous stomatitis
- Hand-foot-mouth disease

Herpes Simplex, Genital

- Human papillomavirus
- Molluscum contagiosum
- HIV infection
- Fungal infections (*Candida*)
- Bacterial infections (syphilis, chancroid, granuloma inguinale)
- Follicular abscess
- Hidradenitis suppurativa
- Vulvar dystrophies
- Cancer of the vulva

Herpes Simplex, Oral

- Impetigo
- Behçet's syndrome
- Coxsackievirus infection
- Stevens-Johnson syndrome
- Herpangina
- Aphthous stomatitis
- Varicella
- Herpes zoster

Herpes Zoster

- Rash: herpes simplex and other viral infections
- Pain from herpes zoster: may be confused with acute myocardial infarction (MI), pulmonary embolism, pleuritis, pericarditis, renal colic

Hiatal Hernia

- Peptic ulcer disease
- Unstable angina
- Esophagitis (e.g., *Candida*, herpes, nonsteroidal anti-inflammatory drugs [NSAIDs])
- Esophageal spasm
- Barrett's esophagus
- Schatzki's ring

- Achalasia
- Zenker's diverticulum
- Esophageal cancer

Hiccups[22]

TRANSIENT HICCUPS
- Sudden excitement, emotion
- Gastric distention
- Esophageal obstruction
- Alcohol ingestion
- Sudden change in temperature

PERSISTENT OR CHRONIC HICCUPS
- Toxic/metabolic: uremia, DM, hyperventilation, hypocalcemia, hypokalemia, hyponatremia, gout, fever
- Drugs: benzodiazepines, steroids, methyldopa, barbiturates
- Surgery/general anesthesia
- Thoracic/diaphragmatic disorders: pneumonia, lung cancer, asthma, pleuritis, pericarditis, myocardial infarction (MI), aortic aneurysm, esophagitis, esophageal obstruction, diaphragmatic hernia or irritation
- Abdominal disorders: gastric ulcer or cancer, hepatobiliary or pancreatic disease, inflammatory bowel disease (IBD), bowel obstruction, intra-abdominal or subphrenic abscess, prostatic infection or cancer
- CNS disorders: traumatic, infectious, vascular, structural
- Ear, nose, and throat disorders: pharyngitis, laryngitis, tumor, irritation of auditory canal
- Psychogenic disorders
- Idiopathic disorders

Hidradenitis Suppurativa

- Folliculitis and other follicular pyodermas, furuncles, pilonidal cysts
- Granuloma inguinale
- Crohn's disease (perianal and vulvar manifestations)

- Bartholin's cyst infection
- Actinomycosis
- Lymphogranuloma venereum
- Furuncle
- Lymphangitis
- Cat-scratch disease
- Tularemia
- Erysipelas
- Ulcerative colitis

Hip Pain, Children[27]

TRAUMA
- Hip or pelvis fractures
- Overuse injuries

INFECTION
- Septic arthritis
- Osteomyelitis

INFLAMMATION
- Transient synovitis
- Juvenile rheumatoid arthritis (JRA)
- Rheumatic fever

NEOPLASM
- Leukemia
- Osteogenic or Ewing's sarcoma
- Metastatic disease

HEMATOLOGIC DISORDERS
- Hemophilia
- Sickle cell anemia

MISCELLANEOUS
- Legg-Calvé-Perthes disease
- Slipped capital femoral epiphysis

Hip Pain, in Different Age Groups[8]

Common causes of hip pain in different age groups:

CHILDHOOD (2–10 YEARS)

Intra-articular
- Developmental dislocation of the hip
- Perthes' disease
- Irritable hip
- Rickets

Periarticular
- Osteomyelitis

Referred
- Abdominal

ADOLESCENCE (10–18 YEARS)

Intra-articular
- Slipped upper femoral epiphysis
- Torn labrum

Periarticular
- Trochanteric bursitis
- Snapping hip
- Osteomyelitis
- Tumors

Referred
- Abdominal
- Lumbar spine

EARLY ADULTHOOD (18–30 YEARS)

Intra-articular
- Inflammatory arthritis
- Torn labrum

Periarticular
- Bursitis

Referred
- Abdominal
- Lumbar spine

ADULTHOOD (30–50 YEARS)

Intra-articular
- Osteoarthritis
- Inflammatory arthritis

- Osteonecrosis
- Transient osteoporosis

Periarticular
- Bursitis

Referred
- Abdominal
- Lumbar spine

OLD AGE (>50 YEARS)
Intra-articular
- Osteoarthritis
- Inflammatory arthritis

Referred
- Abdominal
- Lumbar spine

Hirsutism

- Idiopathic: familial, possibly increased sensitivity to androgens
- Menopause
- Polycystic ovary syndrome
- Drugs: androgens, anabolic steroids, methyltestosterone, minoxidil, diazoxide, phenytoin, glucocorticoids, cyclosporine
- Congenital adrenal hyperplasia
- Adrenal virilizing tumor
- Ovarian virilizing tumor: arrhenoblastoma, hilar cell tumor
- Pituitary adenoma
- Cushing's syndrome
- Hypothyroidism (congenital and juvenile)
- Acromegaly
- Testicular feminization

Histoplasmosis

- Acute pulmonary histoplasmosis: *Mycobacterium tuberculosis*; community-acquired pneumonias caused by *Mycoplasma* and *Chlamydia*; other fungal diseases, such as *Blastomyces dermatitidis* and *Coccidioides immitis*
- Chronic cavitary pulmonary histoplasmosis: *M. tuberculosis*

- Yeast forms of histoplasmosis on tissue section: cysts of *Pneumocystis jiroveci*, which tend to be larger, are extracellular, and do not display budding
- Intracellular parasites of *Leishmania* and *Toxoplasma* species: distinguishable by inability to take up methenamine silver
- Histoplasmomas: true neoplasms

Histrionic Personality

- Borderline personality disorder
- Antisocial personality disorder
- Narcissistic personality disorder
- Dependent personality disorder
- Personality change secondary to general medical condition
- Symptoms may develop in association with chronic substance abuse.

HIV Infection, Anorectal Lesions[27]

COMMON CONDITIONS
- Anal fissure
- Abscess and fistula
- Hemorrhoids
- Pruritus ani
- Pilonidal disease

COMMON STDS
- Gonorrhea
- Chlamydia
- Herpes
- Chancroid
- Syphilis
- Condylomata acuminata

ATYPICAL CONDITIONS
- Infectious: TB, cytomegalovirus (CMV), actinomycosis, cryptococcosis
- Neoplastic: lymphoma, Kaposi's sarcoma, squamous cell carcinoma
- Other: idiopathic and ulcer

HIV Infection, Chest Radiographic Abnormalities[27]

DIFFUSE INTERSTITIAL INFILTRATION
* *Pneumocystis jiroveci*
* Cytomegalovirus
* *Mycobacterium tuberculosis*
* *Mycobacterium avium* complex
* Histoplasmosis
* Coccidioidomycosis
* Lymphoid interstitial pneumonitis

FOCAL CONSOLIDATION
* Bacterial pneumonia
* *Mycoplasma pneumoniae*
* *P. jiroveci*
* *M. tuberculosis*
* *M. avium* complex

NODULAR LESIONS
* Kaposi's sarcoma
* *M. tuberculosis*
* *M. avium* complex
* Fungal lesions
* Toxoplasmosis

CAVITARY LESIONS
* *P. jiroveci*
* *M. tuberculosis*
* Bacterial infection

PLEURAL EFFUSION
* Kaposi's sarcoma
* Small effusion may be associated with any infection.

ADENOPATHY
* Kaposi's sarcoma
* Lymphoma
* *M. tuberculosis*
* *Cryptococcus*

PNEUMOTHORAX
• Kaposi's sarcoma

HIV Infection, Cognitive Impairment[26]

EARLY TO MIDSTAGE HIV DISEASE
• Depression
• Alcohol and substance abuse
• Medication-induced cognitive impairment
• Metabolic encephalopathies
• HIV-related cognitive impairment

ADVANCED HIV DISEASE (CD4+ < 100/MM³)
• Opportunistic infection of CNS
• Neurosyphilis
• CNS lymphoma
• Progressive multifocal leukoencephalopathy
• Depression
• Metabolic encephalopathies
• Medication-induced cognitive impairment
• Stroke
• HIV dementia

HIV Infection, Cutaneous Manifestations[22]

BACTERIAL INFECTION
• Bacillary angiomatosis: numerous angiomatous nodules associated with fever, chills, weight loss
• *Staphylococcus aureus:* folliculitis, ecthyma, impetigo, bullous impetigo, furuncles, carbuncles
• Syphilis: may occur in different forms (primary, secondary, tertiary); chancre may become painful because of secondary infection

FUNGAL INFECTION
• Candidiasis: mucous membranes (oral, vulvovaginal), less commonly *Candida* intertrigo or paronychia
• Cryptococcoses: papules or nodules that strongly resemble molluscum contagiosum; other forms include pustules, purpuric papules, and vegetating plaques

- Seborrheic dermatitis: scaling and erythema in the hair-bearing areas (eyebrows, scalp, chest, and pubic area)

ARTHROPOD INFESTATIONS

- Scabies: pruritus with or without rash, usually generalized but can be limited to a single digit

VIRAL INFECTION

- Herpes simplex: vesicular lesion in clusters; perianal, genital, orofacial, or digital; can be disseminated
- Herpes zoster: painful dermatomal vesicles that may ulcerate or disseminate
- HIV: discrete erythematous macules and papules on the upper trunk, palms, and soles are the most characteristic cutaneous finding of acute HIV infection.
- Human papillomavirus: genital warts (may become unusually extensive)
- Kaposi's sarcoma (herpesvirus): erythematous macules or papules; enlarge at varying rates; violaceous nodules or plaques; occasionally painful
- Molluscum contagiosum: discrete umbilicated papules commonly on the face, neck, and intertriginous sites (axilla, groin, or buttocks)

NONINFECTIOUS

- Drug reactions: more frequent and severe in patients with HIV infection
- Nutritional deficiencies: mainly seen in children and patients with chronic diarrhea; diffuse skin manifestations, depending on the deficiency
- Psoriasis: scaly lesions; diffuse or localized; can be associated with arthritis
- Vasculitis: palpable purpuric eruption (can resemble septic emboli)

HIV Infection, Esophageal Disease

- *Candida* infection
- Cytomegalovirus (CMV) infection
- Aphthous ulcer
- Herpes simplex

HIV Infection, Hepatic Disease[26]

VIRUSES
- Hepatitis A
- Hepatitis B
- Hepatitis C
- Hepatitis D (with hepatitis B virus [HBV])
- Epstein-Barr virus
- Cytomegalovirus (CMV)
- Herpes simplex virus
- Adenovirus
- Varicella-zoster virus

MYCOBACTERIA
- *Mycobacterium avium* complex
- *Mycobacterium tuberculosis*

FUNGI
- *Histoplasma capsulatum*
- *Cryptococcus neoformans*
- *Coccidioides immitis*
- *Candida albicans*
- *Pneumocystis jiroveci*
- *Penicillium marneffei*

PROTOZOA
- *Toxoplasma gondii*
- *Cryptosporidium parvum*
- *Microsporida* spp.
- *Schistosoma*

BACTERIA
- *Bartonella henselae* (peliosis hepatis)

MALIGNANCY
- Kaposi's sarcoma (human herpesvirus 8 [HHV-8])
- Non-Hodgkin's lymphoma
- Hepatocellular carcinoma

MEDICATIONS
- Zidovudine
- Didanosine

- Ritonavir
- Other HIV-1 protease inhibitors
- Fluconazole
- Macrolide antibiotics
- Isoniazid
- Rifampin
- Trimethoprim-sulfamethoxazole

HIV Infection, Lower GI Tract Disease[26]

CAUSES OF ENTEROCOLITIS

Bacteria
- *Campylobacter jejuni* and other spp.
- *Salmonella* spp.
- *Shigella flexneri*
- *Aeromonas hydrophila*
- *Plesiomonas shigelloides*
- *Yersinia enterocolitica*
- *Vibrio* spp.
- *Mycobacterium avium* complex
- *Mycobacterium tuberculosis*
- *Escherichia coli* (enterotoxigenic, enteroadherent)
- Bacterial overgrowth
- *Clostridium difficile* (toxin)

Parasites
- *Clostridium parvum*
- Microsporida *(Enterocytozoon bieneusi, Septata intestinalis)*
- *Isospora belli*
- *Entamoeba histolytica*
- *Giardia lamblia*
- *Cyclospora cayetanensis*

Viruses
- Cytomegalovirus (CMV)
- Adenovirus
- Calicivirus
- Astrovirus
- Picobirnavirus
- HIV

Fungi
- *Histoplasma capsulatum*

CAUSES OF PROCTITIS
Bacteria
- *Chlamydia trachomatis*
- *Neisseria gonorrhoeae*
- *Treponema pallidum*

Viruses
- Herpes simplex
- CMV

HIV Infection, Ocular Manifestations[37]

EYELIDS
- Molluscum contagiosum
- Kaposi's sarcoma

CORNEA/CONJUNCTIVA
- Keratoconjunctivitis sicca
- Bacterial/fungal ulcerative keratitis
- Herpes simplex
- Herpes zoster ophthalmicus
- Conjunctival microvasculopathy
- Kaposi's sarcoma

RETINA, CHOROID, AND VITREOUS
- Microvasculopathy
- Endophthalmitis
- Cytomegalovirus (CMV) retinitis
- Acute retinal necrosis
- Syphilis
- Toxoplasmosis
- *Pneumocystis* choroidopathy
- Cryptococcosis
- Mycobacterial infection
- Intraocular lymphoma
- Candidiasis
- Histoplasmosis

DRUGS ASSOCIATED WITH OCULAR TOXICITY
- Rifabutin
- Didanosine

NEURO-OPHTHALMIC
- Disc edema
- Primary or secondary optic neuropathy
- Cranial nerve palsies

ORBITAL
- Lymphoma
- Infection
- Pseudotumor

HIV Infection, Pulmonary Disease[26]

MYCOBACTERIAL
- *Mycobacterium tuberculosis*
- *Mycobacterium kansasii*
- *Mycobacterium avium* complex
- Other nontuberculous mycobacteria

OTHER BACTERIAL
- *Streptococcus pneumoniae*
- *Staphylococcus aureus*
- *Haemophilus influenzae*
- Enterobacteriaceae
- *Pseudomonas aeruginosa*
- *Moraxella catarrhalis*
- Group A streptococcus
- *Nocardia* species
- *Rhodococcus equi*
- *Chlamydia pneumoniae*

FUNGAL
- *Pneumocystis jiroveci*
- *Cryptococcus neoformans*
- *Histoplasma capsulatum*
- *Coccidioides immitis*
- *Aspergillus* species
- *Bacillus dermatitidis*
- *Penicillium marneffei*

VIRAL

- Cytomegalovirus (CMV)
- Herpes simplex virus
- Adenovirus
- Respiratory syncytial virus
- Influenza viruses
- Parainfluenza virus

OTHER

- *Toxoplasma gondii*
- *Strongyloides stercoralis*
- Kaposi's sarcoma
- Lymphoma
- Lung cancer
- Lymphocytic interstitial pneumonitis
- Nonspecific interstitial pneumonitis
- Bronchiolitis obliterans with organizing pneumonia
- Pulmonary hypertension
- Emphysema-like or bullous disease
- Pneumothorax
- Congestive heart failure (CHF)
- Diffuse alveolar damage
- Pulmonary embolus

Hoarseness

- Allergic rhinitis
- Infections (laryngitis, epiglottitis, tracheitis, croup)
- Vocal cord polyps
- Voice strain
- Irritants (tobacco smoke)
- Vocal cord trauma (intubation, surgery)
- Neoplastic involvement of vocal cord (primary or metastatic)
- Neurologic abnormalities (multiple sclerosis [MS], amyotrophic lateral sclerosis [ALS], parkinsonism)
- Endocrine abnormalities (puberty, menopause, hypothyroidism)
- Other (laryngeal webs or cysts, psychogenic, muscle tension abnormalities)

Hodgkin's Disease

- Non-Hodgkin's lymphoma
- Sarcoidosis
- Infections (e.g., cytomegalovirus [CMV], Epstein-Barr virus, toxoplasma, HIV)
- Drug reaction
- Cat-scratch disease
- Metastatic neoplasm
- Chronic lymphocytic leukemia (CLL)

Hookworm

- Strongyloidiasis
- Ascariasis
- Other causes of iron deficiency anemia and malabsorption

Hordeolum

- Eyelid abscess
- Chalazion
- Allergy or contact dermatitis with conjunctival edema
- Acute dacryocystitis
- Herpes simplex infection
- Cellulitis of the eyelid

Horner's Syndrome

CAUSES OF ANISOCORIA (UNEQUAL PUPILS)
- Normal variant
- Mydriatic use
- Prosthetic eye
- Unilateral cataract
- Iritis

Hot Flashes

- Menopause
- Anxiety disorder

- Idiopathic flushing
- Lymphoma (night sweats)
- Hyperthyroidism
- Carcinoid syndrome
- Medications (e.g., niacin)

Human Granulocytic Ehrlichiosis

- Human monocytic ehrlichiosis (HME)
  - Caused by *Ehrlichia chaffeensis* (vector: tick *Amblyomma americanum*, possibly *Dermacentor variabilis*)
  - Rash more common, sometimes petechial
  - Morulae in monocytes
- Rocky Mountain spotted fever, Colorado tick fever, Q fever, relapsing fever
- Babesiosis
- Leptospirosis
- Typhus
- Lyme disease
- Legionnaires' disease
- Tularemia
- Typhoid fever, paratyphoid fever
- Brucellosis
- Viral hepatitis
- Enteroviral infections
- Meningococcemia
- Influenza
- Adenovirus pneumonia

Human Immunodeficiency Virus Infection

- Acute infection: mononucleosis or other respiratory viral infections
- Late symptoms: similar to those produced by other wasting illnesses, such as neoplasms, TB, disseminated fungal infection, malabsorption, or depression
- HIV-related encephalopathy: confused with Alzheimer's disease or other causes of chronic dementia; myelopathy and neuropathy possibly resembling other demyelinating diseases, such as multiple sclerosis (MS)

Huntington's Disease

- Drug-induced chorea: dopamine, stimulants, anticonvulsants, antidepressants, and oral contraceptives have all been known to cause chorea.
- Sydenham's chorea: decreased incidence with decline of rheumatic fever
- Benign hereditary chorea: autosomal dominant with onset in childhood. There is no progression of symptoms and no associated dementia or behavioral problems.
- Senile chorea
- Wilson's disease: autosomal recessive; tremor, dysarthria, and dystonia are more common presentations than chorea. Of patients with neurologic manifestations, 95% will have Kayser-Fleischer rings.
- Neuroacanthocytosis: autosomal recessive; chorea, dystonia, tics, and orolingual dyskinesias that can result in self-mutilation; must look for acanthocytes in peripheral smear
- Dentatorubropallidoluysian atrophy: autosomal dominant, triplet repeat disease; presentation is variable and includes chorea, myoclonus, dementia, and ataxia; more common in Japan; can be confirmed by genetic testing
- Postinfectious
- Systemic lupus erythematosus (SLE): can be the presenting feature of lupus; occurs in only about 1% of individuals with lupus; pathophysiology unknown
- Chorea gravidarum: presents during first 4 to 5 months of pregnancy and resolves after delivery
- Paraneoplastic: seen most commonly in small cell lung cancer and lymphoma

Hydrocele

- Spermatocele
- Inguinoscrotal hernia
- Testicular tumor
- Varicocele
- Epididymitis

Hydrocephalus

- Head trauma
- Brain neoplasm (primary or metastatic)
- Spinal cord tumor
- Cerebellar infarction
- Exudative or granulomatous meningitis
- Cerebellar hemorrhage
- Subarachnoid hemorrhage
- Aqueductal stenosis
- Third ventricle colloid cyst
- Hindbrain malformation
- Viral encephalitis
- Metastases to leptomeninges

Hydrocephalus, Normal Pressure

- Alzheimer's disease with extrapyramidal features
- Cognitive impairment in the setting of Parkinson's disease or Parkinson's plus syndromes
- Diffuse Lewy body disease
- Frontotemporal dementia
- Cervical spondylosis with cord compromise in setting of degenerative dementia
- Multifactorial gait disorder
- Multi-infarct dementia

Hydronephrosis

- Urinary stones
- Neoplastic disease
- Prostatic hypertrophy
- Neurologic disease
- Urinary reflux
- Urinary tract infection (UTI)
- Medication effects
- Trauma
- Congenital abnormality of urinary tract

Hyperaldosteronism

- Diuretic use
- Hypokalemia from vomiting, diarrhea
- Renovascular hypertension
- Other endocrine neoplasm (pheochromocytoma, deoxycorticosterone-producing tumor, renin-secreting tumor)

Hyperamylasemia

- Pancreatitis (acute or chronic)
- Macroamylasemia
- Salivary gland inflammation
- Mumps
- Pancreatic neoplasm
- Pancreatic abscess
- Pancreatic pseudocyst
- Perforated peptic ulcer
- Intestinal obstruction
- Intestinal infarction
- Acute cholecystitis
- Appendicitis
- Ruptured ectopic pregnancy
- Peritonitis
- Burns
- Diabetic ketoacidosis (DKA)
- Renal insufficiency
- Drugs (morphine)
- Carcinomatosis of lung, esophagus, ovary
- Acute ethanol ingestion
- Prostate tumors
- Post endoscopic retrograde cholangiopancreatography (ERCP)
- Bulimia, anorexia nervosa

Hyperbilirubinemia (Conjugated Bilirubin)

- Hepatocellular disease
- Biliary obstruction
- Drug-induced cholestasis

- Hereditary disorders (Dubin-Johnson syndrome, Rotor's syndrome)
- Advanced neoplastic states

Hyperbilirubinemia, Total

- Liver disease (hepatitis, cirrhosis, cholangitis, neoplasm, biliary obstruction, infectious mononucleosis)
- Hereditary disorders (Gilbert's disease, Dubin-Johnson syndrome)
- Drugs (steroids, diphenylhydantoin, phenothiazines, penicillin, erythromycin, clindamycin, captopril, amphotericin B, sulfonamides, azathioprine, isoniazid, 5-aminosalicylic acid, allopurinol, methyldopa, indomethacin, halothane, oral contraceptives, procainamide, tolbutamide, labetalol)
- Hemolysis
- Pulmonary embolism or infarct
- Hepatic congestion resulting from congestive heart failure (CHF)

Hyperbilirubinemia (Unconjugated Bilirubin)

- Hemolysis
- Liver disease (hepatitis, cirrhosis, neoplasm)
- Hepatic congestion caused by congestive heart failure (CHF)
- Hereditary disorders (Gilbert's disease, Crigler-Najjar syndrome)

Hypercalcemia

- Malignant disease: increased bone resorption via osteoclast-activating factors, secretion of parathyroid hormone (PTH)–like substances, prostaglandin E_2, direct erosion by tumor cells, transforming growth factors, colony-stimulating activity
- Hypercalcemia is common in the following neoplasms:
  - Solid tumors: breast, lung, pancreas, kidneys, ovary
  - Hematologic cancers: myeloma, lymphosarcoma, adult T-cell lymphoma, Burkitt's lymphoma
- Hyperparathyroidism: increased bone resorption, GI absorption, and renal absorption; etiology:
  - Parathyroid hyperplasia, adenoma

- Hyperparathyroidism or renal failure with secondary hyperparathyroidism
- Granulomatous disorders: increased GI absorption (e.g., sarcoidosis)
- Paget's disease: increased bone resorption, seen only during periods of immobilization
- Vitamin D intoxication, milk-alkali syndrome: increased GI absorption
- Thiazides: increased renal absorption
- Other causes: familial hypocalciuric hypercalcemia, thyrotoxicosis, adrenal insufficiency, prolonged immobilization, vitamin A intoxication, recovery from acute renal failure, lithium administration, pheochromocytoma, disseminated systemic lupus erythematosus (SLE)

Hypercalcemia, Malignancy Induced

- Lung carcinoma: 6% frequency, 35% of hypercalcemic cases
- Breast carcinoma: 10% frequency, 25% of hypercalcemic cases
- Multiple myeloma: 33% frequency, 10% of hypercalcemic cases
- Lymphoma: 4% of hypercalcemic cases
- Genitourinary cancer: 6% of hypercalcemic cases

Hypercapnia, Persistent[37]

- Hypercapnia with normal lungs: CNS disturbances (cerebrovascular accident [CVA], parkinsonism, encephalitis), metabolic alkalosis, myxedema, primary alveolar hypoventilation, spinal cord lesions
- Diseases of the chest wall (e.g., kyphoscoliosis, ankylosing spondylitis)
- Neuromuscular disorders (e.g., myasthenia gravis, Guillain-Barré syndrome, amyotrophic lateral sclerosis [ALS], muscular dystrophy, poliomyelitis)
- Chronic obstructive pulmonary disease (COPD)

Hyperchloremia

- Dehydration
- Sodium loss > chloride loss

- Respiratory alkalosis
- Excessive infusion of normal saline solution
- Cystic fibrosis (CF)
- Hyperparathyroidism
- Renal tubular disease
- Metabolic acidosis
- Prolonged diarrhea
- Acetazolamide administration
- Diabetes insipidus (DI)
- Ureterosigmoidostomy

Hypercholesterolemia

- Diet high in cholesterol and saturated fat
- Primary hypercholesterolemia
- Uncontrolled diabetes mellitus
- Nephrotic syndrome
- Hypothyroidism
- Primary biliary cirrhosis
- Third trimester of pregnancy
- Drugs (steroids, phenothiazines, oral contraceptives)
- Biliary obstruction

Hypercoagulable State, Acquired

ANTIPHOSPHOLIPID ANTIBODY SYNDROME (APS)

- Most common cause of acquired thrombophilia
- Can present as arterial or venous thrombosis, recurrent pregnancy loss, and adverse pregnancy outcomes
- Thromboembolic events occur in up to 30% of population; high risk of recurrent thrombosis (up to 70% reported).
- See Antiphospholipid Antibody Syndrome for more information.

HYPERHOMOCYSTEINEMIA

- Can be inherited (most commonly an autosomal recessive mutation in methylene tetrahydrofolate reductase gene) but more frequently acquired; folate, vitamin B_6, or vitamin B_{12} deficiency accounts for two thirds of cases. Other acquired causes include renal disease, hypothyroidism, malignant disease, smoking, and certain medications.

- May be associated with venous thromboembolism (VTE), atherosclerotic disease (cardiovascular, cerebrovascular, and peripheral vascular), and possibly adverse pregnancy outcomes

CONDITIONS ASSOCIATED WITH INCREASED RISK
OF THROMBOSIS
- Prior thrombosis
- Trauma
- Medical illness: heart failure, respiratory failure, infection, diabetes mellitus, obesity, nephrotic syndrome, inflammatory bowel disease, paroxysmal nocturnal hemoglobinuria, sickle cell anemia
- Pregnancy (sixfold increased risk of VTE), post partum, OC use (fourfold increased risk, higher risk with third-generation OCs), transdermal contraceptive patch, HRT (twofold increased risk), tamoxifen, raloxifene
- Immobilization, travel
- Surgery (especially orthopedic), central venous catheters
- Hyperviscosity syndromes
- Myeloproliferative disorders
- Malignancy: disease or treatment related
- Heparin-induced thrombocytopenia and thrombosis
- Smoking

Hypercoagulable State, Associated Disorders[21]

- Systemic lupus erythematosus in association with the presence of a lupus anticoagulant or antiphospholipid antibodies
- Malignant neoplasm
- Disease related: includes migratory superficial thrombophlebitis (Trousseau's syndrome), nonbacterial thrombotic endocarditis, thrombosis associated with chronic DIC, thrombotic microangiopathy
- Treatment related: associated with the administration of various chemotherapeutic agents (asparaginase, mitomycin, some adjuvant chemotherapeutic agents for treatment of breast cancer, thalidomide or lenalidomide in conjunction with high doses of dexamethasone)
- Infusion of prothrombin complex concentrates
- Nephrotic syndrome

- Heparin-induced thrombocytopenia
- Myeloproliferative disorders
- Paroxysmal nocturnal hemoglobinuria

Hypercoagulable State, Inherited

FACTOR V LEIDEN (FVL) MUTATION
- Autosomal dominant mutation with low penetrance
- Causes activated protein C resistance (APCR); 90% of APCR is caused by FVL mutation
- Most common inherited thrombophilia; accounts for 40% to 50% of cases
- OC use in heterozygous carriers is associated with an 8-fold increased risk of VTE compared with noncarriers and a 35-fold increased risk of VTE compared with noncarriers not using OCs.
- May be associated with cardiovascular disease in select high-risk subgroups

PROTHROMBIN G20210A MUTATION
- Autosomal dominant mutation with low penetrance
- OC use in heterozygous carriers is associated with a 16-fold increased risk of VTE compared with noncarriers not using OCs.
- May be associated with cardiovascular disease in select high-risk subgroups and young patients with ischemic stroke

PROTEIN C, PROTEIN S, ANTITHROMBIN (AT) DEFICIENCY
- Autosomal dominant inheritance; many mutations identified for each of these conditions
- Decreased level or abnormal function
- First episode of thrombosis usually in young adults

Protein C and Protein S
- High risk of VTE
- Homozygous condition very rare; usually associated with lethal thrombosis in infancy
- Associated with warfarin-induced skin necrosis, which occurs secondary to depletion of vitamin K–dependent anticoagulant factors sooner than procoagulant factors in the first few days of therapy

AT Deficiency
- Most thrombogenic of the inherited thrombophilias; 50% lifetime risk of thrombosis
- Homozygous condition very rare, probably not compatible with normal fetal development
- Arterial thrombosis can occur rarely
- Can cause heparin resistance

ELEVATED FACTOR VIII LEVEL
- May be an important risk factor for thrombosis in African American population
- Increased risk of recurrent thrombosis
- Genetic etiology suspected but not yet identified
- Other possible causes: dysfibrinogenemia, elevated thrombin-activatable fibrinolysis inhibitor, plasminogen deficiency, elevated factor IX and factor XI levels

Hypercortisolemia

- Ectopic adrenocorticotropic hormone (ACTH) production (e.g., small cell carcinoma of lung)
- Loss of normal diurnal variation
- Pregnancy
- Chronic renal failure
- Iatrogenic
- Stress
- Adrenal or pituitary hyperplasia or adenomas

Hyperemesis Gravidarum

- Pancreatitis
- Cholecystitis
- Hepatitis
- Pyelonephritis

Hypereosinophilia

- Allergy
- Parasitic infestations (trichinosis, aspergillosis, hydatidosis)
- Angioneurotic edema

- Drug reactions
- Warfarin sensitivity
- Collagen-vascular diseases
- Acute hypereosinophilic syndrome
- Eosinophilic nonallergic rhinitis
- Myeloproliferative disorders
- Hodgkin's disease
- Radiation therapy
- Non-Hodgkin's lymphoma
- L-Tryptophan ingestion
- Urticaria
- Pernicious anemia
- Pemphigus
- Inflammatory bowel disease (IBD)
- Bronchial asthma

Hypergastrinemia

- Decreased gastrin release inhibition from medications (proton pump inhibitors [PPIs], H_2 receptor antagonists), vagotomy
- Chronic renal failure
- Hypochlorhydria due to atrophic gastritis, gastric carcinoma, pernicious anemia
- Gastrinoma (Zollinger-Ellison syndrome)
- Pyloric obstruction
- Hyperplasia of antral G cells
- Rheumatoid arthritis (RA)

Hyperglycemia

- Diabetes mellitus (DM)
- Drugs (glucocorticoids, diuretics [thiazides, loop diuretics])
- Impaired glucose tolerance
- Stress
- Infections
- Myocardial infarction (MI)
- Cerebrovascular accident (CVA)
- Cushing's syndrome
- Acromegaly
- Acute pancreatitis

- Glucagonoma
- Hemochromatosis

Hyperhidrosis[4]

CORTICAL
- Emotional
- Familial dysautonomia
- Congenital ichthyosiform erythroderma
- Epidermolysis bullosa
- Nail-patella syndrome
- Jadassohn-Lewandowsky syndrome
- Pachyonychia congenita
- Palmoplantar keratoderma

HYPOTHALAMIC
Drugs
- Antipyretics
- Emetics
- Insulin
- Meperidine

Exercise

Infection
- Defervescence
- Chronic illness

Metabolic
- Debility
- Diabetes mellitus (DM)
- Hyperpituitarism
- Hyperthyroidism
- Hypoglycemia
- Obesity
- Porphyria
- Pregnancy
- Rickets
- Infantile scurvy

Cardiovascular
- Heart failure
- Shock

Vasomotor
- Cold injury
- Raynaud's phenomenon
- Rheumatoid arthritis (RA)

Neurologic
- Abscess
- Familial dysautonomia
- Postencephalitic
- Tumor

Miscellaneous
- Chédiak-Higashi syndrome
- Compensatory
- Phenylketonuria (PKU)
- Pheochromocytoma
- Vitiligo

MEDULLARY
- Physiologic gustatory sweating
- Encephalitis
- Granulosis rubra nasi
- Syringomyelia
- Thoracic sympathetic trunk injury

SPINAL
- Cord transection
- Syringomyelia

CHANGES IN BLOOD FLOW
- Arteriovenous fistula
- Klippel-Trénaunay syndrome
- Glomus tumor
- Blue rubber bleb nevus syndrome

Hyperimmunoglobulinemia

- IgA: lymphoproliferative disorders, Berger's nephropathy, chronic infections, autoimmune disorders, liver disease
- IgE: allergic disorders, parasitic infections, immunologic disorders, IgE myeloma, AIDS, pemphigoid

- IgG: chronic granulomatous infections, infectious diseases, inflammation, myeloma, liver disease
- IgM: primary biliary cirrhosis, infectious diseases (brucellosis, malaria), Waldenström's macroglobulinemia, liver disease

Hyperkalemia

PSEUDOHYPERKALEMIA
- Hemolyzed specimen
- Severe thrombocytosis (platelet count >106 mL)
- Severe leukocytosis (white blood cell count >105 mL)
- Fist clenching during phlebotomy

EXCESSIVE POTASSIUM INTAKE (OFTEN IN SETTING OF IMPAIRED EXCRETION)
- Potassium replacement therapy
- High-potassium diet
- Salt substitutes with potassium
- Potassium salts of antibiotics

DECREASED RENAL EXCRETION
- Potassium-sparing diuretics (e.g., spironolactone, triamterene, amiloride)
- Renal insufficiency
- Mineralocorticoid deficiency
- Hyporeninemic hypoaldosteronism (diabetes mellitus [DM])
- Tubular unresponsiveness to aldosterone (e.g., systemic lupus erythematosus [SLE], multiple myeloma, sickle cell disease)
- Type 4 renal tubular acidosis (RTA)
- Angiotensin-converting enzyme (ACE) inhibitors
- Heparin administration
- Nonsteroidal anti-inflammatory drugs (NSAIDs)
- Trimethoprim-sulfamethoxazole
- β-Blockers
- Pentamidine

REDISTRIBUTION (EXCESSIVE CELLULAR RELEASE)
- Acidemia (each 0.1 decrease in pH increases the serum potassium by 0.4 to 0.6 mEq/L). Lactic acidosis and ketoacidosis cause minimal redistribution.

- Insulin deficiency
- Drugs (e.g., succinylcholine, markedly increased digitalis level, arginine, β-adrenergic blockers)
- Hypertonicity
- Hemolysis
- Tissue necrosis, rhabdomyolysis, burns
- Hyperkalemic periodic paralysis

Hyperkinetic Movement Disorders[31]

- Chorea, choreoathetosis: drug induced, Huntington's chorea, Sydenham's chorea
- Tardive dyskinesia (e.g., phenothiazines)
- Hemiballismus (lacunar cerebrovascular accident [CVA] near subthalamic nuclei in basal ganglia, metastatic lesions, toxoplasmosis [in AIDS])
- Dystonia (idiopathic, familial, drug induced [prochlorperazine, metoclopramide]), Wilson's disease
- Liver failure
- Thyrotoxicosis
- Systemic lupus erythematosus (SLE), polycythemia

Hyperlipoproteinemia, Primary

SECONDARY CAUSES OF HYPERLIPOPROTEINEMIAS
- Diabetes mellitus (DM)
- Glycogen storage diseases
- Lipodystrophies
- Glucocorticoid use/excess
- Alcohol
- Oral contraceptives
- Renal disease
- Hepatic dysfunction
- Diet high in saturated fats

Hypermagnesemia

- Renal failure (decreased glomerular filtration rate [GFR])
- Decreased renal excretion secondary to salt depletion

- Abuse of antacids and laxatives containing magnesium in patients with renal insufficiency
- Endocrinopathies (deficiency of mineralocorticoid or thyroid hormone)
- Increased tissue breakdown (rhabdomyolysis)
- Redistribution: acute diabetic ketoacidosis (DKA), pheochromocytoma
- Other: lithium, volume depletion, familial hypocalciuric hypercalcemia

Hypernatremia

ISOVOLEMIC HYPERNATREMIA

Decreased total body water, normal total body sodium and extracellular fluid
- Diabetes insipidus (neurogenic and nephrogenic)
- Skin loss (hyperemia), iatrogenic, reset osmostat

HYPERVOLEMIC HYPERNATREMIA

Increased total body water, markedly increased total body sodium and extracellular fluid
- Iatrogenic (administration of hypernatremic solutions)
- Mineralocorticoid excess (Conn's syndrome, Cushing's syndrome)
- Salt ingestion

HYPOVOLEMIC HYPERNATREMIA

Loss of H_2O and Na^+ (H_2O Loss > Na^+)
- Renal losses (e.g., diuretics, glycosuria)
- GI, respiratory, skin losses
- Adrenal deficiencies

Hyperosmolality, Serum

- Dehydration
- Hypernatremia
- Diabetes insipidus (DI)
- Uremia
- Hyperglycemia
- Mannitol therapy
- Ingestion of toxins (ethylene glycol, methanol, ethanol), hypercalcemia, diuretics

Hyperosmolality, Urine

- Syndrome of inappropriate antidiuretic hormone (SIADH)
- Dehydration
- Glycosuria
- Adrenal insufficiency
- High-protein diet

Hyperparathyroidism

OTHER CAUSES OF HYPERCALCEMIA
- Malignant disease: neoplasms of breast, lung, kidney, ovary, pancreas; myeloma, lymphoma
- Granulomatous disorders (e.g., sarcoidosis)
- Paget's disease
- Vitamin D intoxication, milk-alkali syndrome
- Thiazide diuretics
- Other: familial hypocalciuric hypercalcemia, thyrotoxicosis, adrenal insufficiency, prolonged immobilization, vitamin A intoxication, recovery from acute renal failure, lithium administration, pheochromocytoma, disseminated systemic lupus erythematosus (SLE)

Hyperphosphatemia

- Excessive phosphate administration
  - Excessive oral intake or IV administration
  - Laxatives containing phosphate (phosphate tablets, phosphate enemas)
- Decreased renal phosphate excretion
  - Acute or chronic renal failure
  - Hypoparathyroidism or pseudohypoparathyroidism
  - Acromegaly, thyrotoxicosis
  - Bisphosphonate therapy
  - Tumor calcinosis
  - Sickle cell anemia
- Transcellular shift out of cells
  - Chemotherapy of lymphoma or leukemia, tumor lysis syndrome, hemolysis
  - Acidosis

- • Rhabdomyolysis, malignant hyperthermia
- Artifact: in vitro hemolysis
- Pseudohyperphosphatemia: hyperlipidemia, paraproteinemia, hyperbilirubinemia

Hyperpigmentation[6]

- Addison's disease
- Arsenic ingestion
- Adrenocorticotropic hormone (ACTH)– or melanocyte-stimulating hormone (MSH)–producing tumors (e.g., small cell carcinoma of the lung)
- Drug induced (e.g., antimalarials, some cytotoxic agents)
- Hemochromatosis ("bronze" diabetes)
- Malabsorption syndrome (Whipple's disease and celiac sprue)
- Melanoma
- Melanotropic hormone injection
- Pheochromocytoma
- Porphyrias (porphyria cutanea tarda and variegate porphyria)
- Pregnancy
- Progressive systemic sclerosis and related conditions
- Psoralen plus ultraviolet A (PUVA) therapy (psoralen administration) for psoriasis and vitiligo

Hyperprolactinemia

- Prolactinomas (level >200 highly suggestive)
- Drugs (phenothiazines, cimetidine, tricyclic antidepressants, metoclopramide, estrogens, antihypertensives [methyldopa, verapamil], haloperidol)
- Post partum
- Stress
- Hypoglycemia
- Hypothyroidism

Hyperproteinemia

- Dehydration
- Sarcoidosis

- Collagen vascular diseases
- Multiple myeloma
- Waldenström's macroglobulinemia

Hypersensitivity Pneumonitis

- Bronchiectasis
- Aspergillosis
- Chronic bronchitis
- Pulmonary embolism
- Asthma
- Aspiration pneumonia
- Recurrent pneumonia
- Bronchiolitis obliterans organizing pneumonia (BOOP)
- Sarcoidosis
- Churg-Strauss syndrome
- Wegener's granulomatosis

Hypersplenism

- Splenic congestion: cirrhosis; congestive heart failure (CHF); portal, splenic, or hepatic vein thrombosis
- Hematologic causes: hemolytic anemia, sickle cell anemia, thalassemia, spherocytosis, elliptocytosis
- Infections: viral (hepatitis, infectious mononucleosis, cytomegalovirus [CMV], HIV), bacterial (endocarditis, TB, brucellosis, Lyme), parasitic (malaria, leishmaniasis, schistosomiasis, toxoplasmosis), fungal
- Malignant disease: leukemia, lymphoma, polycythemia vera, myeloproliferative diseases, metastatic tumors
- Inflammatory diseases: Felty's syndrome, systemic lupus erythematosus (SLE), sarcoidosis
- Infiltrative diseases: amyloidosis, Gaucher's disease, Niemann-Pick disease, glycogen storage disease

Hyperthyroidism

- Anxiety disorder
- Pheochromocytoma
- Metastatic neoplasm

- Diabetes mellitus (DM)
- Premenopausal state

Hypertrichosis[7]

DRUGS
- Dilantin
- Streptomycin
- Hexachlorobenzene
- Penicillamine
- Diazoxide
- Minoxidil
- Cyclosporine

SYSTEMIC ILLNESS
- Hypothyroidism
- Anorexia nervosa
- Malnutrition
- Porphyria
- Dermatomyositis

IDIOPATHIC

Hypertriglyceridemia

- Hyperlipoproteinemias (types I, IIb, III, IV, V)
- Diet high in saturated fats
- Hypothyroidism
- Pregnancy
- Estrogens
- Pancreatitis
- Alcohol intake
- Nephrotic syndrome
- Poorly controlled diabetes mellitus (DM)
- Sedentary lifestyle
- Glycogen storage disease

Hypertrophic Osteoarthropathy

- Paget's disease
- Reiter's syndrome

- Psoriasis
- Osteoarthritis
- Rheumatoid arthritis (RA)
- Osteomyelitis

Hyperuricemia

- Hereditary enzyme deficiency (hypoxanthine-guanine phosphoribosyltransferase)
- Renal failure
- Gout
- Excessive cell lysis (chemotherapeutic agents, radiation therapy, leukemia, lymphoma, hemolytic anemia)
- Acidosis
- Myeloproliferative disorders
- Diet high in purines or protein
- Drugs (diuretics, low doses of aspirin, ethambutol, nicotinic acid)
- Lead poisoning
- Hypothyroidism

Hyperventilation, Persistent[37]

- Fibrotic lung disease
- Metabolic acidosis (e.g., diabetes, uremia)
- CNS disorders (midbrain and pontine lesions)
- Hepatic coma
- Salicylate intoxication
- Fever
- Sepsis
- Psychogenic (e.g., anxiety)

Hyperviscosity, Serum

- Monoclonal gammopathies (Waldenström's macroglobulinemia, multiple myeloma)
- Hyperfibrinogenemia
- Systemic lupus erythematosus (SLE)
- Rheumatoid arthritis (RA)
- Polycythemia
- Leukemia

Hypoalbuminemia

- Liver disease
- Nephrotic syndrome
- Poor nutritional status
- Rapid IV hydration
- Protein-losing enteropathies (inflammatory bowel disease [IBD])
- Severe burns
- Neoplasia
- Chronic inflammatory diseases
- Pregnancy
- Prolonged immobilization
- Lymphomas
- Hypervitaminosis A
- Chronic glomerulonephritis

Hypoaldosteronism

Pseudohypoaldosteronism: renal unresponsiveness to aldosterone. In this condition, both renin and aldosterone levels are elevated. Pseudohypoaldosteronism can be caused by medications (spironolactone), chronic interstitial nephritis, systemic disorders (systemic lupus erythematosus, amyloidosis), or primary mineralocorticoid resistance.

Hypocalcemia

- Renal insufficiency: hypocalcemia caused by
  - Increased calcium deposits in bone and soft tissue secondary to increased serum PO_4^{-3} level
  - Decreased production of 1,25-dihydroxyvitamin D
  - Excessive loss of 25-OHD (nephrotic syndrome)
- Hypoalbuminemia: each decrease in serum albumin (g/L) will decrease serum calcium by 0.8 mg/dL but will not change free (ionized) calcium.
- Vitamin D deficiency
  - Malabsorption (most common cause)
  - Inadequate intake
  - Decreased production of 1,25-dihydroxyvitamin D (vitamin D–dependent rickets, renal failure)

- Decreased production of 25-OHD (parenchymal liver disease)
  - Accelerated 25-OHD catabolism (phenytoin, phenobarbital)
  - End-organ resistance to 1,25-dihydroxyvitamin D
- Hypomagnesemia: hypocalcemia caused by
  - Decreased parathyroid hormone (PTH) secretion
  - Inhibition of PTH effect on bone
- Pancreatitis, hyperphosphatemia, osteoblastic metastases: hypocalcemia is secondary to increased calcium deposits (bone, abdomen).
- Pseudohypoparathyroidism: autosomal recessive disorder characterized by short stature, shortening of metacarpal bones, obesity, and mental retardation; the hypocalcemia is secondary to congenital end-organ resistance to PTH.
- Idiopathic hypoparathyroidism, surgical removal of parathyroids (e.g., neck surgery)
- "Hungry bones syndrome": rapid transfer of calcium from plasma into bones after removal of a parathyroid tumor
- Sepsis
- Massive blood transfusion (as a result of ethylenediaminetetraacetic acid [EDTA] in blood)

Hypocapnia

- Hyperventilation
- Pneumonia, pneumonitis
- Fever, sepsis
- Medications (salicylates, β-adrenergic agonists, progesterone, methylxanthines)
- Pulmonary disease (asthma, interstitial fibrosis)
- Pulmonary embolism
- Hepatic failure
- Metabolic acidosis
- High altitude
- Congestive heart failure (CHF)
- Pregnancy
- Pain
- CNS lesions

Hypochloremia

- Vomiting
- Gastric suction
- Primary aldosteronism
- Congestive heart failure (CHF)
- Syndrome of inappropriate antidiuretic hormone (SIADH)
- Addison's disease
- Salt-losing nephritis
- Continuous infusion of D_5W
- Thiazide diuretic administration
- Diaphoresis
- Diarrhea
- Burns
- Diabetic ketoacidosis (DKA)

Hypochondriasis

- Underlying medical condition, such as multiple sclerosis, hypothyroidism, or systemic lupus erythematosus (SLE)
- Somatization disorder
- Body dysmorphic disorder (restricted to a circumscribed concern about appearance)
- Factitious disorder or malingering
- Generalized anxiety disorder with health concerns as one worry among many others
- Major depressive disorder with health concerns occurring only during depressive episodes
- Psychosis, such as may occur with depression or schizophrenia

Hypogonadism

HYPERGONADOTROPIC HYPOGONADISM
- Hormone resistance (androgen, luteinizing hormone [LH] insensitivity)
- Gonadal defects (e.g., Klinefelter's syndrome, myotonic dystrophy)
- Drug induced (e.g., spironolactone, cytotoxins)
- Alcoholism, radiation induced

- Mumps orchitis
- Anatomic defects, castration

HYPOGONADOTROPIC HYPOGONADISM
- Pituitary lesions (neoplasms, granulomas, infarction, hemochromatosis, vasculitis)
- Drug induced (e.g., glucocorticoids)
- Hyperprolactinemia
- Genetic disorders (Laurence-Moon-Biedl syndrome, Prader-Willi syndrome)
- Delayed puberty
- Other: chronic disease, nutritional deficiency, Kallmann's syndrome, idiopathic isolated LH or follicle-stimulating hormone (FSH) deficiency

Hypoimmunoglobulinemia

- IgA: nephrotic syndrome, protein-losing enteropathy, congenital deficiency, lymphocytic leukemia, ataxia-telangiectasia, chronic sinopulmonary disease
- IgE: hypogammaglobulinemia, neoplasm (breast, bronchial, cervical), ataxia-telangiectasia
- IgG: congenital or acquired deficiency, lymphocytic leukemia, phenytoin, methylprednisolone, nephrotic syndrome, protein-losing enteropathy
- IgM: congenital deficiency, lymphocytic leukemia, nephrotic syndrome

Hypokalemia

- Cellular shift (redistribution) and undetermined mechanisms
- Alkalosis (each 0.1 increase in pH decreases serum potassium by 0.4 to 0.6 mEq/L)
- Insulin administration
- Vitamin B_{12} therapy for megaloblastic anemias, acute leukemias
- Hypokalemic periodic paralysis: rare familial disorder manifested by recurrent attacks of flaccid paralysis and hypokalemia
- β-Adrenergic agonists (e.g., terbutaline), decongestants, bronchodilators, theophylline, caffeine

- Barium poisoning, toluene intoxication, verapamil intoxication, chloroquine intoxication
- Correction of digoxin intoxication with digoxin antibody fragments (Digibind)
- Increased renal excretion secondary to medications: diuretics, including carbonic anhydrase inhibitors (e.g., acetazolamide); amphotericin B; high-dose sodium penicillin, nafcillin, ampicillin, or carbenicillin; cisplatin; aminoglycosides, corticosteroids, mineralocorticoids, foscarnet sodium
- Renal tubular acidosis (RTA): distal (type 1) or proximal (type 2)
- Diabetic ketoacidosis (DKA), ureteroenterostomy
- Magnesium deficiency
- Postobstruction diuresis, diuretic phase of tyrosinase-negative oculocutaneous albinism (ATN)
- Osmotic diuresis (e.g., mannitol)
- Bartter's syndrome: hyperplasia of juxtaglomerular cells leading to increased renin and aldosterone, metabolic alkalosis, hypokalemia, muscle weakness, and tetany (seen in young adults)
- Increased mineralocorticoid activity (primary or secondary aldosteronism), Cushing's syndrome
- Chronic metabolic alkalosis from loss of gastric fluid (increased renal potassium secretion)
- GI loss: vomiting, nasogastric suction, diarrhea, laxative abuse, villous adenoma, fistulas
- Inadequate dietary intake (e.g., anorexia nervosa)
- Cutaneous loss (excessive sweating)
- High dietary sodium intake, excessive use of licorice

Hypomagnesemia

GI AND NUTRITIONAL
- Defective GI absorption (malabsorption)
- Inadequate dietary intake (e.g., alcoholics)
- Parenteral therapy without magnesium
- Chronic diarrhea, villous adenoma, prolonged nasogastric suction, fistulas (small bowel, biliary)

EXCESSIVE RENAL LOSSES
- Diuretics
- Renal tubular acidosis (RTA)

- Diuretic phase of acute tubular necrosis (ATN)
- Endocrine disturbances (diabetic ketoacidosis [DKA], hyperaldosteronism, hyperthyroidism, hyperparathyroidism), syndrome of inappropriate antidiuretic hormone (SIADH), Bartter's syndrome, hypercalciuria, hypokalemia
- Cisplatin, alcohol, cyclosporine, digoxin, pentamidine, mannitol, amphotericin B, foscarnet, methotrexate
- Antibiotics (gentamicin, ticarcillin, carbenicillin)
- Redistribution: hypoalbuminemia, cirrhosis, administration of insulin and glucose, theophylline, epinephrine, acute pancreatitis, cardiopulmonary bypass
- Miscellaneous: sweating, burns, prolonged exercise, lactation, "hungry bones" syndrome

Hyponatremia

HYPOTONIC HYPONATREMIA

Isovolemic Hyponatremia

- Syndrome of inappropriate antidiuretic hormone (SIADH)
- Water intoxication (e.g., schizophrenic patients, primary polydipsia, sodium-free irrigant solutions, multiple tap-water enemas, dilute infant formulas). These entities are rare and often associated with a deranged antidiuretic hormone (ADH) axis.
- Renal failure
- Reset osmostat (e.g., chronic active TB, carcinomatosis)
- Glucocorticoid deficiency (hypopituitarism)
- Hypothyroidism
- Thiazide diuretics, nonsteroidal anti-inflammatory drugs (NSAIDs), carbamazepine, amitriptyline, thioridazine, vincristine, cyclophosphamide, colchicine, tolbutamide, chlorpropamide, angiotensin-converting enzyme (ACE) inhibitors, clofibrate, oxytocin, selective serotonin reuptake inhibitors (SSRIs), amiodarone. With these medications, various drug-induced mechanisms are involved.

Hypovolemic Hyponatremia

- Renal losses (diuretics, partial urinary tract obstruction, salt-losing renal disease)
- Extrarenal losses: GI (vomiting, diarrhea), extensive burns, third spacing (peritonitis, pancreatitis)
- Adrenal insufficiency

Hypervolemic Hyponatremia
- Congestive heart failure (CHF)
- Nephrotic syndrome
- Cirrhosis
- Pregnancy

ISOTONIC HYPONATREMIA
Normal Serum Osmolality
- Pseudohyponatremia (increased serum lipids and serum proteins). Newer sodium assays eliminate this problem.
- Isotonic infusion (e.g., glucose, mannitol)

HYPERTONIC HYPONATREMIA
Increased Serum Osmolality
- Hyperglycemia: each 100 mg/dL increment in blood glucose level above normal decreases plasma sodium concentration by 1.6 mEq/L
- Hypertonic infusions (e.g., glucose, mannitol)

Hypo-osmolality, Serum

- Syndrome of inappropriate antidiuretic hormone (SIADH)
- Hyponatremia
- Overhydration
- Addison's disease
- Hypothyroidism

Hypo-osmolality, Urine

- Diabetes insipidus (DI)
- Excessive water intake
- IV hydration with D_5W
- Acute renal insufficiency
- Glomerulonephritis

Hypophosphatemia

- Decreased intake (prolonged starvation, hyperalimentation, or IV infusion without phosphate)
- Malabsorption
- Phosphate-binding antacids

- Renal loss: renal tubular acidosis (RTA), Fanconi's syndrome, vitamin D–resistant rickets, tyrosine-negative oculocutaneous albinism (ATN) (diuretic phase), hyperparathyroidism (primary or secondary), familial hypophosphatemia, hypokalemia, hypomagnesemia, acute volume expansion, glycosuria, idiopathic hypercalciuria, acetazolamide
- Transcellular shift into cells: alcohol withdrawal, diabetic ketoacidosis (DKA) (recovery phase), glucose-insulin or catecholamine infusion, anabolic steroids, total parenteral nutrition, theophylline overdose, severe hyperthermia, recovery from hypothermia, "hungry bones" syndrome

Hypopigmentation

- Vitiligo
- Tinea versicolor
- Atopic dermatitis
- Chemical leukoderma
- Idiopathic hypomelanosis
- Sarcoidosis
- Systemic lupus erythematosus (SLE)
- Scleroderma
- Oculocutaneous albinism
- Phenylketonuria (PKU)
- Nevoid hypopigmentation

Hypopituitarism

- Congenital: mutations in transcription factors produce multiple hormonal deficiencies. Mutations in genes produce single hormonal deficiency.
- Acquired: the result of destruction of pituitary cells caused by
  - Pituitary apoplexy: hemorrhage or infarction of the pituitary gland. Predisposing factors include diabetes mellitus, anticoagulation therapy, head trauma, and radiation therapy. Sheehan's syndrome: postpartum necrosis, a rare complication after pregnancy.
  - Infiltrative disease, including sarcoidosis, hemochromatosis, histiocytosis X, Wegener's granulomatosis, lymphocytic hypophysitis, and infection of the pituitary (tuberculosis, mycosis, syphilis)

- Primary empty sella syndrome: flattening of the pituitary gland caused by extension of the subarachnoid space and filling of cerebrospinal fluid into the sella turcica
- Pituitary tumors: classified by size (microadenomas, <10 mm; macroadenomas, >10 mm) and function. Prolactin-secreting tumors and nonfunctioning tumors account for the majority of pituitary adenomas.
- Suprasellar tumors: craniopharyngiomas are the most common.

Hypoproteinemia

- Malnutrition
- Cirrhosis
- Nephrosis
- Low-protein diet
- Overhydration
- Malabsorption
- Pregnancy
- Severe burns
- Neoplasms
- Chronic diseases

Hypotension, Postural

- Antihypertensive medications (especially α-blockers, diuretics, angiotensin-converting enzyme [ACE] inhibitors)
- Volume depletion (hemorrhage, dehydration)
- Impaired cardiac output (constrictive pericarditis, aortic stenosis)
- Peripheral autonomic dysfunction (diabetes mellitus [DM], Guillain-Barré)
- Idiopathic orthostatic hypotension
- Central autonomic dysfunction (Shy-Drager syndrome)
- Peripheral venous disease
- Adrenal insufficiency

Hypothermia

- Cerebrovascular accident (CVA)
- Myxedema coma

- Drug intoxication
- Hypoglycemia

Hypothyroidism

- Depression
- Dementia from other causes
- Systemic disorders (e.g., nephrotic syndrome, congestive heart failure [CHF], amyloidosis)
- Chronic fatigue syndrome

Id Reaction

- Atopic dermatitis
- Contact dermatitis
- Drug eruptions
- Dyshidrotic eczema
- Folliculitis
- Scabies
- Dermatophytic infection
- Viral exanthems

Idiopathic Intracranial Hypertension

- The symptoms and signs of IIH are essentially those of raised intracranial pressure (ICP), and the differential diagnosis includes any condition that may be associated with raised ICP. Here we consider only those disease processes in which elevated ICP occurs in the context of normal CSF analysis and normal MRI. (Of note, venous sinus thrombosis [VST] is on this list despite associated MRI findings. VST should be excluded in all individuals with suspected IIH.)
- Medications: vitamin A and retinoids, steroids (both use and withdrawal), oral contraceptives
- Autoimmune disorders: systemic lupus erythematosus, Behçet's disease
- Vascular disease: venous sinus thrombosis
- Other conditions: hypertension, CHF, pregnancy, obesity, uremia, obstructive sleep apnea

Idiopathic Pulmonary Fibrosis

- Sarcoidosis and connective tissue disease
- Other idiopathic interstitial pneumonias: desquamative interstitial pneumonia, interstitial lung disease, acute interstitial pneumonia, nonspecific interstitial pneumonia, cryptogenic organizing pneumonia, bronchiolitis obliterans organizing pneumonia
- Occupational exposures (e.g., asbestos, silica)

IgA Nephropathy

- Henoch-Schönlein purpura
- Hereditary nephritis
- Thin glomerular basement membrane disease
- Lupus nephritis
- Poststreptococcal nephritis
- Secondary causes associated with IgA nephropathy

Iliac Fossa Pain, Left Sided[39]

GASTROINTESTINAL CAUSES OF ACUTE LEFT ILIAC FOSSA PAIN
- Nonspecific left iliac fossa pain including constipation
- Acute gastroenteritis
- Acute diverticulitis
- Colonic carcinoma
- Colonic ischemia
- Localized small bowel perforation

Iliac Fossa Pain, Right Sided[39]

Differential diagnosis of right iliac fossa pain:

GASTROINTESTINAL CAUSES
- Nonspecific right iliac fossa pain
- Acute appendicitis
- Mesenteric adenitis
- Terminal ileitis
- Acute inflammation of Meckel's diverticulum

- Crohn's disease of the terminal ileum
- Cecal carcinoma
- Inflammatory cecal lesion (e.g., diverticulitis in a solitary cecal diverticulum)
- Inflammatory lesion of the terminal ileum (e.g., foreign body perforation)

NONGASTROINTESTINAL CAUSES
- Ruptured ovarian follicle (mittelschmerz)
- Acute salpingitis (pelvic inflammatory disease)
- Rupture/torsion or hemorrhage of an ovarian cyst
- Endometriosis
- Ectopic pregnancy
- Urinary tract infection

Immune Thrombocytopenic Purpura

- Falsely low platelet count (resulting from ethylenediaminetetraacetic acid [EDTA]–dependent or cold-dependent agglutinins)
- Viral infections (e.g., HIV infection, mononucleosis, rubella)
- Drug induced (e.g., heparin, quinidine, sulfonamides)
- Hypersplenism resulting from liver disease
- Myelodysplastic and lymphoproliferative disorders
- Pregnancy, hypothyroidism
- Systemic lupus erythematosus (SLE), thrombotic thrombocytopenic purpura (TTP), hemolytic-uremic syndrome (HUS)
- Congenital thrombocytopenias (e.g., Fanconi's syndrome, May-Hegglin anomaly, Bernard-Soulier syndrome)

Impetigo

- Acute allergic contact dermatitis
- Herpes simplex infection
- Ecthyma
- Folliculitis
- Eczema
- Insect bites
- Scabies

- Tinea corporis
- Pemphigus vulgaris and bullous pemphigoid
- Chickenpox

Impotence[28]

- Psychogenic
- Endocrine: hyperprolactinemia, diabetes mellitus (DM), Cushing's syndrome, hypothyroidism or hyperthyroidism, abnormality of hypothalamic-pituitary-testicular axis
- Vascular: arterial insufficiency, venous leakage, arteriovenous (AV) malformation, local trauma
- Medications
- Neurogenic: autonomic or sensory neuropathy, spinal cord trauma or tumor, cerebrovascular accident (CVA), multiple sclerosis (MS), temporal lobe epilepsy
- Systemic illness: renal failure, chronic obstructive pulmonary disease (COPD), cirrhosis of liver, myotonic dystrophy
- Peyronie's disease
- Prostatectomy

Inappropriate Secretion of Antidiuretic Hormone

- Hyponatremia associated with hypervolemia (congestive heart failure [CHF], cirrhosis, nephrotic syndrome)
- Factitious hyponatremia (hyperglycemia, abnormal proteins, hyperlipidemia)
- Hypovolemia associated with hypovolemia (e.g., burns, GI fluid loss)

Inclusion Body Myositis

- Polymyositis
- Muscular dystrophy
- Diabetic neuropathy
- Trichinosis
- AIDS
- Alcoholic myopathy
- Hypothyroidism

- Hypophosphatemia
- Myasthenia gravis, Eaton-Lambert syndrome
- Amyotrophic lateral sclerosis (ALS)
- Guillain-Barré syndrome

Incontinence, Fecal[39]

NORMAL SPHINCTER
- Diarrhea
- Anorectal conditions
  - Rectal carcinoma
  - Inflammatory bowel disease
  - Hemorrhoids
  - Mucosal prolapse
  - Fissure in ano
  - Abnormal rectal sensation

ABNORMAL SPHINCTER
- Congenital abnormalities
- Anal sepsis
- Neurologic conditions
- Rectal prolapse
- Sphincter trauma

NEUROGENIC (IDIOPATHIC) INCONTINENCE

Infertility, Female[14]

FALLOPIAN TUBE PATHOLOGY
- Pelvic inflammatory disease (PID) or puerperal infection
- Congenital anomalies
- Endometriosis
- Secondary to past peritonitis of nongenital origin
- Amenorrhea, anovulation
- Minor anovulatory disturbances

CERVICAL AND UTERINE FACTORS
- Leiomyomas, polyps
- Uterine anomalies
- Intrauterine synechiae (Asherman's syndrome)
- Destroyed endocervical glands (after surgery or infection)

VAGINAL FACTORS
- Imperforate hymen
- Vaginismus
- Vaginitis
- Congenital absence of vagina

IMMUNOLOGIC FACTORS
- Sperm-immobilizing antibodies
- Sperm-agglutinating antibodies

NUTRITIONAL AND METABOLIC FACTORS
- Thyroid disorders
- Diabetes mellitus (DM)
- Severe nutritional disturbances

Infertility, Male[14]

DECREASED PRODUCTION OF SPERMATOZOA
- Varicocele
- Testicular failure
- Endocrine disorders
- Cryptorchidism
- Stress, smoking, caffeine, nicotine, recreational drugs
- Ductal obstruction
- Epididymal (post infection)
- Ejaculatory duct (post infection)
- Post vasectomy
- Congenital absence of vas deferens

INABILITY TO DELIVER SPERM INTO VAGINA
- Ejaculatory disturbances
- Hypospadias
- Sexual problems (e.g., impotence), medical or psychological

ABNORMAL SEMEN
- Infection
- Abnormal volume
- Abnormal viscosity
- Abnormal sperm motion

IMMUNOLOGIC FACTORS
- Sperm-immobilizing antibodies
- Sperm-agglutinating antibodies

Influenza

- Respiratory syncytial virus
- Adenovirus infection
- Parainfluenza virus infection
- Secondary bacterial pneumonia or mixed bacterial-viral pneumonia

Insomnia[34]

- Anxiety disorder, psychophysiologic insomnia
- Depression
- Drugs (e.g., caffeine, amphetamines, cocaine), hypnotic-dependent sleep disorder
- Pain, fibromyalgia
- Inadequate sleep hygiene
- Restless leg syndrome
- Obstructive sleep apnea
- Sleep bruxism
- Medical illness (e.g., gastroesophageal reflux disease [GERD], sleep-related asthma, parkinsonism, and movement disorders)
- Narcolepsy
- Other: periodic leg movement of sleep, central sleep apnea, rapid eye movement (REM) behavioral disorder

Insulinoma (Differential Diagnosis of Fasting Hypoglycemia)

- Hyperinsulinism
  - Insulinoma
  - Nonpancreatic tumors
  - Severe congestive heart failure
  - Severe renal insufficiency in non–insulin-dependent diabetes
- Hepatic enzyme deficiencies or decreased hepatic glucose output (primarily in infants and children)

- Glycogen storage diseases
- Endocrine hypofunction
- Hypopituitarism
- Addison's disease
- Liver failure
- Alcohol abuse
- Malnutrition
- Exogenous agents
  - Sulfonylureas, biguanides
  - Insulin
  - Other drugs (aspirin, pentamidine)
- Functional fasting hypoglycemia
  - Autoantibodies to insulin receptor or insulin

Interstitial Cystitis

- Chronic pelvic pain
- Overactive bladder
- Recurrent urinary tract infection
- Endometriosis
- Pelvic adhesions
- Vulvar vestibulitis
- Vulvodynia
- Urethral pain syndrome
- Chronic nonbacterial prostatitis
- Frequent vaginitis
- Benign prostatic hyperplasia

Intestinal Pseudo-obstruction[37]

PRIMARY (IDIOPATHIC INTESTINAL PSEUDO-OBSTRUCTION)
- Hollow visceral myopathy: familial, sporadic
- Neuropathic: abnormal myenteric plexus, normal myenteric plexus

SECONDARY
- Scleroderma
- Myxedema
- Amyloidosis

- Muscular dystrophy
- Hypokalemia
- Chronic renal failure
- Diabetes mellitus (DM)
- Drug toxicity caused by anticholinergics, opiate narcotics
- Ogilvie's syndrome

Intracranial Lesion

- Tumor (primary or metastatic)
- Abscess
- Stroke
- Intracranial hemorrhage
- Angioma
- Multiple sclerosis (MS) (initial single lesion)
- Granuloma
- Herpes encephalitis
- Artifact

Intraocular Neoplasm

MALIGNANT
- Retinoblastoma
- Melanoma
- Reticulum cell sarcoma
- Metastatic tumor

BENIGN
- Melanocytic nevus
- Hemangioma
- Reactive lymphoid hyperplasia

Iron Overload[21]

HEREDITARY IRON OVERLOAD
- Hereditary hemochromatosis
  - HFE associated (type 1)
  - Non–HFE associated
  - Transferrin receptor 2 associated (type 3)
  - Juvenile hemochromatosis (type 2)

- Hemojuvelin associated (type 2A)
- Hepcidin associated (type 2B)
- Autosomal dominant hemochromatosis, ferroprotein associated (type 4)
- DMT1-associated hemochromatosis
- Atransferrinemia
- Aceruloplasminemia

ACQUIRED IRON OVERLOAD
- Iron-loading anemias (refractory anemias with hypercellular erythroid marrow)
- Chronic liver disease
- Porphyria cutanea tarda
- Insulin resistance–associated hepatic iron overload
- African dietary iron overload
- Medicinal iron ingestion
- Parenteral iron overload
- Transfusional iron overload
- Inadvertent iron overload from therapeutic injections

PERINATAL IRON OVERLOAD
- Neonatal hemochromatosis
- Trichohepatoenteric syndrome
- Cerebrohepatorenal syndrome
- GRACILE (Fellman) syndrome

FOCAL SEQUESTRATION OF IRON
- Idiopathic pulmonary hemosiderosis
- Renal hemosiderosis
- Associated with neurologic abnormalities
- Pantothenate kinase–associated neurodegeneration (formerly called Hallervorden-Spatz syndrome)
- Neuroferritinopathy
- Friedreich's ataxia
- GRACILE (growth retardation, aminoaciduria, cholestasis, iron overload, lactic acidosis, and early death)

Irritable Bowel Syndrome

- Inflammatory bowel disease (IBD)
- Diverticulitis

- Colon malignant neoplasm
- Endometriosis
- Peptic ulcer disease (PUD)
- Biliary liver disease
- Chronic pancreatitis
- Celiac disease

Ischemic Colitis, Nonocclusive[22]

ACUTE DIMINUTION OF COLONIC INTRAMURAL BLOOD FLOW
Small-Vessel Obstruction
- Collagen-vascular disease
- Vasculitis, diabetes
- Oral contraceptives

Nonocclusive Hypoperfusion
- Hemorrhage
- Congestive heart failure (CHF), myocardial infarction (MI), arrhythmias
- Sepsis
- Vasoconstricting agents: vasopressin, ergot
- Increased viscosity: polycythemia, sickle cell disease, thrombocytosis

INCREASED DEMAND ON MARGINAL BLOOD FLOW
Increased Motility
- Mass lesion, stricture
- Constipation

Increased Intraluminal Pressure
- Bowel obstruction
- Colonoscopy
- Barium enema

Ischemic Necrosis of Cartilage and Bone[14]

- Endocrine/metabolic: ethanol abuse, glucocorticoid therapy, Cushing's disease, diabetes mellitus (DM), hyperuricemia, osteomalacia, hyperlipidemia, storage diseases (e.g., Gaucher's disease)

- Hemoglobinopathies (e.g., sickle cell disease)
- Trauma (e.g., dislocation, fracture)
- HIV infection
- Dysbaric conditions (e.g., caisson disease)
- Collagen-vascular disorders
- Irradiation
- Pancreatitis
- Organ transplantation
- Hemodialysis
- Burns
- Intravascular coagulation
- Idiopathic, familial

Jaundice

PREDOMINANCE OF DIRECT (CONJUGATED) BILIRUBIN

- Extrahepatic obstruction
- Common duct abnormalities: calculi, neoplasm, stricture, cyst, sclerosing cholangitis
- Metastatic carcinoma
- Pancreatic carcinoma, pseudocyst
- Ampullary carcinoma
- Hepatocellular disease: hepatitis, cirrhosis
- Drugs: estrogens, phenothiazines, captopril, methyltestosterone, labetalol

- Cholestatic jaundice of pregnancy
- Hereditary disorders: Dubin-Johnson syndrome, Rotor's syndrome
- Recurrent benign intrahepatic cholestasis

PREDOMINANCE OF INDIRECT (UNCONJUGATED) BILIRUBIN

- Hemolysis: hereditary and acquired hemolytic anemias
- Inefficient marrow production
- Impaired hepatic conjugation: chloramphenicol
- Neonatal jaundice
- Hereditary disorders: Gilbert's syndrome, Crigler-Najjar syndrome

Jaundice in the Adult Patient

PREHEPATIC CAUSES

- Unconjugated hyperbilirubinemia: excessive heme metabolism from hemolysis (e.g., sickle cell disease, spherocytosis, G6PD, immune hemolysis), ineffective erythropoiesis (e.g., thalassemia, folate, severe iron deficiency), or large hematoma reabsorption

INTRAHEPATIC CAUSES

- Unconjugated hyperbilirubinemia: disorders of enzyme metabolism such as Gilbert's disease (common, benign), Crigler-Najjar syndrome (rare, severe), or drugs such as rifampin and probenecid
- Conjugated hyperbilirubinemia: intrahepatic cholestasis

- Viruses: hepatitis A, B, and C; Epstein-Barr
- Alcohol: alcoholic hepatitis, alcoholic cirrhosis
- Autoimmune: primary biliary cirrhosis, primary sclerosing cholangitis
- Drug induced: acetaminophen, penicillins, oral contraceptives, chlorpromazine (Thorazine), steroids (estrogenic or anabolic), some herbals
- Hereditary metabolic: hemochromatosis, Wilson's disease, Dubin-Johnson and Rotor's syndromes, α_1-antitrypsin deficiency
- Systemic disease: sarcoidosis, amyloidosis, glycogen storage diseases, celiac disease, tuberculosis, *Mycobacterium avium-intracellulare*
- Other: sepsis, total parenteral nutrition, pregnancy, graft-versus-host disease, environmental toxins

POSTHEPATIC CAUSES

- Conjugated hyperbilirubinemia: intrinsic or extrinsic obstruction of the biliary system
- Intrinsic blockage: gallstones, cholangitis, strictures, infection (e.g., cytomegalovirus, *Cryptosporidium* in AIDS patients, parasites, cholangiocarcinoma, gallbladder cancer)
- Extrinsic blockage: pancreatitis, pancreatic carcinoma, pancreatic pseudocyst
- Pseudojaundice: caused by an excessive ingestion of foods containing beta-carotene (carrots, melons, squash); does *not* result in hyperbilirubinemia or scleral icterus

Joint Pain, Anterior Hip, Medial Thigh, Knee[29]

ACUTE

- Acute rheumatic fever
- Adductor muscle strain
- Avascular necrosis
- Crystal arthritis
- Femoral artery (pseudo) aneurysm
- Fracture (femoral neck or intertrochanteric)
- Hemarthrosis
- Hernia
- Herpes zoster
- Iliopectineal bursitis

- Iliopsoas tendinitis
- Inguinal lymphadenitis
- Osteomalacia
- Painful transient osteoporosis of hip
- Septic arthritis

SUBACUTE AND CHRONIC
- Adductor muscle strain
- Amyloidosis
- Acute rheumatic fever
- Femoral artery aneurysm
- Hernia (inguinal or femoral)
- Iliopectineal bursitis
- Iliopsoas tendinitis
- Inguinal lymphadenopathy
- Osteochondromatosis
- Osteomyelitis
- Osteitis deformans (Paget's disease)
- Osteomalacia (pseudofracture)
- Postherpetic neuralgia
- Sterile synovitis (e.g., rheumatoid arthritis [RA], psoriatic, systemic lupus erythematosus [SLE])

Joint Pain, Hip, Lateral Thigh[29]

ACUTE
- Herpes zoster
- Iliotibial tendinitis
- Impacted fracture of femoral neck
- Lateral femoral cutaneous neuropathy (meralgia paresthetica)
- Radiculopathy: L4–5
- Trochanteric avulsion fracture (greater trochanter)
- Trochanteric bursitis
- Trochanteric fracture

SUBACUTE AND CHRONIC
- Lateral femoral cutaneous neuropathy (meralgia paresthetica)
- Osteomyelitis
- Postherpetic neuralgia
- Radiculopathy: L4–5
- Tumors

Joint Pain, Polyarticular

- Osteoarthritis
- Rheumatoid arthritis (RA)
- Fibromyalgia
- Viral syndrome (e.g., human parvovirus B19 infection)
- Systemic lupus erythematosus (SLE)
- Psoriatic arthritis
- Ankylosing spondylitis

Joint Pain, Posterior Hips, Thigh, Buttocks[29]

ACUTE
- Gluteal muscle strain
- Herpes zoster
- Ischial bursitis
- Ischial or sacral fracture
- Osteomalacia (pseudofracture)
- Sciatic neuropathy
- Radiculopathy: L5-S1

SUBACUTE AND CHRONIC
- Gluteal muscle strain
- Ischial bursitis
- Lumbar spinal stenosis
- Osteoarthritis of hip
- Osteitis deformans (Paget's disease)
- Osteomyelitis
- Osteochondromatosis
- Osteomalacia (pseudofracture)
- Postherpetic neuralgia
- Radiculopathy: L5-S1
- Tumors

Joint Swelling

- Trauma
- Osteoarthritis
- Gout
- Pyogenic arthritis

- Pseudogout
- Rheumatoid arthritis (RA)
- Viral syndrome

Jugular Venous Distention

- Right-sided heart failure
- Cardiac tamponade
- Constrictive pericarditis
- Goiter
- Tension pneumothorax
- Pulmonary hypertension
- Cardiomyopathy (restrictive)
- Superior vena cava syndrome
- Valsalva maneuver
- Right atrial myxoma
- Chronic obstructive pulmonary disease (COPD)

Juvenile Idiopathic Arthritis

- Infectious causes of fever
- Systemic lupus erythematosus
- Rheumatic fever
- Drug reaction
- Serum sickness
- "Viral arthritis"
- Lyme arthritis

Kaposi's Sarcoma

- Stasis dermatitis
- Pyogenic granuloma
- Capillary hemangiomas
- Granulation tissue
- Postinflammatory hyperpigmentation
- Cutaneous lymphoma
- Melanoma
- Dermatofibroma
- Hematoma
- Prurigo nodularis

Kawasaki's Disease

- Scarlet fever
- Stevens-Johnson syndrome
- Drug eruption
- Henoch-Schönlein purpura
- Toxic shock syndrome
- Measles
- Rocky Mountain spotted fever
- Infectious mononucleosis

Keloid

- Hypertrophic scar
- Dermatofibrosarcoma protuberans
- Sarcoidosis
- Squamous cell carcinoma
- Recurrence of original tumor
- Fibromatosis

Keratitis, Noninfectious

- Collagen-vascular disease
- Atopic keratoconjunctivitis
- Chemical injury
- Thermal injury
- Ectropion/entropion
- Lid defects
- Exophthalmos
- Keratoconjunctivitis sicca
- Erythema multiforme
- Mucous membrane pemphigoid
- DM (delayed epithelial healing)
- Neuroparalytic (cranial nerve VII)
- Neurotrophic (diabetes, cranial nerve V)

Keratoacanthoma

- Squamous cell carcinoma
- Seborrheic keratosis

- Wart
- Molluscum contagiosum
- Basal cell carcinoma

Kidney Enlargement, Unilateral[39]

- Hydronephrosis (may be bilateral)
- Polycystic kidney (may be bilateral)
- Simple cyst of kidney
- Renal cell carcinoma
- Pyonephrosis (may be bilateral)
- Acute renal vein thrombosis

Knee Pain[29]

DIFFUSE

- Articular
- Anterior
  - Prepatellar bursitis
  - Patellar tendon enthesopathy
  - Chondromalacia patellae
  - Patellofemoral osteoarthritis
  - Cruciate ligament injury
  - Medial plica syndrome

MEDIAL

- Anserine bursitis
- Spontaneous osteonecrosis
- Osteoarthritis
- Medial meniscal tear
- Medial collateral ligament bursitis
- Referred pain from hip and L3
- Fibromyalgia

LATERAL

- Iliotibial band syndrome
- Meniscal cyst
- Lateral meniscal tear
- Collateral ligament
- Peroneal tenosynovitis

POSTERIOR
* Popliteal cyst (Baker's cyst)
* Tendinitis
* Aneurysms, ganglions, sarcoma

Knee Pain, in Different Age Groups[8]

Common causes of knee pain in different age groups:

CHILDHOOD (2–10 YEARS)
Intra-articular
* Juvenile arthritis
* Osteochondritis dissecans
* Infection
* Torn discoid meniscus

Periarticular
* Osteomyelitis

Referred
* Perthes' disease
* Irritable hip

ADOLESCENCE (10–18 YEARS)
Intra-articular
* Osteochondritis dissecans
* Torn meniscus
* Anterior knee pain syndrome
* Patellar instability

Periarticular
* Osgood-Schlatter disease
* Sinding-Larsen-Johansson syndrome
* Osteomyelitis
* Bone tumors

Referred
* Slipped upper femoral epiphysis

EARLY ADULTHOOD (18–30 YEARS)
Intra-articular
* Torn meniscus
* Patellar instability

- Anterior knee pain syndrome
- Inflammatory arthritis

Periarticular
- Ligament injuries
- Bursitis

ADULTHOOD (30–50 YEARS)
Intra-articular
- Degenerate meniscal tears
- Osteoarthritis
- Inflammatory arthritis

Periarticular
- Bursitis

Referred
- Osteoarthritis of hip
- Spinal disorders

OLD AGE (>50 YEARS)
Intra-articular
- Osteoarthritis
- Inflammatory arthritis

Referred
- Osteoarthritis of hip
- Spinal disorders

Korsakoff's Psychosis

- Stroke affecting the temporal lobes or hippocampus
- Trauma affecting the temporal lobes or hippocampus
- Tumor affecting the temporal lobes or hippocampus
- Cerebral anoxia
- Transient global amnesia
- Dementing illness

Labyrinthitis

- Acute labyrinthine ischemia (vascular insufficiency)
- Other forms of labyrinthitis (bacterial and syphilitic)

- Labyrinthine fistula
- Benign positional vertigo
- Meniere's disease
- Cholesteatoma
- Drug induced
- Eighth nerve tumor
- Head trauma

Lactose Intolerance

- Inflammatory bowel disease (IBD)
- Irritable bowel syndrome (IBS)
- Pancreatic insufficiency
- Nontropical and tropical sprue
- Cystic fibrosis
- Diverticular disease
- Bowel neoplasm
- Laxative abuse
- Celiac disease
- Parasitic disease (e.g., giardiasis)
- Viral or bacterial infections

Lambert-Eaton Myasthenic Syndrome

- Myasthenia gravis
- Polymyositis
- Primary myopathies
- Carcinomatous myopathies
- Polymyalgia rheumatica
- Botulism
- Guillain-Barré syndrome

Laryngeal Cancer

- Laryngitis
- Allergic and nonallergic rhinosinusitis
- Gastroesophageal reflux
- Voice abuse leading to hoarseness
- Laryngeal papilloma

- Vocal cord paralysis secondary to a neurologic condition or secondary to entrapment of the recurrent laryngeal nerve caused by mediastinal compression
- Tracheomalacia

Laryngitis

YOUNG CHILDREN WITH SIGNS OF AIRWAY OBSTRUCTION
- Supraglottitis (epiglottitis)
- Laryngotracheobronchitis
- Tracheitis
- Foreign body aspiration

ADULTS WITH PERSISTENT HOARSENESS
- Allergic and nonallergic rhinosinusitis
- Gastroesophageal reflux
- Voice abuse leading to hoarseness
- Laryngeal papilloma
- Laryngeal carcinoma
- Vocal cord paralysis secondary to a neurologic condition or secondary to entrapment of the recurrent laryngeal nerve caused by mediastinal compression

Laryngotracheobronchitis

- Spasmodic croup
- Epiglottitis
- Bacterial tracheitis
- Angioneurotic edema
- Diphtheria
- Peritonsillar abscess
- Retropharyngeal abscess
- Smoke inhalation
- Foreign body

Lead Poisoning

- Polyneuropathies from other sources
- Anxiety disorder, attention deficit disorder
- Malabsorption, acute abdomen
- Iron deficiency anemia

Left Axis Deviation[23]

- Normal variation
- Left anterior fascicular block (hemiblock)
- Left bundle branch block
- Left ventricular hypertrophy (LVH)
- Mechanical shifts causing a horizontal heart, high diaphragm, pregnancy, ascites
- Some forms of ventricular tachycardia
- Endocardial cushion defects and other congenital heart disease

Left Bundle Branch Block

- Ischemic heart disease
- Electrolyte abnormalities (e.g., hyperkalemia)
- Cardiomyopathy
  - Idiopathic
  - Left ventricular hypertrophy (LVH)
- Pulmonary embolism
- Cardiac trauma
- Bacterial endocarditis

Leg Cramps, Nocturnal

- Diabetic neuropathy
- Medications
- Electrolyte abnormalities (hypokalemia, hyponatremia, hypocalcemia, hyperkalemia, hypophosphatemia)
- Respiratory alkalosis
- Uremia
- Hemodialysis
- Peripheral nerve injury
- Alcohol use
- Heat cramps
- Vitamin B_{12} deficiency
- Hyperthyroidism
- Contractures
- Deep venous thrombosis (DVT)
- Hypoglycemia
- Peripheral vascular insufficiency

- Baker's cyst
- Amyotrophic lateral sclerosis (ALS)

Leg Length Discrepancies[24]

CONGENITAL
- Proximal femoral local deficiency
- Coxa vara
- Hemiatrophy-hemihypertrophy (anisomelia)
- Development dysplasia of the hip

DEVELOPMENTAL
- Legg-Calvé-Perthes disease (LCPD)

NEUROMUSCULAR
- Polio
- Cerebral palsy (hemiplegia)

INFECTIOUS
- Pyogenic osteomyelitis with physeal damage

TRAUMA
- Physeal injury with premature closure
- Overgrowth
- Malunion (shortening)

TUMOR
- Physeal destruction
- Radiation-induced physeal injury
- Overgrowth

Leg Pain with Exercise

- Shin splints
- Arteriosclerosis obliterans
- Neurogenic (spinal cord compression or ischemia)
- Venous claudication
- Popliteal cyst
- Deep venous thrombosis (DVT)
- Thromboangiitis obliterans
- Adventitial cysts

- Popliteal artery entrapment syndrome
- McArdle's syndrome

Leg Ulcers[29]

VASCULAR

- Arterial: arteriosclerosis, thromboangiitis obliterans, arteriovenous (AV) malformation, cholesterol emboli
- Venous: superficial varicosities, incompetent perforators, deep venous thrombosis (DVT), lymphatic abnormalities

VASCULITIS/HEMATOLOGIC

- Sickle cell anemia, thalassemia, polycythemia vera, leukemia, cold agglutinin disease
- Macroglobulinemia, protein C and protein S deficiency, cryoglobulinemia, lupus anticoagulant, antiphospholipid syndrome

INFECTIOUS

- Fungus: blastomycosis, coccidioidomycosis, histoplasmosis, sporotrichosis
- Bacterial: furuncle, ecthyma, septic emboli
- Protozoal: leishmaniasis

METABOLIC

- Necrobiosis lipoidica diabeticorum
- Localized bullous pemphigoid
- Gout, calcinosis cutis, Gaucher's disease

TUMORS

- Basal cell carcinoma, squamous cell carcinoma, melanoma
- Mycosis fungoides, Kaposi's sarcoma, metastatic neoplasms

TRAUMA

- Burns, cold injury, radiation dermatitis
- Insect bites
- Factitial, excessive pressure

NEUROPATHIC

- Diabetic trophic ulcers
- Tabes dorsalis, syringomyelia

DRUGS
- Warfarin, IV colchicine extravasation, methotrexate, halogens, ergotism, hydroxyurea

PANNICULITIS
- Weber-Christian disease
- Pancreatic fat necrosis, α-antitrypsinase deficiency

Legg-Calvé-Perthes Disease

- Transient synovitis
- Low-grade septic arthritis
- Juvenile rheumatoid arthritis

Leishmaniasis

- Malaria
- African trypanosomiasis
- Brucellosis
- Enteric fever
- Bacterial endocarditis
- Generalized histoplasmosis
- Chronic myelocytic leukemia
- Hodgkin's disease and other lymphomas
- Sarcoidosis
- Hepatic cirrhosis
- Tuberculosis

Lentigo

- Lentigo maligna
- Ephelides
- Actinic keratosis
- Flat seborrheic keratosis
- Melanocytic nevus

Leprosy

- Sarcoidosis
- Rheumatoid arthritis
- Systemic lupus erythematosus

- Lymphomatoid granulomatosis
- Carpal tunnel syndrome
- Cutaneous leishmaniasis
- Fungal infections

Leptomeningeal Lesions

- Metastases
- Multiple sclerosis
- Bacterial or viral meningitis
- Vasculitis
- Lyme disease
- Tuberculosis
- Fungal infections (e.g., *Cryptococcus*)
- Sarcoidosis
- Wegener's granulomatosis
- Neurocysticercosis
- Rheumatoid nodules
- Histiocytosis

Leptospirosis

- Bacterial meningitis
- Viral hepatitis
- Influenza
- Legionnaire's disease

Leukocoria

- Cataract
- Retinal detachment
- Retinoblastoma
- Retinal telangiectasia
- Retrolenticular vascularized membrane
- Familial exudative vitreoretinopathy

Leukocytoclastic Vasculitis

- Wegener's granulomatosis
- Infective endocarditis

- Cherry angiomas
- Insect bites
- Septic vasculitis
- Thrombocytopenia (ITP, TTP)
- Benign pigmented purpura
- Rocky Mountain spotted fever

Leukoplakia, Oral Hairy (Oral Hairy Cell Leukoplakia)

- *Candida albicans*
- Lichen planus
- Idiopathic leukoplakia
- White sponge nevus
- Focal epithelial hyperplasia
- Squamous cell carcinoma

Lichen Planus

- Drug eruption
- Psoriasis
- Bowen's disease
- Leukoplakia
- Candidiasis
- Lupus
- Secondary syphilis
- Seborrheic dermatitis
- Chronic graft-versus-host disease
- Scabies

Lichen Sclerosus

- Localized scleroderma (morphea)
- Cutaneous discoid lupus erythematosus
- Atrophic lichen planus
- Psoriasis
- Bowen's disease
- Vitiligo

Lichen Simplex Chronicus

- Lichen planus
- Psoriasis
- Atopic dermatitis
- Insect bite
- Nummular eczema
- Contact dermatitis
- Stasis dermatitis

Limp

- Degenerative joint disease, osteochondritis dissecans, chondromalacia patellae
- Trauma to extremities, vertebral disk, hips
- Poorly fitting shoes, foreign body in shoe, unequal leg length
- Splinter in foot
- Joint infection (septic arthritis, osteomyelitis), viral arthritis
- Polio, neuromuscular disorders, Guillain-Barré syndrome, multiple sclerosis (MS)
- Osgood-Schlatter disease
- Legg-Calvé-Perthes disease (LCPD)
- Factitious, somatization syndrome
- Neoplasm (local or metastatic)
- Abdominal pain (e.g., appendicitis, incarcerated hernia), testicular torsion
- Other: diskitis, periostitis, sickle cell disease, hemophilia

Limping, Pediatric Age[24]

TODDLER (1–3 YEARS)
- Infection: septic arthritis (hip, knee), osteomyelitis, diskitis
- Occult trauma: toddler's fracture
- Neoplasia

CHILDHOOD (4–10 YEARS)
- Infection: septic arthritis (hip, knee); osteomyelitis; diskitis; transient synovitis, hip
- Legg-Calvé-Perthes disease (LCPD)
- Tarsal coalition

- Rheumatologic disorder: juvenile rheumatoid arthritis (JRA)
- Trauma
- Neoplasia

ADOLESCENCE (11+ YEARS)

- Slipped capital femoral epiphysis (SCFE)
- Rheumatologic disorder: JRA
- Trauma
- Tarsal coalition
- Hip dislocation (developmental dysplasia of the hip [DDH])
- Neoplasia

Listeriosis

- Meningitis caused by other bacteria, mycobacteria, or fungi
- CNS sarcoidosis
- Brain neoplasm or abscess
- Tuberculous and fungal (especially cryptococcal) meningitis
- Cerebral toxoplasmosis
- Lyme disease
- Sarcoidosis

Livedo Reticularis

- Emboli (subacute bacterial endocarditis [SBE], left atrial myxoma, cholesterol emboli)
- Thrombocythemia or polycythemia
- Antiphospholipid antibody syndrome
- Cryoglobulinemia, cryofibrinogenemia
- Leukocytoclastic vasculitis
- Systemic lupus erythematosus (SLE), rheumatoid arthritis (RA), dermatomyositis
- Pancreatitis
- Drugs (quinine, quinidine, amantadine, catecholamines)
- Physiologic (cutis marmorata)
- Congenital

Liver Enzyme Elevation

- Liver disease (e.g., viral hepatitis, cirrhosis, Reye's syndrome)
- Alcohol abuse

- Drugs (e.g., acetaminophen, statins, nonsteroidal anti-inflammatory drugs [NSAIDs], fenofibrates, antibiotics, anabolic steroids, narcotics, heparin, labetalol, amiodarone, chlorpromazine, phenytoin)
- Hepatic congestion
- Infectious mononucleosis, sepsis, cytomegalovirus (CMV) infection, HIV infection
- Liver metastases
- Autoimmune hepatitis
- Myocardial infarction (MI)
- Myocarditis
- Severe muscle trauma
- Dermatomyositis or polymyositis
- Primary liver malignant disease
- Renal and pulmonary infarction
- Convulsions
- Eclampsia
- Dehydration (relative increase)
- Chinese herbs

Liver Lesions, Benign, Often Confused with Malignancy

- Fatty infiltration
- Adenoma
- Hemangioma
- Cysts
- Flow artifacts
- Focal nodular hyperplasia
- Nonenhanced vessels

Low-Voltage Electrocardiogram (ECG)

- Hypothyroidism
- Obesity
- Pericardial effusion
- Anasarca
- Pleural effusion
- Pneumothorax

- Amyloidosis
- Aortic stenosis

Lumbar Disk Syndrome

- Soft tissue strain or sprain
- Tumor
- Degenerative arthritis of hip
- Insufficiency fracture of hip or pelvis

Lung Neoplasm, Primary

- Pneumonia
- Tuberculosis (TB)
- Metastatic carcinoma to the lung
- Lung abscess
- Granulomatous disease
- Carcinoid tumor
- Mycobacterial and fungal diseases
- Sarcoidosis
- Viral pneumonitis
- Benign lesions that simulate thoracic malignant disease
  - Lobar atelectasis: pneumonia, TB, chronic inflammatory disease, allergic bronchopulmonary aspergillosis
  - Multiple pulmonary nodules: septic emboli, Wegener's granulomatosis, sarcoidosis, rheumatoid nodules, fungal disease, multiple pulmonary atrioventricular fistulas
- Mediastinal adenopathy: sarcoidosis, lymphoma, primary TB, fungal disease, silicosis, pneumoconiosis, drug induced (e.g., phenytoin, trimethadione)
- Pleural effusion: congestive heart failure, pneumonia with parapneumonic effusion, TB, viral pneumonitis, ascites, pancreatitis, collagen-vascular disease

Lyme Disease

- Acute viral illnesses
- Babesiosis
- Ehrlichiosis
- Insect bite

- Granuloma annulare
- Seborrheic dermatitis
- Erythema annulare
- Erythema marginatum

Lymphadenopathy[14]

GENERALIZED

- AIDS
- Lymphoma: Hodgkin's disease, non-Hodgkin's lymphoma
- Leukemias, reticuloendotheliosis
- Infectious mononucleosis, cytomegalovirus (CMV) and other viral infections
- Diffuse skin infection: generalized furunculosis, multiple tick bites
- Parasitic infections: toxoplasmosis, filariasis, leishmaniasis, Chagas' disease
- Serum sickness
- Collagen-vascular diseases (rheumatoid arthritis [RA], systemic lupus erythematosus [SLE])
- Sarcoidosis and other granulomatous diseases
- Dengue (arbovirus infection)
- Drugs: isonicotinic acid hydrazide (INH), hydantoin derivatives, antithyroid and antileprosy drugs
- Secondary syphilis
- Hyperthyroidism, lipid storage diseases

LOCALIZED

Cervical Nodes

- Infections of the head, neck, ears, sinuses, scalp, pharynx
- Mononucleosis
- Lymphoma
- TB
- Malignant neoplasm of head and neck
- Rubella

Scalene/Supraclavicular Nodes

- Lymphoma
- Lung neoplasm

- Bacterial or fungal infection of thorax or retroperitoneum
- GI malignant disease

Axillary Nodes
- Infections of hands and arms
- Cat-scratch disease
- Neoplasm (lymphoma, melanoma, breast carcinoma)
- Brucellosis

Epitrochlear Nodes
- Infections of the hand
- Lymphoma
- Tularemia
- Sarcoidosis, secondary syphilis (usually bilateral)

Inguinal Nodes
- Infections of leg or foot, folliculitis (pubic hair)
- Lymphogranuloma venereum (LGV), syphilis
- Lymphoma
- Pelvic malignant neoplasm
- *Pasteurella pestis*

Hilar Nodes
- Sarcoidosis
- TB
- Lung carcinoma
- Fungal infections, systemic

Mediastinal Nodes
- Sarcoidosis
- Lymphoma
- Lung neoplasm
- TB
- Mononucleosis
- Histoplasmosis

Abdominal/Retroperitoneal Nodes
- Lymphoma
- TB
- Exclude other causes of edema (e.g., cirrhosis, nephrosis, congestive heart failure, myxedema, hypoalbuminemia, chronic venous stasis, reflex sympathetic dystrophy, obstruction from abdominal or pelvic malignant neoplasm)

- Neoplasm (ovary, testes, prostate, and other malignant neoplasms)

Lymphangitis[26]

ACUTE
- Group A streptococci
- *Staphylococcus aureus*
- *Pasteurella multocida*

CHRONIC
- *Sporothrix schenckii* (sporotrichosis)
- *Mycobacterium marinum* (swimming pool granuloma)
- *Mycobacterium kansasii*
- *Nocardia brasiliensis*
- *Wuchereria bancrofti*

Lymphedema

- Exclude other causes of edema (e.g., cirrhosis, nephrosis, congestive heart failure)
- Myxedema
- Hypoalbuminemia
- Chronic venous stasis
- Reflex sympathetic dystrophy
- Obstruction from abdominal or pelvic malignant neoplasm

Lymphocytopenia

- HIV infection
- Bone marrow suppression from chemotherapeutic agents or chemotherapy
- Aplastic anemia
- Neoplasms
- Steroids
- Hyperadrenalism
- Neurologic disorders (multiple sclerosis [MS], myasthenia gravis, Guillain-Barré syndrome)

Lymphocytosis

- Chronic infections
- Infectious mononucleosis and other viral infections
- Chronic lymphocytic leukemia (CLL)
- Hodgkin's disease
- Ulcerative colitis
- Hypoadrenalism
- Idiopathic thrombocytopenic purpura (ITP)

Lymphogranuloma Venereum

- Inguinal adenitis
- Chancroid
- Syphilis
- Suppurative adenitis
- Retroperitoneal adenitis
- Proctitis
- Cat-scratch disease
- Schistosomiasis

Lymphoma, Non-Hodgkin's

- Hodgkin's disease
- Viral infections
- Metastatic carcinoma
- Sarcoidosis

Lynch Syndrome

- Familial adenomatous polyposis
- Peutz-Jeghers syndrome
- Juvenile polyposis
- Nonhereditary colorectal cancer
- Gardner's syndrome

Macrocytosis

- Alcohol abuse
- Reticulocytosis

- Vitamin B$_{12}$ deficiency
- Folic acid deficiency
- Liver disease
- Hypothyroidism
- Marrow aplasia
- Myelofibrosis

Macrothrombocytopenia, Inherited[21]

- Bernard-Soulier syndrome
- *MYH9*-related disorders
- May-Hegglin anomaly
- Sebastian syndrome
- Fechtner syndrome
- Epstein syndrome
- Gray platelet syndrome
- Montreal platelet syndrome
- Mediterranean macrothrombocytopenia
- Mediterranean stomatocytosis/macrothrombocytopenia
- *GATA1* mutations
- Sialyl Lewis S antigen deficiency
- Paris-Trousseau syndrome
- Platelet-type von Willebrand disease

Macular Degeneration

- Diabetic retinopathy
- Hypertension
- Histoplasmosis
- Trauma

Malabsorption[39]

Causes of malabsorption:

MORE COMMON
- Celiac disease
- Chronic pancreatitis
- Post gastrectomy
- Crohn's disease

- Small bowel resection
- Small intestinal bacterial overgrowth
- Lactase deficiency

LESS COMMON
- AIDS (*Mycobacterium avium-intracellulare*, AIDS enteropathy)
- Whipple's disease
- Intestinal lymphoma
- Immunoproliferative small intestinal disease (alpha heavy chain disease)
- Irradiation enteritis
- Collagenous sprue
- Tropical sprue
- Nongranulomatous ulcerative jejunoileitis
- Eosinophilic gastroenteritis
- Amyloidosis
- Zollinger-Ellison syndrome
- Intestinal lymphangiectasia
- Systemic mastocytosis
- Chronic mesenteric ischemia
- Abetalipoproteinemia (autosomal recessive)

Malaria

- Typhoid fever
- Dengue fever
- Yellow fever
- Viral hepatitis
- Influenza
- Brucellosis
- Urinary tract infection (UTI)
- Leishmaniasis
- Trypanosomiasis
- Rickettsial diseases
- Leptospirosis

Malignant Hyperthermia

- Neuroleptic malignant syndrome
- Fever
- Heat stroke

- Thyrotoxicosis
- Pheochromocytoma
- Central nervous system infection or space-occupying lesion
- MDMA (ecstasy), cocaine, alcohol withdrawal, or amphetamine use
- Serotonin syndrome
- Adverse reaction to monoamine oxidase inhibitor or anticholinergic drug
- Strychnine poisoning

Mallory-Weiss Tear

- Esophageal or gastric varices
- Esophagitis/esophageal ulcers (peptic or pill induced)
- Gastric erosions
- Gastric or duodenal ulcer
- Arteriovenous malformations
- Neoplasms (usually gastric)

Mastocytosis (Urticaria Pigmentosa)

- Insect bites
- Nevi and congenital pigment abnormalities
- Café au lait spots
- Granuloma annulare
- Lentigo
- Drug eruption
- Sarcoidosis

Mastitis

- Plugged lactiferous ducts
- Breast abscess
- Inflammatory breast cancer
- Mastitis as a symptom of hyperprolactinemia or galactorrhea
- Other cancers; 3% of women diagnosed with breast cancer are lactating
- Granulomatous mastitis can be a manifestation of systemic disease, including sarcoidosis, Wegener's granulomatosis, giant cell arteritis, polyarteritis nodosa, tuberculosis, and syphilis

Mastoiditis

CHILDREN
- Rhabdomyosarcoma
- Histiocytosis X
- Leukemia
- Kawasaki's disease

ADULTS
- Fulminant otitis externa
- Histiocytosis X
- Metastatic disease

Measles (Rubeola)

- Other viral infections by enteroviruses, adenoviruses, human parvovirus B19, rubella
- Scarlet fever
- Allergic reaction
- Kawasaki's disease

Meckel's Diverticulum

- Appendicitis
- Crohn's disease
- All causes of lower GI bleeding (polyp, colon cancer, arteriovenous [AV] malformation, diverticulosis, hemorrhoids)
- Mesenteric adenitis

Mediastinal Masses or Widening on Chest Radiograph

- Lymphoma: Hodgkin's disease and non-Hodgkin's lymphoma
- Sarcoidosis
- Vascular: aortic aneurysm, ectasia or tortuosity of aorta or other thoracic vessels
- Carcinoma: lungs, esophagus
- Esophageal diverticula
- Hiatal hernia
- Achalasia

- Prominent pulmonary outflow tract: pulmonary hypertension, pulmonary embolism, right-to-left shunts
- Trauma: mediastinal hemorrhage
- Pneumomediastinum
- Lymphadenopathy caused by silicosis and other pneumoconioses
- Leukemias
- Infections: TB, viral (rare), *Mycoplasma* (rare), fungal, tularemia
- Substernal thyroid
- Thymoma
- Teratoma
- Bronchogenic cyst
- Pericardial cyst
- Neurofibroma, neurosarcoma, ganglioneuroma

Mediastinitis, Acute[26]

- Esophageal perforation
- Iatrogenic
- Esophagogastroduodenoscopy, esophageal dilation, esophageal variceal sclerotherapy, nasogastric tube, Sengstaken-Blakemore tube, endotracheal intubation, esophageal surgery, paraesophageal surgery, transesophageal echocardiography, anterior stabilization of cervical vertebral bodies
- Swallowed foreign bodies
- Trauma
- Spontaneous perforation (e.g., emesis, carcinoma)
- Head and neck infections (e.g., tonsillitis, pharyngitis, parotitis, epiglottitis, odontogenic)
- Infections originating at another site (e.g., TB; pneumonia; pancreatitis; osteomyelitis of sternum, clavicle, ribs)
- Cardiothoracic surgery (median sternotomy) (e.g., CABG, valve replacement, other types of cardiothoracic surgery)

Meigs' Syndrome

- Abdominal-ovarian malignant disease
- Gynecologic disorders
  - Uterus: endometrial tumor, sarcoma, leiomyoma ("pseudo-Meigs' syndrome")

- Fallopian tube: hydrosalpinx, granulomatous salpingitis, fallopian tube malignant neoplasm
- Ovary: benign, serous, mucinous, endometrioid, clear cell, Brenner tumor, granulosa, stromal, dysgerminoma, fibroma, metastatic tumor
- Nongynecologic causes of pelvic mass
  - Ascites
  - Portal vein obstruction
  - Inferior vena cava (IVC) obstruction
  - Hypoproteinemia
  - Thoracic duct obstruction
  - TB
  - Amyloidosis
  - Pancreatitis
  - Neoplasm
  - Ovarian hyperstimulation
  - Pleural effusion
  - Congestive heart failure (CHF)
  - Malignant disease
  - Collagen-vascular disease
  - Pancreatitis
  - Cirrhosis

Melanocytic Nevi (Moles)

- Actinic keratosis
- Melanoma
- Lentigines
- Ephelides
- Seborrheic keratosis
- Basal cell carcinoma

Melanoma

- Dysplastic nevi
- Lentigo
- Vascular lesions
- Blue nevus
- Basal cell carcinoma
- Seborrheic keratosis

- Cherry hemangioma
- Keratoacanthoma
- Pyogenic granuloma
- Dermatofibroma
- Squamous cell carcinoma
- Subungual hematoma

Melanonychia

- Pregnancy
- Trauma
- Medications (e.g., AZT, 5-fluorouracil, doxorubicin, psoralens)
- Nail matrix nevus
- HIV infection
- Onychomycosis
- Melanocyte hyperplasia
- Verrucae
- Pustular psoriasis
- Lichen planus
- Basal cell carcinoma
- Nail matrix melanoma
- Subungual keratosis
- Addison's disease
- Bowen's disease

Melasma (Chloasma)

- Postinflammatory hyperpigmentation
- Photolichenoid drug reaction
- Poikiloderma of Civatte

Memory Loss Symptoms, Elderly Patients

- Age-related mild cognitive impairment
- Depression (pseudodementia)
- Medications (e.g., anticholinergics, sedatives)
- Hypothyroidism
- Chronic hypoxia
- Cerebrovascular infarcts
- Alzheimer's disease

- B_{12} deficiency
- Hepatic disease
- Chronic renal failure
- Hyperthyroidism
- Frontotemporal dementia
- Lewy body dementia

Meniere's Disease

- Acoustic neuroma
- Migrainous vertigo
- Multiple sclerosis (MS)
- Autoimmune inner ear syndrome
- Otitis media
- Vertebrobasilar disease
- Viral labyrinthitis

Meningioma

OTHER WELL-CIRCUMSCRIBED INTRACRANIAL TUMORS
- Acoustic schwannoma (typically at the pontocerebellar junction)
- Ependymoma, lipoma, and metastases within the spinal cord

BRAIN OR SPINAL CORD ABSCESS
- Metastatic disease from lymphoma or adenocarcinoma, inflammatory disease, or infections such as tuberculosis

Meningitis, Bacterial

- Other infectious meningitides (e.g., viral or fungal meningitis)
- Endocarditis, bacteremia
- Intracranial tumor
- Lyme disease
- Brain abscess
- Partially treated bacterial meningitis
- Medications
- Systemic lupus erythematosus (SLE)
- Seizures
- Acute mononucleosis
- Neuroleptic malignant syndrome

- Subdural empyema
- Rocky Mountain spotted fever

Meningitis, Chronic[27]

- TB
- Fungal CNS infection
- Tertiary syphilis
- CNS neoplasm
- Metabolic encephalopathies
- Multiple sclerosis
- Chronic subdural hematoma
- Systemic lupus erythematosus (SLE) cerebritis
- Encephalitides
- Sarcoidosis
- Nonsteroidal anti-inflammatory drugs (NSAIDs)
- Behçet's syndrome
- Anatomic defects (traumatic, congenital, postoperative)
- Granulomatous angiitis

Meningitis, Recurrent[26]

- Drug induced (with rechallenge)
- Parameningeal focus
- Infection (sinusitis, mastoiditis, osteomyelitis, brain abscess)
- Tumor (epidermoid cyst, craniopharyngioma)
- Posttraumatic (bacterial)
- Mollaret's meningitis
- SLE
- Herpes simplex virus

Meningitis, Viral

- Bacterial meningitis
- Meningitis secondary to Lyme disease, TB, syphilis, amebiasis, leptospirosis
- Rickettsial illnesses: Rocky Mountain spotted fever
- Migraine headache
- Medications
- Systemic lupus erythematosus (SLE)

- Acute mononucleosis/Epstein-Barr virus
- Seizures
- Carcinomatous meningitis

Menopause

- Hypothalamic dysfunction
- Hypothyroidism
- Pituitary tumors
- Adrenal abnormalities
- Ovarian abnormalities
- Polycystic ovary syndrome
- Pregnancy
- Ovarian neoplasm
- Asherman's syndrome
- TB

Mesenteric Adenitis

- Acute appendicitis (5% to 10% of patients admitted to hospitals with a diagnosis of appendicitis are discharged with a diagnosis of mesenteric adenitis)
- Viral syndrome
- Irritable bowel syndrome (IBS)
- Crohn's disease

Mesenteric Ischemia, Nonocclusive[27]

- Cardiovascular disease resulting in low-flow states (congestive heart failure [CHF], cardiogenic shock, post cardiopulmonary bypass, dysrhythmias)
- Septic shock
- Drug induced (cocaine, vasopressors, ergot alkaloid poisoning)

Mesenteric Venous Thrombosis[27]

- Hypercoagulable states (protein C or S deficiency, antithrombin III deficiency, factor V Leyden, malignant neoplasm, polycythemia vera, sickle cell disease, homocystinemia, lupus anticoagulant, cardiolipin antibody)

- Trauma (operative venous injury, abdominal trauma, post splenectomy)
- Inflammatory conditions (pancreatitis, diverticulitis, appendicitis, cholangitis)
- Other: CHF, renal failure, portal hypertension, decompression sickness

Metabolic Syndrome

- Other causes of weight gain or obesity (Cushing's syndrome, hypothyroidism)
- Other causes of hyperlipidemia (familial hyperlipidemia, hypothyroidism)
- Other causes of hypertension (Cushing's syndrome, hyperaldosteronism)
- Other forms of diabetes (type 1)

Metastatic Neoplasms

TO BONE
- Breast
- Lung
- Prostate
- Thyroid
- Kidney
- Bladder
- Endometrium
- Cervix
- Melanoma

TO BRAIN
- Lung
- Breast
- Melanoma
- GU tract
- Colon
- Sinuses
- Sarcoma
- Skin
- Thyroid

TO LIVER
- Colon
- Stomach
- Pancreas
- Breast
- Lymphomas
- Bronchus
- Lung
- Sarcoma
- Choriocarcinoma

TO LUNG
- Breast
- Colon
- Kidney
- Testis
- Stomach
- Thyroid
- Melanoma

Metatarsalgia

- Splayfoot
- Osteoarthritis, rheumatoid arthritis
- Freiberg's disease (avascular necrosis of second metatarsal head)
- Cavus foot (high arch)
- Bunion deformity
- Hallux rigidus
- MTP synovitis
- Morton's neuroma

Microcephaly[4]

PRIMARY (GENETIC)
- Familial (autosomal recessive)
- Autosomal dominant
- Syndromes: Down (21 trisomy), Edwards (18 trisomy), cri du chat (5p–), Cornelia de Lange, Rubinstein-Taybi, Smith-Lemli-Opitz

SECONDARY (NONGENETIC)
- Radiation
- Congenital infections: cytomegalovirus (CMV), rubella, toxoplasmosis
- Drugs: fetal alcohol, fetal hydantoin
- Meningitis/encephalitis
- Malnutrition
- Metabolic
- Hyperthermia
- Hypoxic-ischemic encephalopathy

Microcytosis

- Iron deficiency
- Anemia of chronic disease
- Thalassemia trait or syndrome, other hemoglobinopathies
- Sideroblastic anemia
- Chronic renal failure
- Lead poisoning

Micropenis[28]

HYPOGONADOTROPIC HYPOGONADISM
- Kallmann's syndrome: autosomal dominant; associated with hyposmia
- Prader-Willi syndrome: hypotonia, mental retardation, obesity, small hands and feet
- Rud's syndrome: hyposomia, ichthyosis, mental retardation
- de Morsier's syndrome (septo-optic dysplasia): hypopituitarism, hypoplastic optic discs, absent septum pellucidum

HYPERGONADOTROPIC HYPOGONADISM
- Primary testicular defect: disorders of testicular differentiation or inborn errors of testosterone synthesis
- Klinefelter's syndrome
- Other X polysomies (i.e., XXXXY, XXXY)
- Robinow's syndrome: brachymesomelic dwarfism, dysmorphic facies

PARTIAL ANDROGEN INSENSITIVITY
- Idiopathic
- Defective morphogenesis of the penis

Mild Cognitive Impairment

- Delirium
- Dementia
- Depression
- "Reversible" cognitive impairment
  - Medication related (anticholinergics)
  - Hypothyroidism
  - Vitamin B_{12} deficiency
- Reversible CNS conditions
  - Subdural hematoma
  - Normal-pressure hydrocephalus
- Metastatic disease

Miliaria

- Viral exanthem
- Drug eruption
- Candidiasis
- Insect bites
- Milia
- Folliculitis

Miosis

- Medications (e.g., morphine, pilocarpine)
- Neurosyphilis
- Congenital
- Iritis
- CNS pontine lesion
- CNS infections
- Cavernous sinus thrombosis
- Inflammation/irritation of cornea or conjunctiva

Mitral Regurgitation

- Hypertrophic cardiomyopathy
- Pulmonary regurgitation
- Tricuspid regurgitation
- Ventricular septal defect (VSD)

Mitral Stenosis

- Left atrial myxoma
- Other valvular abnormalities (e.g., tricuspid stenosis, mitral regurgitation)
- Atrial septal defect

Mitral Valve Prolapse

- Other valvular abnormalities
- Constrictive pericarditis
- Ventricular aneurysm

Molluscum Contagiosum

- Verruca plana (flat warts): no central umbilication, not dome shaped, irregular surface, can involve palms and soles
- Herpes simplex: lesions become rapidly umbilicated
- Varicella: blisters and vesicles are present
- Folliculitis: no central umbilication, presence of hair piercing the pustule or papule
- Cutaneous cryptococcosis in AIDS patients: budding yeasts will be present on cytologic examination of the lesions
- Basal cell carcinoma: multiple lesions are absent

Mongolian Spot

- Nevus of Ito
- Dermal melanocytic hamartoma (macular blue nevus)
- Late-onset dermal melanosis
- Trauma
- Acquired bilateral nevus of Ota-like macules

Monoarthritis, Acute

- Overuse
- Trauma
- Gout
- Pseudogout
- Osteoarthritis
- Infectious arthritis (e.g., gonococcal, Lyme disease, viral, mycobacteria, fungi)
- Osteomyelitis
- Avascular necrosis of bone
- Hemarthrosis
- Bowel disease–associated arthritis
- Bone malignant neoplasm
- Psoriatic arthritis
- Juvenile RA
- Sarcoidosis
- Hemoglobinopathies
- Vasculitic syndromes
- Behçet's syndrome
- Foreign body synovitis
- Hypertrophic pulmonary osteoarthropathy
- Amyloidosis, familial Mediterranean fever

Monocytosis

- Viral diseases
- Parasites
- Neoplasms
- Inflammatory bowel disease (IBD)
- Monocytic leukemia
- Lymphomas
- Myeloma
- Sarcoidosis

Mononeuropathy

- Herpes zoster
- Herpes simplex
- Vasculitis

- Trauma, compression
- Diabetes
- Postinfectious or postinflammatory

Mononucleosis

- Heterophil-negative infectious mononucleosis caused by cytomegalovirus (CMV); although clinical presentation may be similar, CMV more frequently follows transfusion.
- Bacterial and viral causes of pharyngitis
- Toxoplasmosis
- Acute retroviral syndrome of HIV, lymphoma

Morphea

- Granuloma annulare
- Lichen sclerosus
- Hypertrophic scar
- Scleroderma
- Eosinophilic fasciitis
- Porphyria cutanea tarda
- Atrophoderma
- Nephrogenic fibrosing dermopathy
- Necrobiosis lipoidica

Morton's Neuroma

- Diabetic neuropathy
- Alcoholic neuropathy
- Nutritional neuropathy
- Toxic neuropathy
- Osteoarthritis
- Trauma (e.g., fracture)
- Gouty arthritis
- Rheumatoid arthritis (RA)

Motion Sickness

- Acute labyrinthitis
- Gastroenteritis

- Metabolic disorders
- Viral syndrome
- Anxiety

Mucormycosis

- Infection of the site by other organisms (bacterial [including TB and leprosy], viral, fungal, or protozoan)
- Noninfectious tissue necrosis (e.g., neoplasia, vasculitis, degenerative) of the site

Multifocal Atrial Tachycardia

- Atrial fibrillation
- Atrial flutter
- Sinus tachycardia
- Paroxysmal atrial tachycardia
- Extrasystoles

Multiple Myeloma

- Metastatic carcinoma
- Lymphoma
- Bone neoplasms (e.g., sarcoma)
- Monoclonal gammopathy of undetermined significance (MGUS)

Multiple Sclerosis (MS)

- Autoimmune: acute disseminated encephalomyelitis (ADEM), postvaccination encephalomyelitis
- Degenerative: subacute combined degeneration (vitamin B_{12} deficiency), inherited spastic paraparesis
- Infections: progressive multifocal leukoencephalopathy, Lyme disease, syphilis, HIV infection, human T-cell lymphotropic virus type 1 (HTLV-1), Whipple's syndrome, expanded differential in immunocompromised patients
- Inflammatory: systemic lupus erythematosus (SLE), Sjögren's syndrome, Behçet's syndrome, vasculitis, sarcoidosis, celiac disease
- Inherited metabolic disorders: leukodystrophies

- Mitochondrial: Leber's hereditary optic neuropathy; mitochondrial encephalopathy, lactic acidosis, and stroke-like episodes (MELAS)
- MS variants: recurrent optic neuropathy, neuromyelitis optica (Devic's), acute tumor-like lesion (Marburg's variant), Baló's concentric sclerosis, myelinoclastic diffuse sclerosis (Schilder's disease)
- Neoplasms: metastases, CNS lymphoma
- Vascular: subcortical infarcts, Binswanger's disease

Mumps

- Other viruses that may cause acute parotitis: parainfluenza types 1 and 3, coxsackieviruses, influenza A, cytomegalovirus (CMV)
- Suppurative parotitis
- Other conditions that may occur with parotid enlargement or swelling: Sjögren's syndrome, leukemia, diabetes mellitus (DM), uremia, malnutrition, cirrhosis
- Drugs that cause parotid swelling: phenothiazines, phenylbutazone, thiouracil, iodides
- Conditions that cause unilateral swelling: tumors, cysts, stones causing obstruction, strictures causing obstruction

Munchausen's Syndrome

- Malingering: a clear secondary gain (e.g., financial gain or avoidance of unwanted duties) is present.
- Somatoform disorders or hypochondriasis: similar presentations, but the disorder is not under the patient's control.
- Self-injurious behavior is common in many other psychiatric conditions (e.g., borderline personality disorder, psychoses, or nonfatal suicide attempt as may occur in depression); in those conditions, the patients confess the intentional self-harm and describe motivating factors.
- Munchausen's by proxy: a mother (86% of the time) or other caregiver induces illness in a child (52% between the ages of 3 and 13 years) for the purpose of obtaining medical attention without other secondary gain.

Muscle Weakness

- Physical deconditioning
- Impaired cardiac output (e.g., mitral stenosis, mitral regurgitation)
- Uremia, liver failure
- Electrolyte abnormalities (hypokalemia, hyperkalemia, hypophosphatemia, hypercalcemia, hypoglycemia)
- Drug induced (e.g., statin myopathy)
- Muscular dystrophies
- Steroid myopathy
- Alcoholic myopathy
- Myasthenia gravis, Lambert-Eaton syndrome
- Infections (polio, botulism, HIV, hepatitis, diphtheria, tick paralysis, neurosyphilis, brucellosis, TB, trichinosis)
- Pernicious anemia, other anemias, beriberi
- Psychiatric illness (depression, somatization syndrome)
- Organophosphate or arsenic poisoning
- Inflammatory myopathies (e.g., collagen-vascular disease, rheumatoid arthritis [RA], sarcoidosis)
- Endocrinopathies (e.g., adrenal insufficiency, hypothyroidism), diabetic neuropathy
- Other: motor neuron disease, mitochondrial myopathy, L-tryptophan (eosinophilia-myalgia), rhabdomyolysis, glycogen storage disease, lipid storage disease

Muscle Weakness, Lower Motor Neuron Versus Upper Motor Neuron[40]

LOWER MOTOR NEURON
- Weakness, usually severe
- Marked muscle atrophy
- Fasciculations
- Decreased muscle stretch reflexes
- Clonus not present
- Flaccidity
- No Babinski's sign
- Asymmetric and may involve one limb only in the beginning to become generalized as the disease progresses

UPPER MOTOR NEURON
- Weakness, usually less severe
- Minimal disuse muscle atrophy
- No fasciculations
- Increased muscle stretch reflexes
- Clonus may be present
- Spasticity
- Babinski's sign
- Often initial impairment of only skilled movements
- In the limbs, the following muscles may be the only ones weak or weaker than the others: triceps; wrist and finger extensors; interossei; iliopsoas; hamstrings; and foot dorsiflexors, inverters, and extroverters

Muscular Dystrophy

- Myasthenia gravis
- Inflammatory myopathy
- Metabolic myopathy
- Endocrine myopathy
- Toxic myopathy
- Mitochondrial myopathy

Mushroom Poisoning

- Food poisoning
- Overdose of prescription or illegal drug
- Other intoxications (e.g., alcohol)
- Viral infection

Myasthenia Gravis

- Lambert-Eaton myasthenic syndrome
- Botulism
- Medication-induced myasthenia
- Chronic progressive external ophthalmoplegia
- Congenital myasthenic syndromes
- Thyroid disease
- Basilar meningitis
- Intracranial mass lesion with cranial neuropathy
- Miller-Fisher variant of Guillain-Barré syndrome

Mycosis Fungoides

- Contact dermatitis
- Atopic dermatitis
- Nummular dermatitis
- Parapsoriases
- Superficial fungal infections
- Drug eruptions
- Psoriasis
- Photodermatitis
- Alopecia mucinosa
- Lymphomatoid papulosis

Mydriasis

- Coma
- Medications (e.g., cocaine, atropine, epinephrine)
- Glaucoma
- Cerebral aneurysm
- Ocular trauma
- Head trauma
- Optic atrophy
- Cerebral neoplasm
- Iridocyclitis

Myelin Disorders

- Multiple sclerosis
- Vitamin B_{12} deficiency
- Irradiation
- Hypoxia
- Toxicity from carbon monoxide, alcohol, mercury
- Progressive multifocal encephalopathy
- Acute disseminated encephalomyelitis
- Acute hemorrhagic leukoencephalopathy
- Phenylketonuria
- Adrenoleukodystrophy
- Krabbe's disease

Myelodysplastic Syndrome

- Hereditary dysplasias (e.g., Fanconi's anemia, Diamond-Blackfan syndrome)
- Vitamin B_{12}/folate deficiency
- Exposure to toxins (e.g., drugs, alcohol, chemotherapy)
- Renal failure
- Irradiation
- Autoimmune disease
- Infections (TB, viral infections)
- Paroxysmal nocturnal hemoglobinuria

Myelopathy and Myelitis[37]

INFLAMMATORY
- Infectious: spirochetal, TB, zoster, rabies, HIV, polio, rickettsial, fungal, parasitic
- Noninfectious: idiopathic transverse myelitis, multiple sclerosis

TOXIC/METABOLIC
- Diabetes mellitus (DM), pernicious anemia, chronic liver disease, pellagra, arsenic

TRAUMA, COMPRESSION
- Spinal neoplasm, cervical spondylosis, epidural abscess, epidural hematoma

VASCULAR
- Arteriovenous (AV) malformation, systemic lupus erythematosus (SLE), periarteritis nodosa, dissecting aortic aneurysm

PHYSICAL AGENTS
- Electrical injury, irradiation

NEOPLASTIC
- Spinal cord tumors, paraneoplastic myelopathy

Myocardial Ischemia[37]

- Atherosclerotic obstructive coronary artery disease
- Nonatherosclerotic coronary artery disease

- Coronary artery spasm
- Congenital coronary artery anomalies
- Anomalous origin of coronary artery from pulmonary artery
- Aberrant origin of coronary artery from aorta or another coronary artery
- Coronary arteriovenous fistula
- Coronary artery aneurysm
- Acquired disorders of coronary arteries
  - Coronary artery embolism
  - Dissection: surgical, during percutaneous coronary angioplasty, aortic dissection, spontaneous (e.g., during pregnancy)
- Extrinsic compression: tumors, granulomas, amyloidosis
- Collagen-vascular disease: polyarteritis nodosa, temporal arteritis, rheumatoid arthritis, systemic lupus erythematosus, scleroderma
- Miscellaneous disorders: irradiation, trauma, Kawasaki's disease
- Syphilis
- Hereditary disorders: pseudoxanthoma elasticum, gargoylism, progeria, homocystinuria, primary oxaluria
- "Functional" causes of myocardial ischemia in absence of anatomic coronary artery disease: syndrome X, hypertrophic cardiomyopathy, dilated cardiomyopathy, muscle bridge, hypertensive heart disease, pulmonary hypertension, valvular heart disease; aortic stenosis, aortic regurgitation

Myocarditis

- Cardiomyopathy
- Acute myocardial infarction
- Valvulopathy
- Viral syndrome
- Pleuritis
- Anxiety disorder

Myoclonus

- Physiologic (e.g., exercise or anxiety induced)
- Renal failure
- Hepatic failure
- Hyponatremia
- Hypoglycemia or severe hyperglycemia

- Post dialysis
- Epileptic myoclonus
- Post encephalitis
- CNS lesion (stroke, neoplasm)
- CNS trauma
- Parkinson's disease
- Medications (e.g., tricyclics, levodopa)
- Friedreich's ataxia
- Ataxia-telangiectasia
- Wilson's disease
- Huntington's disease
- Progressive supranuclear palsy
- Heavy metal poisoning
- Benign familial

Myoglobinuria

- Severe trauma
- Hyperthermia
- Polymyositis or dermatomyositis
- Carbon monoxide poisoning
- Drugs (narcotic and amphetamine toxicity)
- Hypothyroidism
- Muscle ischemia

Myopathies, Infectious

- HIV infection
- Viral myositis
- Trichinosis
- Toxoplasmosis
- Cysticercosis

Myopathies, Inflammatory

- Systemic lupus erythematosus (SLE), rheumatoid arthritis
- Sarcoidosis
- Paraneoplastic syndrome
- Polymyositis, dermatomyositis
- Polyarteritis nodosa

- Mixed connective tissue disease
- Scleroderma
- Inclusion body myositis
- Sjögren's syndrome
- Cimetidine, D-penicillamine

Myopathies, Toxic[1]

- Inflammatory: cimetidine, D-penicillamine
- Noninflammatory necrotizing or vacuolar: statins, chloroquine, colchicine
- Acute muscle necrosis and myoglobinuria: statins, alcohol, cocaine
- Malignant hyperthermia: halothane, ethylene, others; succinylcholine
- Mitochondrial: zidovudine
- Myosin loss: nondepolarizing neuromuscular blocking agents; glucocorticoids

Myositis, Inflammatory[1]

INFECTIOUS

- Viral myositis: retroviruses (HIV, HTLV-1), enteroviruses (echovirus, coxsackievirus), other viruses (influenza, hepatitis A and B, Epstein-Barr)
- Bacterial: pyomyositis
- Parasites: trichinosis, cysticercosis
- Fungi: candidiasis

IDIOPATHIC

- Granulomatous myositis (sarcoid, giant cell)
- Eosinophilic myositis
- Eosinophilia-myalgia syndrome

ENDOCRINE/METABOLIC DISORDERS

- Hypothyroidism
- Hyperthyroidism
- Hypercortisolism
- Hyperparathyroidism
- Hypoparathyroidism

- Hypocalcemia
- Hypokalemia

METABOLIC MYOPATHIES
- Myophosphorylase deficiency (McArdle's disease)
- Phosphofructokinase deficiency
- Myoadenylate deaminase deficiency
- Acid maltase deficiency
- Lipid storage diseases
- Acute rhabdomyolysis

DRUG-INDUCED MYOPATHIES
- Alcohol
- D-Penicillamine
- Zidovudine
- Colchicine
- Chloroquine, hydroxychloroquine
- Statins
- Cyclosporine
- Cocaine, heroin, barbiturates
- Corticosteroids

NEUROLOGIC DISORDERS
- Muscular dystrophies
- Congenital myopathies
- Motor neuron disease
- Guillain-Barré syndrome
- Myasthenia gravis

Myotonia

- Myotonia congenita (Thomsen's disease)
  - May be autosomal dominant or recessive (two distinct varieties)
  - The disease is limited to muscles and causes hypertrophy and stiffness after rest. Muscle function normalizes with exercise. There is no weakness. Symptoms are exacerbated by exposure to cold.
- Paramyotonia congenita
  - Autosomal dominant disease
  - Weakness and stiffness of facial muscles and distal upper extremities, especially or exclusively on cold exposure

- Muscular dystrophies
- Inflammatory myopathies (polymyositis)
- Metabolic muscle diseases
- Myasthenic syndromes
- Motor neuron disease

Myxedema Coma

- Severe depression, primary psychosis
- Drug overdose
- Cerebrovascular accident (CVA)
- Liver failure
- Renal failure
- Hypoglycemia
- Carbon dioxide (CO_2) narcosis
- Encephalitis

Nail Clubbing

- Chronic obstructive pulmonary disease (COPD)
- Pulmonary malignant neoplasm
- Cirrhosis
- Inflammatory bowel disease
- Chronic bronchitis
- Congenital heart disease
- Endocarditis
- Arteriovenous (AV) malformations
- Asbestosis
- Trauma
- Idiopathic

Nail, Horizontal White Lines (Beau's Lines)

- Malnutrition
- Idiopathic
- Trauma
- Prolonged systemic illnesses
- Pemphigus
- Raynaud's disease

Nail, Koilonychia

- Trauma
- Iron deficiency
- Systemic lupus erythematosus (SLE)
- Hemochromatosis
- Raynaud's disease
- Nail-patella syndrome
- Idiopathic

Nail, Onycholysis

- Infection
- Trauma
- Psoriasis
- Connective tissue disorders
- Sarcoidosis
- Hyperthyroidism
- Amyloidosis
- Nutritional deficiencies

Nail Pitting

- Psoriasis
- Alopecia areata
- Reiter's syndrome
- Trauma
- Idiopathic

Nail Splinter Hemorrhage

- Subacute bacterial endocarditis (SBE)
- Trauma
- Malignant neoplasms
- Oral contraceptives
- Pregnancy
- Systemic lupus erythematosus (SLE)
- Antiphospholipid syndrome
- Psoriasis

- Rheumatoid arthritis
- Peptic ulcer disease

Nail Striations

- Psoriasis
- Alopecia areata
- Trauma
- Atopic dermatitis
- Vitiligo

Nail Telangiectasia

- Rheumatoid arthritis
- Scleroderma
- Trauma
- Systemic lupus erythematosus (SLE)
- Dermatomyositis

Nail Whitening (Terry's Nails)

- Malnutrition
- Trauma
- Liver disease (e.g., cirrhosis, hepatic failure)
- Diabetes mellitus
- Hyperthyroidism
- Idiopathic

Nail Yellowing

- Tobacco abuse
- Nephrotic syndrome
- Chronic infections (TB, sinusitis)
- Bronchiectasis
- Lymphedema
- Raynaud's disease
- Rheumatoid arthritis
- Pleural effusions
- Thyroiditis
- Immunodeficiency

Narcissistic Personality

- Mania and hypomania, which are characterized by an episodic course and impairments
- Dysthymia and major depressive episode, which cause depressed mood and feelings of worthlessness without criticism or perceived slight
- Substance-induced euphoria, especially cocaine abuse
- Histrionic, borderline, antisocial, and paranoid personality disorders share common features and are often comorbid.
- Personality changes due to a general medical condition, including CNS processes in the frontal-temporal regions of the brain

Narcolepsy

- Sleep apnea
- Inadequate sleep time
- Insomnia
- Hypothyroidism
- Drugs and alcohol
- Seizures
- Sleep fragmentation (multiple causes)
- Chronic fatigue syndrome
- Depression

Nausea and Vomiting

- Infections (viral, bacterial)
- Intestinal obstruction
- Metabolic (e.g., uremia, electrolyte abnormalities, diabetic ketoacidosis [DKA], acidosis)
- Severe pain
- Anxiety, fear
- Psychiatric disorders (bulimia, anorexia nervosa)
- Pregnancy
- Medications (e.g., NSAIDs, erythromycin, morphine, codeine, aminophylline, chemotherapeutic agents)
- Withdrawal from substance abuse (drugs, alcohol)
- Head trauma
- Vestibular or middle ear disease

- Migraine headache
- CNS neoplasms
- Radiation sickness
- Peptic ulcer disease (PUD)
- Carcinoma of GI tract
- Reye's syndrome
- Eye disorders
- Abdominal trauma

Neck and Arm Pain

- Cervical disk syndrome
- Trauma, musculoskeletal strain
- Rotator cuff syndrome
- Bicipital tendinitis
- Glenohumeral arthritis
- Acromioclavicular arthritis
- Thoracic outlet syndrome
- Infection (cellulitis, abscess)
- Angina pectoris
- Pancoast tumor

Neck Mass[29]

- Congenital anomalies: thyroglossal duct cyst, bronchial apparatus anomalies, teratomas, ranula, dermoid cysts, hemangioma, laryngoceles, cystic hygroma
- Non-neoplastic inflammatory etiologies: folliculitis, adenopathy secondary to peritonsillar abscess, retropharyngeal or parapharyngeal abscess, salivary gland infections, viral infections (mononucleosis, HIV, cytomegalovirus [CMV]), TB, cat-scratch disease, toxoplasmosis, *Actinomyces*, atypical mycobacterium, jugular vein thrombus
- Neoplasm (primary or metastatic): lipoma

Neck Pain[29]

INFLAMMATORY DISEASES
- Rheumatoid arthritis (RA)
- Spondyloarthropathies
- Juvenile rheumatoid arthritis (JRA)

NONINFLAMMATORY DISEASE
- Cervical osteoarthritis
- Discogenic neck pain
- Diffuse idiopathic skeletal hyperostosis
- Fibromyalgia or myofascial pain

INFECTIOUS CAUSES
- Meningitis
- Osteomyelitis
- Infectious diskitis

NEOPLASMS
- Primary
- Metastatic

REFERRED PAIN
- Temporomandibular joint pain
- Cardiac pain
- Diaphragmatic irritation
- Gastrointestinal sources (gastric ulcer, gallbladder, pancreas)

Necrobiosis Lipoidica

- Xanthoma
- Morphea
- Granuloma annulare
- Vasculitis
- Lichen sclerosus

Nephritic Syndrome, Acute[1]

LOW SERUM COMPLEMENT LEVEL
- Acute postinfectious glomerulonephritis
- Membranoproliferative glomerulonephritis
- Systemic lupus erythematosus (SLE)
- Subacute bacterial endocarditis
- Visceral abscess "shunt" nephritis
- Cryoglobulinemia

NORMAL SERUM COMPLEMENT LEVEL
- IgA nephropathy
- Idiopathic rapidly progressive glomerulonephritis

- Anti–glomerular basement membrane disease
- Polyarteritis nodosa
- Wegener's glomerulonephritis
- Henoch-Schönlein purpura
- Goodpasture's syndrome

Nephroblastoma

- Other renal malignant neoplasms: hypernephroma, transitional cell carcinoma, lymphoma, clear cell sarcoma, rhabdoid tumor of the kidney
- Renal cyst
- Other intra-abdominal or retroperitoneal tumors

Nephrocalcinosis

- Sarcoidosis
- Hyperparathyroidism
- Chronic glomerulonephritis
- Milk-alkali syndrome
- Distal renal tubular acidosis
- Medullary sponge kidney
- Bartter's syndrome
- Hypervitaminosis D
- Idiopathic hypercalciuria
- Hyperoxaluria
- Cortical necrosis
- Tuberculosis
- Idiopathic hypercalciuria
- Rapidly progressive osteoporosis

Nephrotic Syndrome

- Other edema states (congestive heart failure [CHF], cirrhosis)
- Primary renal disease (e.g., focal glomerulonephritis, membranoproliferative glomerulonephritis)
- Carcinoma
- Infections
- Malignant hypertension
- Polyarteritis nodosa

- Serum sickness
- Toxemia of pregnancy

Neuroblastoma

- Other small, round, blue cell childhood tumors, such as lymphoma, rhabdomyosarcoma, soft tissue sarcoma, and primitive neuroectodermal tumors (PNETs)
- Wilms' tumor
- Hepatoblastoma

Neurofibromatosis

- Abdominal neurofibromatosis
- Myxoid lipoma
- Nodular fasciitis
- Fibrous histiocytoma
- Segmental NF

Neurogenic Bladder[30]

SUPRATENTORIAL
- Cerebrovascular accident (CVA)
- Parkinson's disease
- Alzheimer's disease
- Cerebral palsy

SPINAL CORD
- Spinal cord injury
- Spinal stenosis
- Central cord syndrome
- Amyotrophic lateral sclerosis (ALS)
- Multiple sclerosis
- Myelodysplasia

PERIPHERAL NEUROPATHY
- Diabetes
- Alcohol
- Shingles
- Syphilis

Neuroleptic Malignant Syndrome

- Heat stroke, drug-induced states and overdose (ecstasy abuse, phencyclidine), thyrotoxicosis, pheochromocytoma, serotonin syndrome
- Malignant hyperthermia, catatonia, acute psychosis with agitation
- CNS or systemic infections, including sepsis

Neurologic Deficit, Focal[27]

TRAUMATIC: INTRACRANIAL, INTRASPINAL
- Subdural hematoma
- Intraparenchymal hemorrhage
- Epidural hematoma
- Traumatic hemorrhagic necrosis

INFECTIOUS
- Brain abscess
- Epidural and subdural abscesses
- Meningitis

NEOPLASTIC
- Primary CNS tumors
- Metastatic tumors
- Syringomyelia
- Vascular
- Thrombosis
- Embolism
- Spontaneous hemorrhage: arteriovenous malformation, aneurysm, hypertensive

METABOLIC
- Hypoglycemia
- Vitamin B_{12} deficiency
- Post seizure
- Hyperosmolar nonketotic

OTHER
- Migraine
- Bell's palsy
- Psychogenic

Neurologic Deficit, Multifocal[27]

- Acute disseminated encephalomyelitis: postviral or postimmunization
- Infectious encephalomyelitis: poliovirus, enteroviruses, arbovirus, herpes zoster, Epstein-Barr virus
- Granulomatous encephalomyelitis: sarcoid
- Autoimmune: systemic lupus erythematosus (SLE)
- Other: familial spinocerebellar degenerations

Neuropathic Bladder

- Diabetes
- Stroke
- Multiple sclerosis
- Parkinson's disease
- Dementia
- Encephalopathy
- Brain trauma
- Spinal cord trauma
- Pelvic surgery
- Spina bifida

Neuropathies, Painful[40]

MONONEUROPATHIES
- Compressive neuropathy (carpal tunnel, meralgia paresthetica)
- Trigeminal neuralgia
- Ischemic neuropathy
- Polyarteritis nodosa
- Diabetic mononeuropathy
- Herpes zoster
- Idiopathic and familial brachial plexopathy

POLYNEUROPATHIES
- Diabetes mellitus
- Paraneoplastic sensory neuropathy
- Nutritional neuropathy
- Multiple myeloma
- Amyloid

- Dominantly inherited sensory neuropathy
- Toxic (arsenic, thallium, metronidazole)
- AIDS-associated neuropathy
- Tangier disease
- Fabry's disease

Neuropathies with Facial Nerve Involvement

- Sarcoidosis
- HIV infection
- Lyme disease
- Guillain-Barré syndrome
- Others: chronic inflammatory polyneuropathy, Tangier disease, amyloidosis

Neuropathy, Hereditary

- Charcot-Marie-Tooth (CMT) disease; other genetic, metabolic, and multisystem disorders including
  - Spinocerebellar ataxias
  - Friedreich's ataxia
  - Leukodystrophies
  - Refsum's disease (elevated serum phytanic acid)
  - Distal spinal muscular atrophies and distal myopathies, which can present with pes cavus and other foot deformities
- Chronic inflammatory demyelinating polyneuropathy (CIDP)
- Hereditary neuropathy with liability to pressure-sensitive palsies (HNPP)
  - Hereditary neuralgic amyotrophy (HNA), which typically is painful rather than painless. In addition, in HNA, there is no evidence of generalized polyneuropathy.
- Multifocal motor neuropathy with conduction block (MMNCB): autoimmune mediated and pure motor
- Neuropathy associated with renal failure
- Lead neuropathy
- Neuropathy relating to paraproteinemia (demyelinating pathophysiology)

Neutropenia

- Viral infections
- Aplastic anemias
- Immunosuppressive drugs
- Radiation therapy to bone marrow
- Agranulocytosis
- Drugs (antibiotics, antithyroidals)
- Lymphocytic and monocytic leukemias

Neutrophilia[21]

PRIMARY (NO OTHER EVIDENT ASSOCIATED DISEASE)
- Hereditary neutrophilia
- Chronic idiopathic neutrophilia
- Chronic myelogenous leukemia (CML) and other myeloproliferative diseases
- Familial myeloproliferative disease
- Congenital anomalies and leukemoid reaction
- Leukocyte adhesion factor deficiency (LAD)
- Familial cold urticaria and leukocytosis

SECONDARY
- Infection
- Stress neutrophilia
- Chronic inflammation
- Drug induced
- Nonhematologic malignant neoplasm
- Generalized marrow stimulation as in hemolysis
- Asplenia and hyposplenism

Nevus Flammeus

- Capillary hemangioma
- Salmon patch
- Cherry angiomas
- Glomus tumor
- Lymphocytoma cutis

Nevus of Ota and Ito

- Melanoma
- Blue nevus
- Melasma
- Late-onset dermal melanosis

Nipple Lesions

- Contact dermatitis
- Trauma
- Paget's disease
- Sebaceous hyperplasia
- Neurofibroma
- Accessory nipple
- Papillary adenoma
- Nevoid hyperkeratosis
- Cellulitis

Nocardiosis

- Tuberculosis
- Lung abscess
- Lung tumor
- Other causes of pneumonia
- Actinomycosis
- Mycosis
- Cellulitis
- Coccidioidomycosis
- Histoplasmosis
- Kaposi's sarcoma
- Aspergillosis

Nodular Lesions, Skin

- Lipoma
- Cherry angioma
- Angiokeratoma
- Hemangioma
- Classic Kaposi's sarcoma

- Nodular melanoma
- Pyogenic granuloma
- Angiosarcoma
- Eccrine poroma

Nodules, Painful

- Arthropod bite or sting
- Erythema nodosum
- Glomus tumor
- Neuroma
- Leiomyoma
- Angiolipoma
- Dermatofibroma
- Osler's node
- Blue rubber bleb nevus
- Vasculitis
- Sweet's syndrome

Nonalcoholic Fatty Liver

- Alcohol-induced liver disease (A daily alcohol intake of 20 g in women and 30 g in men [three 12-oz beers or 12 oz of wine] may be enough to cause alcohol-induced liver disease.)
- Viral hepatitis
- Autoimmune hepatitis
- Toxin- or drug-induced liver disease

Nummular Eczema

- Psoriasis
- Atopic dermatitis
- Contact dermatitis
- Stasis dermatitis
- Tinea infection
- Scabies

Nystagmus

- Medications (e.g., meperidine, barbiturates, phenytoin, phenothiazines)

- Multiple sclerosis
- Congenital
- Neoplasm (cerebellar, brainstem, cerebral)
- Labyrinthine or vestibular lesions
- CNS infections
- Optic atrophy
- Other: Arnold-Chiari malformation, syringobulbia, chorioretinitis, meningeal cysts

Nystagmus, Monocular

- Amblyopia
- Strabismus
- Multiple sclerosis
- Monocular blindness
- Internuclear ophthalmoplegia
- Lid fasciculations
- Brainstem infarct

Obesity

- Hypothalamic disorders
- Hypothyroidism
- Cushing's syndrome
- Insulinoma
- Chronic corticosteroid use
- Nephrotic syndrome
- Cirrhosis
- Congestive heart failure (CHF)

Obsessive-Compulsive Disorder (OCD)

- Other psychiatric disorders in which obsessive thoughts occur (e.g., body dysmorphic disorder or phobias)
- Other conditions in which compulsive behaviors are seen (e.g., trichotillomania)
- Major depression, hypochondriasis, and several anxiety disorders with predominant obsessions or compulsions; however, in these disorders, the thoughts are not anxiety provoking or extremes of normal concern

- Delusions or psychosis, which may be mistaken for obsessive thoughts; distinguished from OCD in that the individual recognizes the ideas are not real
- Tics and stereotypic movements that appear compulsive but are not driven by the desire to neutralize an obsession
- Paraphilias or pathologic gambling; distinguished from compulsions in that they are usually enjoyable

Ocular Foreign Body

- Corneal abrasion
- Corneal ulceration
- Glaucoma
- Herpes ulcers
- Infection
- Other keratitis

Odynophagia[39]

Causes of odynophagia:

INFECTIONS
- Herpes simplex virus
- Cytomegalovirus
- Candidiasis

CHEMICAL, INFLAMMATORY
- Gastroesophageal reflux
- Drug induced (Slow-K, tetracyclines, quinidine)
- Irradiation
- Graft-versus-host disease
- Crohn's disease
- Dermatologic diseases (pemphigus and pemphigoid)

Onychomycosis (Tinea Unguium)

- Psoriasis
- Contact dermatitis
- Lichen planus
- Subungual keratosis
- Paronychia

- Infection (e.g., *Pseudomonas*)
- Trauma
- Peripheral vascular disease
- Yellow nail syndrome

Ophthalmoplegia[1]

BILATERAL
- Botulism
- Myasthenia gravis
- Wernicke's encephalopathy
- Acute cranial polyneuropathy
- Brainstem stroke

UNILATERAL
- Carotid, posterior (third cranial nerve, pupil involved, communicating aneurysm)
- Diabetic, idiopathic (third or sixth cranial nerve, pupil spared)
- Myasthenia gravis
- Brainstem stroke

Opioid Dependence

- Psychiatric disorders (e.g., anxiety, depression, bipolar disorder)
- Acute medical illness (e.g., hypoglycemia, seizure disorder, sepsis, renal or hepatic insufficiency) may mimic opiate withdrawal symptoms.

Opsoclonus*

- Multiple sclerosis
- Encephalitis
- CNS lymphoma
- Hydrocephalus
- Pontine hemorrhage
- Thalamic disorder (glioma, hemorrhage)

---

*Spontaneous, multivector, chaotic eye movement.

- Hyperosmolar coma
- Carcinoma, paraneoplastic
- Cocaine
- Medications (e.g., phenytoin, haloperidol, amitriptyline, diazepam, vidarabine)

Optic Atrophy

- Nutritional, toxic, and hereditary causes are usually bilateral.
- Unilateral optic atrophy in a young person is more commonly MS.
- Postviral atrophy may be seen in childhood.

Optic Neuritis

- Inflammatory: sarcoidosis, systemic lupus erythematosus (SLE), Behçet's syndrome, postinfectious, postvaccination
- Infectious: syphilis, TB, Lyme disease, *Bartonella*, HIV
- Ischemic: giant cell arteritis, anterior and posterior ischemic optic neuropathies, diabetic papillopathy, branch or central retinal artery or vein occlusion
- Mitochondrial: Leber's hereditary optic neuropathy
- Mass lesion: aneurysm, meningioma, glioma, metastases
- Retinal migraine
- Ocular: optic drusen, retinal detachment, vitreous hemorrhage, posterior scleritis, neuroretinitis, maculopathies and retinopathies
- Acute papilledema
- Toxic/nutritional: vitamin B_{12} deficiency, tobacco-alcohol amblyopia, methanol, ethambutol

Oral Mucosa, Erythematous Lesions[9]

- Allergy
- Erythroplakia
- Candidiasis
- Geographic tongue
- Stomatitis areata migrans
- Plasma cell gingivitis
- Pemphigus vulgaris

Oral Mucosa, Pigmented Lesions[9]

- Racial pigmentation
- Oral melanotic macule
- Peutz-Jeghers syndrome
- Neurofibromatosis
- Albright's syndrome
- Addison's disease
- Chloasma
- Drug reaction: quinacrine, minocycline, chlorpromazine, busulfan
- Amalgam tattoo
- Lead line
- Smoker's melanosis
- Nevi
- Melanoma

Oral Mucosa, Punctate Erosive Lesions[9]

- Viral lesion: herpes simplex, coxsackievirus (A, B, A16), herpes zoster
- Aphthous stomatitis
- Sutton's disease (giant aphthae)
- Behçet's syndrome
- Reiter's syndrome
- Neutropenia
- Acute necrotizing ulcerative gingivostomatitis (ANUG)
- Drug reaction
- Inflammatory bowel disease
- Contact allergy

Oral Mucosa, White Lesions[9]

- Leukoplakia
- White, hairy leukoplakia
- Squamous cell carcinoma
- Lichen planus
- Stomatitis nicotinica
- Benign intraepithelial dyskeratosis
- White spongy nevus

- Leukoedema
- Darier-White disease
- Pachyonychia congenita
- Candidiasis
- Allergy
- Systemic lupus erythematosus (SLE)

Oral Ulcers, Acute

- Trauma (including thermal trauma)
- Aphthous stomatitis
- Syphilis
- Herpes simplex infection
- Herpes zoster

Oral Vesicles and Ulcers[1]

- Aphthous stomatitis
- Primary herpes simplex infection
- Vincent's stomatitis
- Syphilis
- Coxsackievirus A (herpangina)
- Fungi (histoplasmosis)
- Behçet's syndrome
- Systemic lupus erythematosus (SLE)
- Reiter's syndrome
- Crohn's disease
- Erythema multiforme
- Pemphigus
- Pemphigoid

Orbital Lesions, Calcified

- Chronic inflammation
- Phlebolith
- Dermoid cyst
- Mucocele walls
- Tumors (lacrimal gland, fibro-osseous)
- Meningioma (optic sheath)
- Lymphangioma
- Orbital varix

Orbital Lesions, Cystic

- Sweat gland cyst
- Dermoid cyst
- Lacrimal gland cyst
- Abscess
- Conjunctival cyst
- Lymphangioma
- Schwannoma

Orchitis

- Epididymo-orchitis, gonococcal
- Autoimmune disease
- Vasculitis
- Epididymitis
- Mumps, with or without parotitis
- Neoplasm
- Hematoma
- Spermatic cord torsion

Orgasm Dysfunction[12]

- Anorgasmia: inadequate stimulation or learning
- Spinal cord lesion or injury
- Multiple sclerosis (MS)
- Alcoholic neuropathy
- Amyotrophic lateral sclerosis (ALS)
- Spinal cord accident
- Spinal cord trauma
- Peripheral nerve damage
- Radical pelvic surgery
- Herniated lumbar disk
- Hypothyroidism
- Addison's disease
- Cushing's disease
- Acromegaly
- Hypopituitarism
- Pharmacologic agents (e.g., selective serotonin reuptake inhibitors [SSRIs], β-blockers)
- Psychogenic

Orofacial Pain

- Dental abscess
- Sinusitis
- Otitis media
- Otitis externa
- Wisdom tooth eruption
- Sialoadenitis
- Herpes zoster
- Trigeminal neuralgia
- Parotitis
- Anxiety disorder
- Malingering

Orthostatic Hypotension

COMMON

- Medications: antihypertensives, antidepressants (tricyclics), antipsychotics (phenothiazines), alcohol, narcotics, barbiturates, insulin, nitrates
- Reduced intravascular volume (hemorrhage, dehydration, hyperglycemia, hypoalbuminemia)
- Postprandial effect (especially in the elderly)
- Vasovagal syncope
- Deconditioning
- Peripheral autonomic dysfunction (diabetes mellitus, Guillain-Barré syndrome)

UNCOMMON

- Central autonomic dysfunction (Shy-Drager syndrome)
- Postganglionic autonomic dysfunction: impaired norepinephrine release
- Autoimmune autonomic dysfunction: nicotinic acetylcholine receptor autoantibodies
- Paraneoplastic autonomic dysfunction: anti-Hu antibodies (in small cell lung cancer)
- Postural tachycardia syndrome (POTS): usually occurs in young women; an abnormally large increase in heart rate is observed in the upright position caused by increased venous pooling from autonomic dysfunction of the lower extremities, but blood

pressure is not affected because of an excess of plasma norepinephrine.
- Impaired cardiac output
- Cerebrovascular accident
- Adrenal insufficiency
- Deconditioning
- Carotid sinus hypersensitivity
- Anxiety, panic attacks
- Seizures
- Idiopathic

Osgood-Schlatter Disease

- Referred hip pain (any child with hip pain should have a thorough clinical hip examination)
- Patellar tendinitis

Osler-Rendu-Weber Disease

- Generalized essential telangiectasia
- Unilateral nevoid telangiectasia
- Scleroderma with CREST syndrome
- Rosacea
- Actinic keratosis
- Ataxia-telangiectasia
- Venous hypertension
- Cushing's syndrome

Osteoarthritis

- Bursitis, tendinitis
- Radicular spine pain
- Inflammatory arthritides
- Infectious arthritis
- Rheumatoid arthritis
- Neoplasm (myeloma, primary or metastatic bone cancer)

Osteomyelitis

- Brodie's abscess
- Gaucher's disease

- Bone infarction
- Charcot's joint
- Gout
- Fracture

Osteoporosis

- Malignant disease (multiple myeloma, lymphoma, leukemia, metastatic carcinoma)
- Primary hyperparathyroidism
- Osteomalacia
- Paget's disease
- Osteogenesis imperfecta: types I, III, and IV

Osteoporosis, Secondary Causes

- Medication induced (e.g., glucocorticoids, anticonvulsants, heparin, LHRH agonists or antagonists)
- Hyperparathyroidism
- Hyperthyroidism
- Prolonged immobilization
- Chronic renal failure
- Sickle cell disease
- Multiple myeloma
- Myeloproliferative diseases
- Leukemias and lymphomas
- Acromegaly
- Prolactinoma
- DM
- Total parenteral nutrition
- Malabsorption
- Chronic hypophosphatemia
- Connective tissue disorders (e.g., osteogenesis imperfecta, Marfan syndrome, Ehlers-Danlos syndrome)
- Hepatobiliary disease
- Post gastrectomy
- Aluminum-containing antacids
- Systemic mastocytosis
- Homocystinuria

Otitis Externa

- Acute otitis media
- Bullous myringitis
- Mastoiditis
- Foreign bodies
- Neoplasms

Otitis Media

- Otitis externa
- Referred pain: mouth, nasopharynx, tonsils, other parts of the upper respiratory tract

Otosclerosis

HEARING LOSS FROM ANY CAUSE
- Cochlear otosclerosis
- Polyps
- Granulomas
- Tumors
- Osteogenesis imperfecta
- Chronic ear infections
- Trauma

Ovarian Cancer

- Primary peritoneal cancer
- Benign ovarian tumor
- Functional ovarian cyst
- Endometriosis
- Ovarian torsion
- Pelvic kidney
- Pedunculated uterine fibroid
- Primary cancer from breast, GI tract, or other pelvic organ metastasized to the ovary

Ovarian Mass

- Ovarian torsion
- Malignant neoplasm: ovary, fallopian tube, colon
- Uterine fibroid
- Diverticular abscess/diverticulitis
- Appendiceal abscess/appendicitis (especially in children)
- Tubo-ovarian abscess
- Paraovarian cyst
- Distended bladder
- Pelvic kidney
- Ectopic pregnancy
- Retroperitoneal cyst/neoplasm
- Non-neoplastic tumors of ovary: germinal inclusion cyst, follicle cyst, corpus luteum cyst, pregnancy luteoma, theca lutein cysts, sclerocystic ovaries, endometrioma

Ovulatory Dysfunction[22]

HYPERANDROGENIC ANOVULATION
- Polycystic ovary syndrome
- Late-onset congenital adrenal hyperplasias
- Ovarian hyperthecosis
- Androgen-producing ovarian tumors
- Androgen-producing adrenal tumors
- Cushing's syndrome

HYPOESTROGENIC ANOVULATION (HYPOTHALAMIC OR PITUITARY ETIOLOGY)
Hypogonadotropic Hypoestrogenic States
- Reversible
  - Functional hypothalamic amenorrhea: eating disorders (anorexia nervosa, excessive weight loss), excessive athletic training
  - Neoplastic: craniopharyngioma, pituitary stalk compression
  - Infiltrative diseases: histiocytosis X, sarcoidosis
  - Hypophysitis
  - Pituitary adenomas: hyperprolactinemia, euprolactinemic galactorrhea

- Endocrinopathies: hypothyroidism/hyperthyroidism, Cushing's disease
- Irreversible
  - Kallmann's syndrome
  - Isolated gonadotropin deficiency (hypothalamic or pituitary origin)
  - Panhypopituitarism/pituitary insufficiency: Sheehan's syndrome, pituitary apoplexy, pituitary irradiation or ablation

Hypergonadotropic Hypoestrogenic States

- Physiologic states: menopause, perimenopause
- Premature ovarian failure
- Immune related: radiation therapy/chemotherapy induced
- Ovarian dysgenesis
- Turner's syndrome
- 46XX with mutations of X
- Androgen insensitivity syndrome

MISCELLANEOUS
- Endometriosis
- Luteal phase defect

Paget's Disease of Bone

- Fibrous dysplasia
- Skeletal neoplasm (primary or metastatic)
- Osteomyelitis
- Hyperparathyroidism
- Vertebral hemangioma

Paget's Disease of Breast

- Chronic dermatitis
- Florid papillomatosis of the nipple or nipple adenoma
- Eczema
- Lichen simplex
- Bowen's disease
- Intertrigo
- Melanoma
- Basal cell carcinoma

- Contact dermatitis
- Seborrheic dermatitis

Pain, Midfoot

MEDIAL ASPECT
- Tendinitis of posterior tibialis
- Tendinitis of flexor digitorum longus
- Tendinitis of flexor hallucis longus
- Infection (osteomyelitis, septic arthritis, cellulitis) of foot
- Peripheral vascular insufficiency
- Fracture
- Osteoarthritis
- Gout, pseudogout
- Neuropathy
- Tumor

LATERAL ASPECT
- Peroneus longus tendinitis
- Peroneus brevis tendinitis
- Infection (osteomyelitis, septic arthritis, cellulitis) of foot
- Peripheral vascular insufficiency
- Fracture
- Osteoarthritis
- Gout, pseudogout
- Neuropathy
- Tumor

Pain, Plantar Aspect, Heel

- Plantar fasciitis
- Tarsal tunnel syndrome
- Neuroma
- Infection (osteomyelitis, septic arthritis, cellulitis) of foot
- Peripheral vascular insufficiency
- Fracture
- Bone cyst
- Osteoarthritis
- Gout, pseudogout
- Neuropathy

- Tumor
- Heel pad atrophy
- Plantar fascia rupture

Pain, Posterior Heel

- Achilles tendinitis
- Retrocalcaneal bursitis
- Retroachilles bursitis
- Infection (osteomyelitis, septic arthritis, cellulitis) of foot
- Peripheral vascular insufficiency
- Fracture
- Osteoarthritis
- Gout, pseudogout
- Neuropathy
- Tumor

Palindromic Rheumatism[5]

- Palindromic rheumatoid arthritis
- Essential palindromic rheumatism
- Crystal synovitis (gout, calcium pyrophosphate dihydrate [CPPD], pseudogout, calcific periarthritis)
- Lyme borreliosis, stages 2 and 3
- Sarcoidosis
- Whipple's disease
- Acute rheumatic fever
- Reactive arthritis (rare)

Palmoplantar Hyperkeratosis

- Superficial skin infection
- Chronic eczema
- Repeated trauma
- Psoriasis
- Reiter's syndrome
- Paraneoplastic acrokeratosis

Palpitations[34]

- Anxiety
- Electrolyte abnormalities (hypokalemia, hypomagnesemia)
- Exercise
- Hyperthyroidism
- Ischemic heart disease
- Ingestion of stimulant drugs (cocaine, amphetamines, caffeine)
- Medications (digoxin, β-blockers, calcium channel antagonists, hydralazines, diuretics, minoxidil)
- Hypoglycemia in type 1 diabetes mellitus (DM)
- Mitral valve prolapse
- Wolff-Parkinson-White (WPW) syndrome
- Sick sinus syndrome

Pancreatic Calcifications

- Chronic pancreatitis
- Hyperparathyroidism
- Metastatic neoplasm
- Pseudocyst
- Hereditary pancreatitis
- Cystadenoma
- Cystadenocarcinoma
- Cavernous lymphangioma
- Hemorrhage
- Acute pancreatitis (saponification)

Pancreatic Cancer (Exocrine)

- Common duct cholelithiasis
- Cholangiocarcinoma
- Common duct stricture
- Sclerosing cholangitis
- Primary biliary cirrhosis
- Drug-induced cholestasis (e.g., phenothiazines)
- Chronic hepatitis
- Sarcoidosis
- Other pancreatic tumors (islet cell tumor, cystadenocarcinoma, epidermoid carcinoma, sarcomas, lymphomas)

Pancreatitis, Acute

- Peptic ulcer disease (PUD)
- Acute cholangitis, biliary colic
- High intestinal obstruction
- Early acute appendicitis
- Mesenteric vascular obstruction
- Diabetic ketoacidosis (DKA)
- Pneumonia (basilar)
- Myocardial infarction (inferior wall)
- Renal colic
- Ruptured or dissecting aortic aneurysm

Pancreatitis, Chronic

- Pancreatic cancer
- Peptic ulcer disease (PUD)
- Cholelithiasis with biliary obstruction
- Malabsorption from other causes
- Recurrent acute pancreatitis

Pancytopenia[21]

PANCYTOPENIA WITH HYPOCELLULAR BONE MARROW

- Acquired aplastic anemia
- Inherited aplastic anemia (Fanconi's anemia and others)
- Some myelodysplasia syndromes
- Rare aleukemic leukemia (acute myelogenous leukemia)
- Some acute lymphoblastic leukemias
- Some lymphomas of bone marrow

PANCYTOPENIA WITH CELLULAR BONE MARROW

- Primary bone marrow diseases
- Myelodysplasia syndromes
- Paroxysmal nocturnal hemoglobinuria
- Myelofibrosis
- Some aleukemic leukemias
- Myelophthisis
- Bone marrow lymphoma
- Hairy cell leukemia
- Secondary to systemic diseases

- Systemic lupus erythematosus, Sjögren's syndrome
- Hypersplenism
- Vitamin B_{12}, folate deficiency (familial defect)
- Overwhelming infection
- Alcohol
- Brucellosis, ehrlichiosis, sarcoidosis, tuberculosis,* and atypical mycobacteria

HYPOCELLULAR BONE MARROW ± CYTOPENIA

- Q fever
- Legionnaires' disease
- *Mycobacteria tuberculosis*
- Anorexia nervosa, starvation
- Hypothyroidism

Panic Disorder

MEDICAL CONDITIONS

- Endocrinopathies
  - Hyperthyroidism
  - Hyperparathyroidism
  - Pheochromocytoma
  - Carcinoid tumor
- Cardiac and respiratory diseases
  - Arrhythmias
  - Myocardial infarction
  - Chronic obstructive pulmonary disease
  - Asthma
- Metabolic
  - Hypoglycemia
  - Electrolyte imbalances
  - Porphyria
- Seizure disorders
- Psychiatric disorders (NOTE: Panic attacks are common in a variety of psychiatric disorders. Panic disorder could be conceptualized as a phobia of the somatic sensations or situations that have become paired with panic attacks.)

---

*Pancytopenia in tuberculosis is only rarely associated with a hypocellular bone marrow at biopsy or autopsy. Marrow failure in the setting of tuberculosis is almost always fatal; exceptional patients probably had underlying myelodysplasia or acute leukemia.

- Phobias (e.g., specific phobia or social phobia)
- Obsessive-compulsive disorder (cued by exposure to the object of the obsession)
- Post-traumatic stress disorder (cued by recall of a stressor)
- Therapeutic (theophylline, steroids) and recreational (cocaine, amphetamine, caffeine, diet pills) drugs and drug withdrawal (alcohol, barbiturates, benzodiazepines)

Papilledema

- CNS infections (viral, bacterial, fungal)
- Medications (e.g., lithium, cisplatin, corticosteroids, tetracycline)
- Head trauma
- CNS neoplasm (primary or metastatic)
- Pseudotumor cerebri
- Cavernous sinus thrombosis
- Systemic lupus erythematosus (SLE)
- Sarcoidosis
- Subarachnoid hemorrhage
- Carbon dioxide retention
- Arnold-Chiari malformation and other developmental or congenital malformations
- Orbital lesions
- Central retinal vein occlusion
- Hypertensive encephalopathy
- Metabolic abnormalities

Papulosquamous Diseases[14]

- Psoriasis
- Pityriasis rubra pilaris
- Pityriasis rosea
- Lichen planus
- Lichen nitidus
- Secondary syphilis
- Pityriasis lichenoides
- Parapsoriasis
- Mycosis fungoides
- Dermatophytosis
- Tinea versicolor

Paraneoplastic Neurologic Syndromes

- Lambert-Eaton myasthenic syndrome
- Myasthenia gravis
- Guillain-Barré syndrome
- Amyotrophic lateral sclerosis
- Dermatomyositis
- Carcinoid myopathy
- Cerebellar degeneration
- Encephalomyelitis
- Optic neuritis, uveitis, retinopathy
- Stiff-man syndrome
- Autonomic neuropathy
- Brachial neuritis
- Sensory neuropathy
- Progressive multifocal leukoencephalopathy

Paraneoplastic Syndromes, Endocrine[37]

- Hypercalcemia
- Syndrome of inappropriate secretion of antidiuretic hormone (SIADH)
- Hypoglycemia
- Zollinger-Ellison syndrome
- Ectopic secretion of human chorionic gonadotropin (hCG)
- Cushing's syndrome

Paraneoplastic Syndromes, Nonendocrine[37]

CUTANEOUS
- Dermatomyositis
- Acanthosis nigricans
- Sweet's syndrome
- Erythema gyratum repens
- Systemic nodular panniculitis (Weber-Christian disease)

RENAL
- Nephrotic syndrome
- Nephrogenic diabetes insipidus

NEUROLOGIC

- Subacute cerebellar degeneration
- Progressive multifocal leukoencephalopathy
- Subacute motor neuropathy
- Sensory neuropathy
- Ascending acute polyneuropathy (Guillain-Barré syndrome)
- Myasthenic syndrome (Eaton-Lambert syndrome)

HEMATOLOGIC

- Microangiopathic hemolytic anemia
- Migratory thrombophlebitis (Trousseau's syndrome)
- Anemia of chronic disease

RHEUMATOLOGIC

- Polymyalgia rheumatica
- Hypertrophic pulmonary osteoarthropathy

Paranoid Personality Disorder

- Schizophrenia (paranoid type), delusional disorder (paranoid type), and mood disorder with psychotic symptoms: require presence of persistent positive psychotic symptoms such as delusions and hallucinations. To give an additional diagnosis of paranoid personality disorder (PPD), the personality disorder must be present before the onset of psychotic symptoms and must persist when the psychotic symptoms are in remission.
- Substance-induced paranoia, especially in the context of cocaine or methamphetamine abuse or dependence
- Personality changes due to a general medical condition that affects the central nervous system
- Paranoid traits associated with a sensory disability, for example, hearing impairment
- The most common co-occurring personality disorders are schizotypal, schizoid, narcissistic, avoidant, and borderline:
  - Schizotypal personality disorder includes magical thinking and unusual perceptual experiences.
  - Schizoid and borderline personality disorders do not have prominent paranoid ideation.
  - Avoidant personality disorder includes fear of embarrassment.
  - Narcissistic personality disorder includes the fear that hidden "flaws" or "inferiority" may be revealed.

Paraplegia

- Trauma: penetrating wounds to motor cortex, fracture-dislocation of vertebral column with compression of spinal cord or cauda equina, prolapsed disk, electrical injuries
- Neoplasm: parasagittal region, vertebrae, meninges, spinal cord, cauda equina; Hodgkin's disease, non-Hodgkin's lymphoma (NHL), leukemic deposits, pelvic neoplasms
- Multiple sclerosis (MS) and other demyelinating disorders
- Mechanical compression of spinal cord, cauda equina, or lumbosacral plexus: Paget's disease, kyphoscoliosis, herniation of intervertebral disk, spondylosis, ankylosing spondylitis, rheumatoid arthritis (RA), aortic aneurysm
- Infections: spinal abscess, syphilis, TB, poliomyelitis, leprosy
- Thrombosis of superior sagittal sinus
- Polyneuritis: Guillain-Barré syndrome, diabetes, alcohol, beriberi, heavy metals
- Heredofamilial muscular dystrophies
- Amyotrophic lateral sclerosis (ALS)
- Congenital and familial conditions: syringomyelia, myelomeningocele, myelodysplasia
- Hysteria

Paresthesias

- Multiple sclerosis (MS)
- Nutritional deficiencies (thiamine, vitamin B_{12}, folic acid)
- Compression of spinal cord or peripheral nerves
- Medications (e.g., isonicotinic acid hydrazide [INH], lithium, nitrofurantoin, gold, cisplatin, hydralazine, amitriptyline, sulfonamides, amiodarone, metronidazole, dapsone, disulfiram, chloramphenicol)
- Toxic chemicals (e.g., lead, arsenic, cyanide, mercury, organophosphates)
- Diabetes mellitus (DM)
- Myxedema
- Alcohol
- Sarcoidosis
- Neoplasms

- Infections (HIV, Lyme disease, herpes zoster, leprosy, diphtheria)
- Charcot-Marie-Tooth syndrome and other hereditary neuropathies
- Guillain-Barré neuropathy

Parkinson's Disease

- Multisystem atrophy: distinguishing features of autonomic dysfunction, including urinary incontinence, orthostatic hypotension, and erectile dysfunction; parkinsonism, cerebellar signs, and normal cognition
- Diffuse Lewy body disease: parkinsonism with concomitant dementia. Patients often have early hallucinations and fluctuations in level of alertness and mental status.
- Corticobasal degeneration: often begins asymmetrically with apraxia, cortical sensory loss in one limb, and sometimes alien limb phenomenon
- Progressive supranuclear palsy: tends to have axial rigidity greater than appendicular (limb) rigidity. These patients have early and severe postural instability. Hallmark is supranuclear gaze palsy that usually involves vertical gaze before horizontal.
- Essential tremor
- Secondary (acquired) parkinsonism
- Postinfectious parkinsonism: von Economo's encephalitis
- Parkinson's pugilistica: after repeated head trauma
- Iatrogenic: any of the neuroleptics and antipsychotics. The high-potency D_2 blocker neuroleptics are most likely to cause parkinsonism.
- Toxins (e.g., 1-methyl-4-phenyl-1,2,3,6-tetrahydropyridine [MPTP], manganese, carbon monoxide)
- Cerebrovascular disease (basal ganglia infarcts)

Parkinson's Plus Syndromes

- Parkinson's disease
- Shy-Drager syndrome
- Corticobasal degeneration
- Olivopontocerebellar atrophy

- Dementia with Lewy bodies
- Progressive supranuclear palsy
- Striatonigral degeneration

Paronychia

- Herpetic whitlow
- Pyogenic granuloma
- Viral warts
- Ganglions
- Squamous cell carcinoma

Parotid Swelling[3]

INFECTIOUS
- Mumps
- Parainfluenza
- Influenza
- Cytomegalovirus infection
- Coxsackievirus infection
- Lymphocytic choriomeningitis
- Echovirus infection
- Suppuration (bacterial)
- *Actinomyces* infection
- Mycobacterial infection
- Cat-scratch disease

NONINFECTIOUS
- Drug hypersensitivity (thiouracil, phenothiazines, thiocyanate, iodides, copper, isoprenaline, lead, mercury, phenylbutazone)
- Sarcoidosis
- Tumors, mixed
- Hemangioma, lymphangioma
- Sialectasis
- Sjögren's syndrome
- Mikulicz's syndrome (scleroderma, mixed connective tissue disease, systemic lupus erythematosus)
- Recurrent idiopathic parotitis
- Pneumoparotitis

- Trauma
- Sialolithiasis
- Foreign body
- Cystic fibrosis
- Malnutrition (marasmus, alcohol cirrhosis)
- Dehydration
- Diabetes mellitus
- Waldenström's macroglubulinemia
- Reiter's syndrome
- Amyloidosis

NONPAROTID SWELLING
- Hypertrophy of masseter muscle
- Lymphadenopathy
- Rheumatoid mandibular joint swelling
- Tumors of jaw
- Infantile cortical hyperostosis

Paroxysmal Cold Hemoglobinuria (PCH)

OTHER CAUSES OF RED OR BROWN URINE
- Beet ingestion
- Medications (e.g., phenazopyridine)
- Myoglobinuria
- Hematuria

OTHER CAUSES OF HEMOLYSIS
- Hemoglobinopathies
- Erythrocyte membrane defects
- Medications, toxins
- Microangiopathy
- Other forms of autoimmune hemolysis

Pediculosis

- Seborrheic dermatitis
- Scabies
- Eczema
- Other: pilar casts, trichonodosis (knotted hair), monilethrix

Pedophilia

- Psychosis: may present with unusual ideas or statements that may rarely be confused with pedophilia; but statements or behaviors of psychotic individuals are usually disorganized and relatively short-lived.
- Incest: some is not based in pedophilia but may instead reflect a dysfunctional family unit.
- Paraphilic sexual behavior in the setting of another condition, such as mental retardation, brain injury, or drug intoxication

Pelvic Inflammatory Disease

- Ectopic pregnancy
- Appendicitis
- Ruptured ovarian cyst
- Endometriosis
- Urinary tract infection (cystitis or pyelonephritis)
- Renal calculus
- Adnexal torsion
- Proctocolitis

Pelvic Mass

- Hemorrhagic ovarian cyst
- Simple ovarian cyst (follicle or corpus luteum)
- Ovarian carcinoma, carcinoma of fallopian tube, colorectal carcinoma, metastatic carcinoma, prostate carcinoma, bladder carcinoma, lymphoma, Hodgkin's disease
- Cystadenoma, teratoma, endometrioma
- Diverticulitis, diverticular abscess
- Appendiceal abscess, tubo-ovarian abscess
- Ectopic pregnancy, intrauterine pregnancy
- Paraovarian cyst
- Hydrosalpinx
- Leiomyoma
- Leiomyosarcoma

Pelvic Pain, Chronic[7]

GYNECOLOGIC DISORDERS
- Primary dysmenorrhea
- Endometriosis
- Adenomyosis
- Adhesions
- Fibroids
- Retained ovary syndrome after hysterectomy
- Previous tubal ligation
- Chronic pelvic infection

MUSCULOSKELETAL DISORDERS
- Myofascial pain syndrome

GASTROINTESTINAL DISORDERS
- Irritable bowel syndrome
- Inflammatory bowel disease

URINARY TRACT DISORDERS
- Interstitial cystitis
- Nonbacterial urethritis

Pelvic Pain, Genital Origin[27]

PERITONEAL IRRITATION
- Ruptured ectopic pregnancy
- Ovarian cyst rupture
- Ruptured tubo-ovarian abscess
- Uterine perforation

TORSION
- Ovarian cyst or tumor
- Pedunculated fibroid

INTRATUMOR HEMORRHAGE OR INFARCTION
- Ovarian cyst
- Solid ovarian tumor
- Uterine leiomyoma

INFECTION

- Endometritis
- Pelvic inflammatory disease (PID)
- *Trichomonas* cervicitis or vaginitis
- Tubo-ovarian abscess

PREGNANCY RELATED

First Trimester

- Ectopic pregnancy
- Abortion
- Corpus luteum hematoma

Late Pregnancy

- Placental problems
- Preeclampsia
- Premature labor

MISCELLANEOUS

- Endometriosis
- Foreign objects
- Pelvic adhesions
- Pelvic neoplasm
- Primary dysmenorrhea

Pemphigus Vulgaris

- Bullous pemphigoid
- Cicatricial pemphigoid
- Behçet's syndrome
- Erythema multiforme
- Systemic lupus erythematosus
- Aphthous stomatitis
- Dermatitis herpetiformis
- Drug eruptions

Penile Rash

- Herpes simplex 2
- Balanitis *(Candida)*
- Condylomata acuminata
- Molluscum contagiosum

- Scabies
- Pediculosis pubis
- Pearly penile papules
- Lichen nitidus
- Fox-Fordyce disease (follicular papules)

Peptic Ulcer Disease

- Gastroesophageal reflux disease (GERD)
- Cholelithiasis syndrome
- Pancreatitis
- Gastritis
- Nonulcer dyspepsia
- Neoplasm (gastric carcinoma, lymphoma, pancreatic carcinoma)
- Angina pectoris, myocardial infarction (MI), pericarditis
- Dissecting aneurysm
- Other: high small bowel obstruction, pneumonia, subphrenic abscess, early appendicitis

Perianal Pain[39]

- Fissure in ano
- Anal sepsis
- Anal abscess–anal fistula
- Hemorrhoids
  - Internal hemorrhoids
  - External hemorrhoids
- Pruritus ani
- Proctalgia fugax
- Chronic perianal pain syndromes
  - Coccygodynia
  - Descending perineum syndrome
  - Levator ani syndrome
  - Idiopathic perineal pain

Pericardial Effusion

- Pericarditis
- Uremia
- Myxedema

- Neoplasm (leukemia, lymphoma, metastatic)
- Hemorrhage (trauma, leakage of thoracic aneurysm)
- Systemic lupus erythematosus (SLE), rheumatoid disease
- Myocardial infarction

Pericarditis

- Angina pectoris
- Pulmonary infarction
- Dissecting aneurysm
- GI abnormalities (e.g., hiatal hernia, esophageal rupture)
- Pneumothorax
- Hepatitis
- Cholecystitis
- Pneumonia with pleurisy

Periodic Paralysis, Hyperkalemic

- Chronic renal failure
- Renal insufficiency with excessive potassium supplementation
- Potassium-sparing diuretics
- Endocrinopathies (hypoaldosteronism, adrenal insufficiency)

Periodic Paralysis, Hypokalemic

- Chronic diarrhea (laxative abuse, sprue, villous adenoma)
- Potassium-depleting diuretics
- Medications (amphotericin B, corticosteroids)
- Chronic licorice ingestion
- Thyrotoxicosis
- Renal tubular acidosis
- Conn's syndrome
- Bartter's syndrome
- Barium intoxication

Peripheral Arterial Disease

- Spinal stenosis
- Degenerative joint disease of the lumbar spine and hips
- Muscle cramps
- Compartment syndrome

Peritoneal Carcinomatosis[14]

- Primary disorders of the peritoneum: mesothelioma
- Metastatic spread from
  - Stomach
  - Colon
  - Pancreas
  - Carcinoid
  - Other intra-abdominal organs
  - Ovary
  - Pseudomyxoma peritonei
- Extra-abdominal primary tumors
  - Breast
  - Lung
- Hematologic malignant neoplasm
  - Lymphoma

Peritoneal Effusion[19]

TRANSUDATES
*Increased Hydrostatic Pressure or Decreased
Plasma Oncotic Pressure*

- Congestive heart failure (CHF)
- Hepatic cirrhosis
- Hypoproteinemia

EXUDATES
*Increased Capillary Permeability or Decreased
Lymphatic Resorption*

- Infections (TB, spontaneous bacterial peritonitis, secondary bacterial peritonitis)
- Neoplasms (hepatoma, metastatic carcinoma, lymphoma, mesothelioma)
- Trauma
- Pancreatitis
- Bile peritonitis (e.g., ruptured gallbladder)

CHYLOUS EFFUSION
Damage or Obstruction to Thoracic Duct

- Trauma
- Lymphoma

- Carcinoma
- Tuberculosis
- Parasitic infection

Peritonitis, Secondary

- Postoperative: abscess, sepsis, bowel obstruction, injury to internal organs
- Gastrointestinal: perforated viscus, appendicitis, inflammatory bowel disease (IBD), infectious colitis, diverticulitis, acute cholecystitis, peptic ulcer perforation, pancreatitis, bowel obstruction
- Gynecologic: ruptured ectopic pregnancy, pelvic inflammatory disease (PID), ruptured hemorrhagic ovarian cyst, ovarian torsion, degenerating leiomyoma
- Urologic: nephrolithiasis, interstitial cystitis
- Miscellaneous: abdominal trauma, penetrating wounds, infections secondary to intraperitoneal dialysis
- Spontaneous bacterial peritonitis

Peritonitis, Spontaneous Bacterial

- Appendicitis (in children)
- Perforated peptic ulcer
- Secondary peritonitis
- Peritoneal abscess
- Splenic, hepatic, or pancreatic abscess
- Cholecystitis
- Cholangitis

Peritonsillar Abscess

- Tonsillitis
- Infectious mononucleosis
- Peritonsillar cellulitis
- Retropharyngeal abscess
- Epiglottitis
- Dental abscess
- Lymphoma

Periumbilical Swelling

- Umbilical hernia
- Lipoma
- Epigastric hernia
- Umbilical granuloma
- Omphalocele
- Gastroschisis
- Caput medusae

Pertussis

- Croup
- Epiglottitis
- Foreign body aspiration
- Bacterial pneumonia

Peutz-Jeghers Syndrome

- Familial adenomatous polyposis
- Juvenile polyposis
- Turcot's syndrome
- Cowden disease

Pheochromocytoma

- Anxiety disorder
- Thyrotoxicosis
- Amphetamine or cocaine abuse
- Carcinoid
- Essential hypertension

Phobias

- Panic attacks: anxiety symptoms seen in specific phobia may resemble panic attacks, but the stimulus in specific phobias or social phobias is clear, whereas panic attacks seem more random.
- Generalized anxiety disorder: difficult to distinguish from social phobia; but in social phobia, the cognitive focus is fear of

embarrassment or humiliation, whereas in generalized anxiety disorder, the focus is more internal on the subjective sensations of discomfort.

Photodermatoses[14]

- Polymorphous light eruption
- Chronic actinic dermatitis
- Solar urticaria
- Phototoxicity and photoallergy
- Porphyrias

Photosensitivity

- Solar urticaria
- Photoallergic reaction
- Phototoxic reaction
- Polymorphous light eruption
- Porphyria cutanea tarda
- Systemic lupus erythematosus (SLE)
- Drug induced (e.g., tetracyclines)

Pilar Cyst (Wen)

- Epidermoid cyst
- Lipoma
- Sebaceous cyst
- Dermoid cyst
- Pilomatricoma

Pilonidal Disease

- Perianal abscess arising from the posterior midline crypt
- Hidradenitis suppurativa
- Carbuncle
- Furuncle
- Osteomyelitis
- Anal fistula
- Coccygeal sinus

Pinworms

- Perianal itching related to poor hygiene
- Hemorrhoidal disease and anal fissures
- Perineal yeast/fungal infections

Pituitary Adenoma

PROLACTINOMA

- Pregnancy
- Postpartum puerperium
- Primary hypothyroidism
- Breast disease
- Breast stimulation
- Drug ingestion (especially phenothiazines, antidepressants, haloperidol, methyldopa, reserpine, opiates, amphetamines, and cimetidine)
- Chronic renal failure
- Liver disease
- Polycystic ovary disease
- Chest wall disorders
- Spinal cord lesions
- Previous cranial irradiation

ACROMEGALY

- Ectopic production of GH-releasing hormone from a carcinoid or other neuroendocrine tumor

CUSHING'S DISEASE

- Diseases that cause ectopic sources of ACTH overproduction (including small cell carcinoma of the lung, bronchial carcinoid, intestinal carcinoid, pancreatic islet cell tumor, medullary thyroid carcinoma, and pheochromocytoma)
- Adrenal adenomas, adrenal carcinoma
- Nelson's syndrome

THYROTROPIN-SECRETING PITUITARY ADENOMAS

- Primary hypothyroidism

NONSECRETORY PITUITARY ADENOMA

- Non-neoplastic mass lesions of various etiologies (e.g., infectious, granulomatous)

Pityriasis Alba

- Eczema
- Tinea
- Vitiligo
- Psoriasis
- Chemical leukoderma

Pityriasis Rosea

- Tinea corporis (can be ruled out by potassium hydroxide examination)
- Secondary syphilis (absence of herald patch, positive serologic test result for syphilis)
- Psoriasis
- Nummular eczema
- Drug eruption
- Viral exanthem
- Eczema
- Lichen planus
- Tinea versicolor (the lesions are more brown and the borders are not as ovoid)

Placenta Previa

- Placenta accreta
- Placenta percreta
- Placenta increta
- Vasa previa
- Abruptio placentae
- Vaginal or cervical trauma
- Labor
- Local malignant neoplasm

Plantar Fasciitis

- Other regional tendinitis
- Stress fracture
- Tarsal tunnel syndrome
- Tumor, infection

Pleural Effusions

EXUDATIVE

- Neoplasm: bronchogenic carcinoma, breast carcinoma, mesothelioma, lymphoma, ovarian carcinoma, multiple myeloma, leukemia, Meigs' syndrome
- Infections: viral pneumonia, bacterial pneumonia, *Mycoplasma*, TB, fungal and parasitic diseases, extension from subphrenic abscess
- Trauma
- Collagen-vascular diseases: systemic lupus erythematosus (SLE), rheumatoid arthritis (RA), scleroderma, polyarteritis, Wegener's granulomatosis
- Pulmonary infarction
- Pancreatitis
- Postcardiotomy/Dressler's syndrome
- Drug-induced lupus erythematosus (hydralazine, procainamide)
- Post abdominal surgery
- Ruptured esophagus
- Chronic effusion secondary to congestive failure

TRANSUDATIVE

- Congestive heart failure (CHF)
- Hepatic cirrhosis
- Nephrotic syndrome
- Hypoproteinemia from any cause
- Meigs' syndrome

Pleural Effusions, Malignant Disease Associated

- Lung cancer (30% to 40%)
- Breast cancer (20% to 25%)
- Lymphoma (10% to 15%)
- Leukemia (5% to 10%)
- GI tract (5%)
- GU tract (5%)
- Reproductive (3%)

Pneumonia, Bacterial

- Exacerbation of chronic bronchitis
- Pulmonary embolism or infarction
- Lung neoplasm
- Bronchiolitis
- Sarcoidosis
- Hypersensitivity pneumonitis
- Pulmonary edema
- Drug-induced lung injury
- Viral pneumonias
- Fungal pneumonias
- Parasitic pneumonias
- Atypical pneumonia
- Tuberculosis

Pneumonia, *Mycoplasma*

- *Chlamydia pneumoniae*
- *Chlamydia psittaci*
- *Legionella* spp.
- *Coxiella burnetii*
- Several viral agents
- Q fever
- *Streptococcus pneumoniae*
- Pleuritic pain
- Pulmonary embolism/infarction

Pneumonia, *Pneumocystis jiroveci*

OTHER OPPORTUNISTIC RESPIRATORY INFECTIONS
- Tuberculosis
- Histoplasmosis
- Cryptococcosis

NONOPPORTUNISTIC INFECTIONS
- Bacterial pneumonia
- Viral pneumonia
- Mycoplasmal pneumonia
- Legionellosis

Pneumonia, Recurrent

- Mechanical obstruction from neoplasm
- Chronic aspiration (tube feeding, alcoholism, cerebrovascular accident [CVA], neuromuscular disorders, seizure disorder, inability to cough)
- Bronchiectasis
- Kyphoscoliosis
- Chronic obstructive pulmonary disease (COPD), congestive heart failure (CHF), asthma, silicosis, pulmonary fibrosis, cystic fibrosis
- Pulmonary TB, chronic sinusitis
- Immunosuppression (HIV infection, corticosteroids, leukemia, chemotherapy, splenectomy)

Pneumonia, Viral

- Bacterial pneumonia, which frequently complicates (i.e., can follow or be simultaneous with) viral (especially influenza) pneumonia
- Other causes of atypical pneumonia: *Mycoplasma*, *Chlamydia*, *Coxiella*, legionnaires' disease
- Acute respiratory distress syndrome (ARDS)
- Pulmonary emboli

Pneumothorax, Spontaneous

- Pleurisy
- Pulmonary embolism
- Myocardial infarction
- Pericarditis
- Asthma
- Pneumonia

Poliomyelitis

- Guillain-Barré syndrome
- Cerebrovascular accident (CVA)
- Spinal cord compression
- Other enteroviruses

Polyarteritis Nodosa

- Cryoglobulinemia
- Systemic lupus erythematosus (SLE)
- Infections (e.g., subacute bacterial endocarditis [SBE], trichinosis, rickettsia)
- Lymphoma

Polycystic Kidney Disease

- Simple cysts
- Tuberous sclerosis
- von Hippel–Lindau syndrome
- Acquired cystic kidney disease

Polycystic Ovary Syndrome (PCOS)

CAUSES OF AMENORRHEA
Primary (unusual in PCOS)
- Genetic disorder (Turner's syndrome)
- Anatomic abnormality (e.g., imperforate hymen)

Secondary
- Pregnancy
- Functional (cause unknown; anorexia nervosa; stress, excessive exercise; hyperthyroidism, less commonly hypothyroidism; adrenal dysfunction, pituitary dysfunction; severe systemic illness; drugs such as oral contraceptives, estrogens, or dopamine agonists)
- Abnormalities of the genital tract (uterine tumor, endometrial scarring, ovarian tumor)

CAUSES OF HIRSUTISM

Polycythemia Vera

- Smoking: polycythemia is secondary to increased carboxyhemoglobin, resulting in left shift in the Hgb dissociation curve. Laboratory evaluation shows increased hematocrit (Hct), red blood cell (RBC) mass, erythropoietin level, and carboxyhemoglobin. Splenomegaly is not present on physical examination.

- Hypoxemia (secondary polycythemia): living for prolonged periods at high altitudes, pulmonary fibrosis, congenital cardiac lesions with right-to-left shunts. Laboratory evaluation shows decreased arterial oxygen saturation and elevated erythropoietin level. Splenomegaly is not present on physical examination.
- Erythropoietin-producing disorders: renal cell carcinoma, hepatoma, cerebral hemangioma, uterine fibroids, polycystic kidneys. The erythropoietin level is elevated in these patients; the arterial oxygen saturation is normal. Splenomegaly may be present with metastatic neoplasms.
- Stress polycythemia (Gaisböck's syndrome, relative polycythemia): laboratory evaluation demonstrates normal RBC mass, arterial oxygen saturation, and erythropoietin level; plasma volume is decreased. Splenomegaly is not present on physical examination.
- Hemoglobinopathies associated with high oxygen affinity: an abnormal oxyhemoglobin dissociation curve (P50) is present.

Polymorphous Light Eruption

- Reticular erythematous mucinosis (clinically, polymorphous light eruption resolves once exposure to sunlight has ceased, in contrast to the persistent lesions of reticular erythematous mucinosis)
- Lymphocytic infiltration (on histologic examination, marked papillary edema favors polymorphic light eruption)
- SLE (most cases of polymorphic light eruption are negative with immunofluorescence testing)

Polymyalgia Rheumatica

- Rheumatoid arthritis (RA): rheumatoid factor is absent in polymyalgia
- Polymyositis: enzyme studies are normal in polymyalgia
- Fibromyalgia
- Viral syndrome

Polymyositis

- Dermatomyositis
- Muscular dystrophies

- Amyotrophic lateral sclerosis (ALS)
- Myasthenia gravis or Eaton-Lambert syndrome
- Guillain-Barré syndrome
- Alcoholic myopathy
- Fibromyalgia
- Drug-induced myopathies (e.g., HMG reductase inhibitors, gemfibrozil)
- Diseases associated with polymyositis (e.g., sarcoidosis, HIV infection)
- Inclusion body myositis

Polyneuropathy[40]

PREDOMINANTLY MOTOR
- Guillain-Barré syndrome
- Porphyria
- Diphtheria
- Lead
- Hereditary sensorimotor neuropathy, types I and II
- Paraneoplastic neuropathy

PREDOMINANTLY SENSORY
- Diabetes
- Amyloidosis
- Leprosy
- Lyme disease
- Paraneoplastic neuropathy
- Vitamin B_{12} deficiency
- Hereditary sensory neuropathy, types I-IV

PREDOMINANTLY AUTONOMIC
- Diabetes
- Amyloidosis
- Alcoholic neuropathy
- Familial dysautonomias

MIXED SENSORIMOTOR
- Systemic diseases: renal failure, hypothyroidism, acromegaly, rheumatoid arthritis, periarteritis nodosa, systemic lupus erythematosus (SLE), multiple myeloma, macroglobulinemia, remote effect of malignant neoplasm

- Medications: isoniazid, nitrofurantoin, ethambutol, chloramphenicol, chloroquine, vincristine, vinblastine, dapsone, disulfiram, diphenylhydantoin, cisplatin, L-tryptophan
- Environmental toxins: *n*-hexane, methyl *n*-butyl ketone, acrylamide, carbon disulfide, carbon monoxide, hexachlorophene, organophosphates
- Deficiency disorders: malabsorption, alcoholism, vitamin B_1 deficiency, Refsum's disease, metachromatic leukodystrophy

Polyneuropathy, Drug Induced[40]

DRUGS IN ONCOLOGY
- Vincristine
- Procarbazine
- Cisplatin
- Misonidazole
- Metronidazole (Flagyl)
- Taxol

DRUGS IN INFECTIOUS DISEASES
- Isoniazid
- Nitrofurantoin
- Dapsone
- ddC (dideoxycytidine)
- ddI (dideoxyinosine)

DRUGS IN CARDIOLOGY
- Hydralazine
- Perhexiline maleate
- Procainamide
- Disopyramide

DRUGS IN RHEUMATOLOGY
- Gold salts
- Chloroquine

DRUGS IN NEUROLOGY AND PSYCHIATRY
- Diphenylhydantoin
- Glutethimide
- Methaqualone

MISCELLANEOUS
- Disulfiram (Antabuse)
- Vitamin: pyridoxine (megadoses)

Polyneuropathy, Symmetric[40]

ACQUIRED NEUROPATHIES
- Toxic: drugs, industrial toxins, heavy metals, abused substances
- Metabolic/endocrine: diabetes, chronic renal failure, hypothyroidism, polyneuropathy of critical illness
- Nutritional deficiency: vitamin B_{12} deficiency, alcoholism, vitamin E deficiency
- Paraneoplastic: carcinoma, lymphoma
- Plasma cell dyscrasia: myeloma, typical, atypical, and solitary forms; primary systemic amyloidosis
- Idiopathic chronic inflammatory demyelinating polyneuropathies
- Polyneuropathies associated with peripheral nerve autoantibodies
- AIDS

INHERITED NEUROPATHIES
- Neuropathies with biochemical markers: Refsum's disease, Bassen-Kornzweig disease, Tangier disease, metachromatic leukodystrophy, Krabbe's disease, adrenomyeloneuropathy, Fabry's disease
- Neuropathies without biochemical markers or systemic involvement: hereditary motor neuropathy, hereditary sensory neuropathy, hereditary sensorimotor neuropathy

Polyuria

- Diabetes mellitus (DM)
- Diabetes insipidus
- Primary polydipsia (compulsive water drinking)
- Hypercalcemia
- Hypokalemia
- Postobstructive uropathy
- Diuretic phase of renal failure
- Drugs: diuretics, caffeine, alcohol, lithium

- Sickle cell trait or disease, chronic pyelonephritis (failure to concentrate urine)
- Anxiety, cold weather

Popliteal Swelling

- Phlebitis (superficial)
- Lymphadenitis
- Trauma: fractured tibia or fibula, contusion, traumatic neuroma
- Deep venous thrombosis (DVT)
- Ruptured varicose vein
- Baker's cyst
- Popliteal abscess
- Osteomyelitis
- Ruptured tendon
- Aneurysm of popliteal artery
- Neoplasm: lipoma, osteogenic sarcoma, neurofibroma, fibrosarcoma

Porphyria Cutanea Tarda (PCT)

- Pseudoporphyria
- Porphyria variegata
- Polymorphous light eruption
- Bullous pemphigoid
- Bullous lupus

Portal Hypertension[1]

INCREASED RESISTANCE TO FLOW

- Presinusoidal: portal or splenic vein occlusion (thrombosis, tumor), schistosomiasis, congenital hepatic fibrosis, sarcoidosis
- Sinusoidal: cirrhosis (all causes), alcoholic hepatitis
- Postsinusoidal: veno-occlusive disease, Budd-Chiari syndrome, constrictive pericarditis

INCREASED PORTAL BLOOD FLOW

- Splenomegaly not due to liver disease
- Arterioportal fistula

Postconcussive Syndrome

- Headache (vascular or tension)
- Epidural hematoma
- Subdural hematoma
- Skull fracture
- Cervical spine disk disease
- Whiplash
- Seizure
- Cerebrovascular accident
- Depression
- Anxiety

Postmenopausal Bleeding

- Hormone replacement therapy
- Neoplasm (uterine, ovarian, cervical, vaginal, vulvar)
- Atrophic vaginitis
- Vaginal infection
- Polyp
- Extragenital (GI, urinary)
- Tamoxifen
- Trauma

Postpoliomyelitis Syndrome

- Amyotrophic lateral sclerosis
- Cervical and lumbosacral radiculopathy
- Adult spinal muscular atrophy
- Diabetic amyotrophy
- Multifocal motor neuropathy with conduction block
- Chronic inflammatory demyelinating polyneuropathy
- Entrapment neuropathies
- Inflammatory and metabolic myopathies
- Vasculitis
- Connective tissue disease–associated myopathies

Post-traumatic Stress Disorder

- Adjustment disorders are distinguished from PTSD in that the precipitating stress is less catastrophic and the psychological reaction less specific.
- Acute stress disorder, if symptoms last between 48 hours and 4 weeks after trauma
- Delayed-onset PTSD, if symptoms develop >6 months after the event
- Major depression; up to 30% of primary care patients with depression also have PTSD

Postural Hypotension, Non-neurologic Causes

- Diuretics and hypertensive agents
- GI hemorrhage
- Alcohol
- Excessive heat
- Rapid volume loss from diarrhea, vomiting
- Hemodialysis
- Extensive burns
- Pyrexia
- Aortic stenosis (impaired output)
- Constrictive pericarditis, atrial myxoma (impaired cardiac filling)
- Adrenal insufficiency
- Diabetes insipidus
- Vasodilatory agents (e.g., nitrates)

Precocious Puberty

- Most common diagnoses to consider: premature thelarche and premature adrenarche
- Gonadotropin hormone–releasing hormone (GnRH)–dependent precocious puberty: idiopathic, CNS tumors, hypothalamic hamartomas, neurofibromatosis, tuberous sclerosis, hydrocephalus, post acute head injury, ventricular cysts, post CNS infection

- GnRH-independent precocious puberty: congenital adrenal hyperplasia, adrenocortical tumors (males), McCune-Albright syndrome (females), gonadal tumors, ectopic human chorionic gonadotropin (hCG)–secreting tumors (chorioblastoma, hepatoblastoma), exposure to exogenous sex steroids, severe hypothyroidism

Preeclampsia

- Acute fatty liver of pregnancy
- Appendicitis
- Diabetic ketoacidosis
- Gallbladder disease
- Gastroenteritis
- Glomerulonephritis
- Hemolytic-uremic syndrome
- Hepatic encephalopathy
- Hyperemesis gravidarum
- Idiopathic thrombocytopenia
- Thrombotic thrombocytopenic purpura
- Nephrolithiasis
- Pyelonephritis
- Peptic ulcer disease (PUD)
- Systemic lupus erythematosus (SLE)

Premature Graying, Scalp Hair

- Chemical exposure (e.g., phenol/catechol derivatives, sulfhydryls, arsenic)
- Physical agents (e.g., ionizing radiation, lasers)
- Hyperthyroidism
- Vitamin B_{12} deficiency
- Down syndrome
- Chronic and severe protein deficiency
- Vitiligo
- Idiopathic
- Myotonic dystrophy
- Ataxia-telangiectasia
- Progeria
- Wermer's syndrome

Premenstrual Dysphoric Disorder

- Premenstrual syndrome
- Dysthymic syndrome
- Personality disorder
- Panic disorder
- Major depressive disorder
- Hyperthyroidism
- Polycystic ovary syndrome

Progressive Supranuclear Palsy

- Parkinson's disease: differs from PSP in that the latter is characterized by prominence of early falls, tremor being unusual, and little response to levodopa.
- Cortical basal ganglionic degeneration: differentiated from PSP by presence of cortical sensory signs and asymmetric limb apraxia.
- Multiple systems atrophy: differs from PSP by the presence of prominent autonomic symptoms or cerebellar signs.
- Dementia with Lewy bodies (DLB): in PSP, visual hallucinations typically occur only if provoked by dopaminergic therapy; whereas in DLB, there are prominent visual hallucinations that may be spontaneous or provoked.

Prolactinoma

- Drugs: phenothiazines, methyldopa, reserpine, monoamine oxidase (MAO) inhibitors, androgens, progesterone, cimetidine, tricyclic antidepressants, haloperidol, meprobamate, chlordiazepoxide, estrogens, narcotics, metoclopramide, verapamil, amoxapine, cocaine, oral contraceptives
- Hepatic cirrhosis, renal failure, primary hypothyroidism
- Ectopic prolactin-secreting tumors (hypernephroma, bronchogenic carcinoma)
- Infiltrating diseases of the pituitary (sarcoidosis, histiocytosis)
- Head trauma, chest wall injury, spinal cord injury
- Polycystic ovary disease, pregnancy, nipple stimulation
- Idiopathic hyperprolactinemia, stress, exercise

Pronator Syndrome

- Carpal tunnel syndrome
- Cervical disk syndrome with radiculopathy
- Tendon rupture
- Tendinitis

Proptosis[31]

- Thyrotoxicosis
- Orbital pseudotumor
- Optic nerve tumor
- Cavernous sinus arteriovenous (AV) fistula, cavernous sinus thrombosis
- Cellulitis
- Metastatic tumor to orbit

Proptosis and Palatal Necrotic Ulcers

- Cavernous sinus thrombosis
- Bacterial orbital cellulitis
- Metastatic neoplasm
- Rhinocerebral mucormycosis
- Ecthyma gangrenosum
- CNS aspergillosis

Prostate Cancer

- Benign prostatic hypertrophy
- Prostatitis
- Prostate stones
- Metastatic neoplasm

Prostatic Hyperplasia, Benign

- Prostatitis
- Prostate cancer
- Strictures (urethral)
- Medication interfering with the muscle fibers in the prostate and also with bladder

Proteinuria

- Nephrotic syndrome as a result of primary renal diseases
- Malignant hypertension
- Malignant neoplasms: multiple myeloma, leukemias, Hodgkin's disease
- Congestive heart failure (CHF)
- Diabetes mellitus (DM)
- Systemic lupus erythematosus (SLE), rheumatoid arthritis (RA)
- Sickle cell disease
- Goodpasture's syndrome
- Malaria
- Amyloidosis, sarcoidosis
- Tubular lesions: cystinosis
- Functional (after heavy exercise)
- Pyelonephritis
- Pregnancy
- Constrictive pericarditis
- Renal vein thrombosis
- Toxic nephropathies: heavy metals, drugs
- Irradiation nephritis
- Orthostatic (postural) proteinuria
- Benign proteinuria: fever, heat, or cold exposure

Pruritus

- Dry skin
- Drug-induced eruption, fiberglass exposure
- Scabies
- Skin diseases
- Myeloproliferative disorders: mycosis fungoides, Hodgkin's disease, multiple myeloma, polycythemia vera
- Cholestatic liver disease
- Endocrine disorders: diabetes mellitus (DM), thyroid disease, carcinoid, pregnancy
- Carcinoma: breast, lung, gastric
- Chronic renal failure
- Iron deficiency
- AIDS

- Neurosis
- Sjögren's syndrome

Pruritus Ani[27]

FECAL IRRITATION
- Poor hygiene
- Anorectal conditions (fissure, fistula, hemorrhoids, skin tags, perianal clefts)
- Spicy foods, citrus foods, caffeine, colchicine, quinidine

CONTACT DERMATITIS
- Anesthetic agents, topical corticosteroids, perfumed soap

DERMATOLOGIC DISORDERS
- Psoriasis, seborrhea, lichen simplex or sclerosus

SYSTEMIC DISORDERS
- Chronic renal failure, myxedema, diabetes mellitus (DM), thyrotoxicosis, polycythemia vera, Hodgkin's disease

SEXUALLY TRANSMITTED DISEASES
- Syphilis, herpes simplex virus, human papillomavirus

OTHER INFECTIOUS AGENTS
- Pinworms
- Scabies
- Bacterial infection, viral infection

Pruritus Vulvae

- Vulvitis
- Vaginitis
- Lichen sclerosus
- Squamous cell hyperplasia
- Pinworms
- Vulvar cancer
- Syringoma of the vulva

Pseudocyanosis, Etiology

- Medications: amiodarone, minocycline, chlorpromazine
- Heavy metals

- Gold (systemic absorption)
- Silver (systemic absorption)
- Local contact with color dyes, gold, silver

Pseudofolliculitis Barbae (Ingrown Hairs, Razor Bumps)

- Acne
- Folliculitis
- Tinea barbae
- Rosacea

Pseudogout

- Gouty arthritis
- Rheumatoid arthritis
- Osteoarthritis
- Neuropathic joint
- Infectious arthritis
- Osteomyelitis
- Trauma

Pseudohermaphroditism, Female

- Congenital adrenal hyperplasia
- Maternal use of testosterone or related steroids
- Virilizing ovarian or adrenal tumor
- Virilizing luteoma of pregnancy
- Disturbances in differentiation of urogenital structures, non–androgen related
- Maternal virilizing adrenal hyperplasia
- Fetal P450 aromatase deficiency

Pseudohermaphroditism, Male

- Maternal ingestion of progestogens
- End-organ resistance to androgenic hormones
- 5α-Reductase 2 deficiency
- XY gonadal dysgenesis
- Testicular regression syndrome

- Defects in testosterone metabolism by peripheral tissues
- Testosterone biosynthesis defects

Pseudoinfarction[23]

- Cardiac tumors, primary and secondary
- Cardiomyopathy (particularly hypertrophic and dilated)
- Chagas' disease
- Chest deformity
- Chronic obstructive pulmonary disease (COPD) (particularly emphysema)
- HIV infection
- Hyperkalemia
- Left anterior fascicular block
- Left bundle branch block
- Left ventricular hypertrophy
- Myocarditis and pericarditis
- Normal variant
- Pneumothorax
- Poor R wave progression, rotational changes, and lead placement
- Pulmonary embolism
- Trauma to chest (nonpenetrating)
- Wolff-Parkinson-White syndrome
- Rare causes: pancreatitis, amyloidosis, sarcoidosis, scleroderma

Pseudomembranous Colitis

- GI bacterial infections (e.g., *Salmonella, Shigella, Campylobacter, Yersinia*)
- Enteric parasites (e.g., *Cryptosporidium, Entamoeba histolytica*)
- Inflammatory bowel disease (IBD)
- Celiac sprue
- Irritable bowel syndrome

Pseudoxanthoma Elasticum

- Ehlers-Danlos syndrome
- Actinic keratosis
- Xanthomas

- Amyloidosis
- Marfan syndrome

Psittacosis

- *Legionella*
- *Mycoplasma*
- *Chlamydia pneumoniae*
- Viral respiratory infections
- Bacterial pneumonia
- Typhoid fever
- Viral hepatitis
- Aseptic meningitis
- Fever of unknown origin
- Mononucleosis

Psoriasis

- Contact dermatitis
- Atopic dermatitis
- Stasis dermatitis
- Tinea
- Nummular dermatitis
- Candidiasis
- Mycosis fungoides
- Cutaneous systemic lupus erythematosus (SLE)
- Secondary and tertiary syphilis
- Drug eruption

Psychosis[29]

PRIMARY
- Schizophrenia related*
- Major depression
- Dementia
- Bipolar disorder

---

*Includes schizophrenia, schizophreniform disorder, brief reactive psychosis.

SECONDARY
- Drug use*
- Drug withdrawal[†]
- Drug toxicity[‡]
- Charles Bonnet syndrome
- Infections (pneumonia)
- Electrolyte imbalance
- Syphilis
- Congestive heart failure (CHF)
- Parkinson's disease
- Trauma to temporal lobe
- Postpartum psychosis
- Hypothyroidism/hyperthyroidism
- Hypomagnesemia
- Epilepsy
- Meningitis
- Encephalitis
- Brain abscess
- Herpes encephalopathy
- Hypoxia
- Hypercapnia
- Hypoglycemia
- Thiamine deficiency
- Postoperative states

Ptosis

- Third nerve palsy
- Myasthenia gravis
- Horner's syndrome
- Senile ptosis

---

*Includes hypnotics, glucocorticoids, marijuana, phencyclidine, atropine, dopaminergic agents (e.g., amantadine, bromocriptine, levodopa), immunosuppressants.

[†]Includes alcohol, barbiturates, benzodiazepines.

[‡]Includes digitalis, theophylline, cimetidine, anticholinergics, glucocorticoids, catecholaminergic agents.

Puberty, Delayed[28]

- Normal or low serum gonadotropin levels
- Constitutional delay in growth and development
- Hypothalamic or pituitary disorders
  - Isolated deficiency of growth hormone
  - Isolated deficiency of gonadotropin-releasing hormone (GnRH)
  - Isolated deficiency of luteinizing hormone (LH) or follicle-stimulating hormone (FSH)
  - Multiple anterior pituitary hormone deficiencies
  - Associated with congenital anomalies: Kallmann's syndrome, Prader-Willi syndrome, Laurence-Moon-Biedl syndrome, Friedreich's ataxia
  - Trauma
  - Post infection
  - Hyperprolactinemia
  - Post irradiation
  - Infiltrative disease (histiocytosis)
  - Tumor
  - Autoimmune hypophysitis
  - Idiopathic
  - Functional: chronic endocrinologic or systemic disorders; emotional disorders; drugs: cannabis
- Increased serum gonadotropin levels
  - Gonadal abnormalities: congenital
  - Gonadal dysgenesis
  - Klinefelter's syndrome
  - Bilateral anorchism
  - Resistant ovary syndrome
  - Myotonic dystrophy in males
  - 17-Hydroxylase deficiency in females
  - Galactosemia
- Acquired
  - Bilateral gonadal failure resulting from trauma or infection or after surgery, irradiation, or chemotherapy
  - Oophoritis: isolated or with other autoimmune disorders
  - Uterine or vaginal disorders

- Absence of uterus or vagina
- Testicular feminization: complete or incomplete androgen insensitivity

Puberty, Precocious

- Idiopathic
- Congenital virilizing adrenal hyperplasia
- Hypothalamic tumors
- Head trauma
- Hydrocephalus
- Degenerative CNS disease
- Arachnoid cyst
- Sex chromosome abnormalities (e.g., 47,XXY, 48,XXXY)
- Perinatal asphyxia
- CNS infection (e.g., meningitis, encephalitis)

Pulmonary Crackles

- Pneumonia
- Left ventricular failure
- Asbestosis, silicosis, interstitial lung disease
- Chronic bronchitis
- Alveolitis (allergic, fibrosing)
- Neoplasm

Pulmonary Embolism

- Myocardial infarction
- Pericarditis
- Pneumonia
- Pneumothorax
- Chest wall pain
- GI abnormalities (e.g., peptic ulcer, esophageal rupture, gastritis)
- Congestive heart failure (CHF)
- Pleuritis
- Anxiety disorder with hyperventilation
- Pericardial tamponade
- Dissection of aorta
- Asthma

Pulmonary Hypertension, Primary

SECONDARY PULMONARY HYPERTENSION CAUSED
BY UNDERLYING PULMONARY AND CARDIAC
CONDITIONS, INCLUDING

- Pulmonary thromboembolic disease
- Chronic obstructive pulmonary disease (COPD)
- Interstitial lung disease
- Obstructive sleep disorder
- Neuromuscular diseases causing hypoventilation (e.g., amyotrophic lateral sclerosis [ALS])
- Collagen-vascular disease (e.g., systemic lupus erythematosus [SLE], calcinosis, Raynaud's phenomenon, sclerodactyly, telangiectasia, CREST, systemic sclerosis)
- Pulmonary venous disease
- Left ventricular failure resulting from hypertension, coronary artery disease (CAD), aortic stenosis, and cardiomyopathy
- Valvular heart disease (e.g., mitral stenosis, mitral regurgitation)
- Congenital heart disease with left-to-right shunting (e.g., atrial septal defect [ASD])

Pulmonary Lesions

- TB
- *Legionella* pneumonia
- *Mycoplasma* pneumonia
- Viral pneumonia
- *Pneumocystis jiroveci*
- Hypersensitivity pneumonitis
- Aspiration pneumonia
- Fungal disease (aspergillosis, histoplasmosis)
- Acute respiratory distress syndrome (ARDS) associated with pneumonia
- Psittacosis
- Sarcoidosis
- Septic emboli
- Metastatic cancer
- Multiple pulmonary emboli
- Rheumatoid nodules

Pulmonary Nodule, Solitary

- Bronchogenic carcinoma
- Granuloma from histoplasmosis
- TB granuloma
- Granuloma from coccidioidomycosis
- Metastatic carcinoma
- Bronchial adenoma
- Bronchogenic cyst
- Hamartoma
- Arteriovenous (AV) malformation
- Other: fibroma, intrapulmonary lymph node, sclerosing hemangioma, bronchopulmonary sequestration

Pulseless Electrical Activity (Electromechanical Dissociation [EMD]), Differential Diagnosis

- Pseudo-EMD
- Idioventricular rhythm
- Post defibrillation idioventricular rhythm
- Ventricular escape rhythm
- Bradyasystolic rhythm

Pulseless Electrical Activity, Etiology

- Hypovolemia
- Hypoxia
- Hyperkalemia
- Acidosis
- Cardiac tamponade
- Tension pneumothorax
- Pulmonary embolus
- Drug overdose
- Hypothermia

Pupillary Dilation, Poor Response to Darkness

- Drugs (narcotics, general anesthetics, cholinergics)
- Acute trauma (spasm from prostaglandin release)

- Inflammation, infection (interruption of inhibitory fibers to the Edinger-Westphal nucleus)
- Old age (loss of inhibition at midbrain from reticular activating formation)
- Horner's syndrome (sympathetic neuron interruption)
- Adie's syndrome tonic pupil
- Lymphoma
- Congenital miosis

Purpura

- Trauma
- Septic emboli, atheromatous emboli
- Disseminated intravascular coagulation (DIC)
- Thrombocytopenia
- Meningococcemia
- Rocky Mountain spotted fever
- Hemolytic-uremic syndrome
- Viral infection: echovirus, coxsackievirus
- Scurvy
- Other: left atrial myxoma, cryoglobulinemia, vasculitis, hyperglobulinemic purpura

Pyelonephritis

- Nephrolithiasis
- Appendicitis
- Ovarian cyst torsion or rupture
- Acute glomerulonephritis
- Pelvic inflammatory disease (PID)
- Endometritis
- Other causes of acute abdomen
- Perinephric abscess
- Hydronephrosis

Pyoderma Gangrenosum

- Insect (spider) bite
- Vasculitis
- Traumatic ulceration

- Vascular insufficiency
- Antiphospholipid antibody syndrome

Pyogenic Granuloma

- Amelanotic melanoma
- Bacillary angiomatosis
- Glomus tumor
- Hemangioma
- Irritated nevus
- Wart
- Kaposi's sarcoma

QT Interval Prolongation[23]

- Drugs
  - Class I antiarrhythmics (e.g., disopyramide, procainamide, quinidine)
  - Class III antiarrhythmics
  - Tricyclic antidepressants
  - Phenothiazines
  - Astemizole
  - Terfenadine
  - Adenosine
  - Antibiotics (e.g., erythromycin and other macrolides)
  - Antifungal agents
  - Pentamidine, chloroquine
- Ischemic heart disease
- Cerebrovascular disease
- Rheumatic fever
- Myocarditis
- Mitral valve prolapse
- Electrolyte abnormalities
- Hypocalcemia
- Hypothyroidism
- Liquid protein diets
- Organophosphate insecticides
- Congenital prolonged QT syndrome

Rabies

- Delirium tremens
- Tetanus
- Hysteria
- Psychiatric disorders
- Other viral encephalitides
- Guillain-Barré syndrome
- Poliomyelitis

Ramsay Hunt Syndrome

- Herpes simplex
- External otitis
- Impetigo
- Enteroviral infection
- Bell's palsy of other etiologies
- Acoustic neuroma (before appearance of skin lesions)

Rash, Febrile Child

- Bacteremia
- Dermatomyositis
- Drug exanthem, including serum sickness
- Erysipelas
- Henoch-Schönlein purpura
- Kawasaki's syndrome
- Lupus erythematosus
- Lyme disease
- Rocky Mountain spotted fever
- Scarlet fever
- Staphylococcal scalded skin syndrome
- Still's disease
- Urticaria
- Viral exanthem

Rash, Pruritic, Child

- Atopic dermatitis
- Contact dermatitis

- Diaper dermatitis
- Eczema, especially xerotic
- Histiocytosis
- Impetigo
- Insect bite
- Dermatosis pilaris
- Pediculosis, especially capitis
- Pityriasis rosea
- Scabies
- Seborrheic dermatitis
- Tinea corporis and tinea capitis

Raynaud's Phenomenon

- Neurogenic thoracic outlet syndrome or carpal tunnel syndrome
- Frostbite or cold weather injury
- Medication reaction (ergotamine, chemotherapeutic agents)
- Atherosclerosis, thromboembolic disease
- Buerger's disease, embolic disease
- Acrocyanosis
- Livedo reticularis
- Injury from repetitive motion

Rectal Mass, Palpable[39]

- Rectal carcinoma
- Rectal polyp
- Hypertrophied anal papilla
- Diverticular phlegmon (prolapsing into the pouch of Douglas)
- Sigmoid colon carcinoma (prolapsing into the pouch of Douglas)
- Metastatic deposits at the pelvic reflection (Blumer's shelf)
- Primary pelvic malignant neoplasm (uterine, ovarian, prostatic, or cervical)
- Mesorectal lymph nodes
- Endometriosis
- Solitary rectal ulcer syndrome
- Foreign body
- Feces (indent)
- Presacral cyst

- Amebic granuloma
- Vaginal tampon and even the pubic bone may be mistaken for a rectal mass

Rectal Pain

- Anal fissure
- Thrombosed hemorrhoid
- Anorectal abscess
- Foreign bodies
- Fecal impaction
- Endometriosis
- Neoplasms (primary or metastatic)
- Pelvic inflammatory disease (PID)
- Inflammation of sacral nerves
- Compression of sacral nerves
- Prostatitis
- Other: proctalgia fugax, uterine abnormalities, myopathies, coccygodynia

Red Blood Cell Aplasia, Acquired, Etiology

- Idiopathic (>50% of cases)
- Medications (most frequent with phenytoin)
- Non-Hodgkin's lymphoma
- Viral infections (parvovirus B19, EB virus, mumps, hepatitis)
- Myelodysplastic syndromes
- Thymoma
- Autoimmune diseases
- Allogenic bone marrow transplant from ABO-incompatible donor
- Pregnancy

Red Eye

- Infectious conjunctivitis (bacterial, viral)
- Allergic conjunctivitis
- Acute glaucoma
- Keratitis (bacterial, viral)
- Iritis
- Trauma

Red Hot Joint

- Trauma
- Gout
- Infection (septic joint)
- Pseudogout (calcium pyrophosphate dehydrate crystal deposition)
- Psoriatic arthropathy
- Reactive arthritis
- Palindromic rheumatism

Red Urine

- Hematuria
- Porphyrins
- Hemoglobinuria
- Myoglobinuria
- Medications (aminosalicylic acid, deferoxamine, phenazopyridine, phenolphthalein, NSAIDs, rifampin, phenytoin, methyldopa, doxorubicin, phenacetin)
- Foods (beets, berries, maize)
- Urate crystalluria

Reiter's Syndrome

- Ankylosing spondylitis
- Psoriatic arthritis
- Rheumatoid arthritis
- Gonococcal arthritis-tenosynovitis
- Rheumatic fever

Renal Artery Occlusion, Causes

- Atrial fibrillation
- Angiography or stent placement
- Abdominal aortic surgery
- Trauma
- Renal artery aneurysm/dissection
- Vasculitis
- Thrombosis in patient with fibromuscular dysplasia

- Atherosclerosis
- Septic embolism
- Mural thrombus thromboembolism
- Atrial myxoma thromboembolism
- Mitral stenosis thromboembolism
- Prosthetic valve thromboembolism
- Renal cell carcinoma

Renal Cell Adenocarcinoma

- Transitional cell carcinomas of the renal pelvis (8% of all renal cancers)
- Wilms' tumor
- Other rare primary renal carcinomas and sarcomas
- Renal cysts
- Retroperitoneal tumors

Renal Cystic Disorders

- Simple cysts
- Acquired cystic kidney disease
- Autosomal dominant polycystic kidney disease
- Autosomal recessive polycystic kidney disease
- Medullary cystic disease
- Medullary sponge kidney

Renal Failure, Intrinsic or Parenchymal Causes[37]

ABNORMALITIES OF THE VASCULATURE
- Renal arteries: atherosclerosis, thromboembolism, arteritis
- Renal veins: thrombosis
- Microvasculature: vasculitis, thrombotic microangiopathy

ABNORMALITIES OF GLOMERULI
(ACUTE GLOMERULONEPHRITIS)
- Anti–glomerular membrane disease (Goodpasture's syndrome)
- Immune complex glomerulonephritis: SLE, postinfectious, idiopathic, membranoproliferative

ABNORMALITIES OF INTERSTITIUM (ACUTE INTERSTITIAL NEPHRITIS)

- Drugs (e.g., antibiotics, NSAIDs, diuretics, anticonvulsants, allopurinol)
- Infectious pyelonephritis
- Infiltrative: lymphoma, leukemia, sarcoidosis

ABNORMALITIES OF TUBULES

- Physical obstruction (uric acid, oxalate, light chains)
- Acute tubular necrosis
  - Ischemic
  - Toxic (antibiotics, chemotherapy, immunosuppressives, radiocontrast dyes, heavy metals, myoglobin, hemolyzed RBCs)

Renal Failure, Postrenal Causes[37]

URETER AND RENAL PELVIS

- Intrinsic obstruction: blood clots; stones; sloughed papillae: diabetes, sickle cell disease, analgesic nephropathy; inflammatory: fungus ball
- Extrinsic obstruction: malignant neoplasm, retroperitoneal fibrosis; iatrogenic: inadvertent ligation of ureters

BLADDER

- Prostatic hypertrophy or malignant neoplasm
- Neuropathic bladder
- Blood clots
- Bladder cancer
- Stones

URETHRAL

- Strictures
- Congenital valves

Renal Failure, Prerenal Causes[37]

DECREASED CARDIAC OUTPUT

- Congestive heart failure (CHF)
- Arrhythmias
- Pericardial constriction or tamponade
- Pulmonary embolism

HYPOVOLEMIA

- GI tract loss (vomiting, diarrhea, nasogastric suction)
- Blood losses (trauma, GI tract surgery)
- Renal losses (diuretics, mineralocorticoid deficiency, postobstructive diuresis)
- Skin losses (burns)

VOLUME REDISTRIBUTION

- Decrease in effective blood volume
  - Hypoalbuminemic states (cirrhosis, nephrosis)
  - Sequestration of fluid in "third" space (ischemic bowel, peritonitis, pancreatitis)
  - Peripheral vasodilation (sepsis, vasodilators, anaphylaxis)

ALTERED RENAL VASCULAR RESISTANCE

- Increase in afferent vascular resistance (nonsteroidal anti-inflammatory drugs [NSAIDs], liver disease, sepsis, hypercalcemia, cyclosporine)
- Decrease in efferent arteriolar tone (angiotensin-converting enzyme [ACE] inhibitors)

Renal Tubular Acidosis

- Diarrhea with significant bicarbonate loss
- Other causes of metabolic acidosis
- Respiratory acidosis

Renal Vein Thrombosis, Causes

- Nephrotic syndrome
- Renal cell carcinoma
- Aortic aneurysm causing compression
- Lymphadenopathy
- Retroperitoneal fibrosis
- Estrogen therapy
- Pregnancy
- Renal cell carcinoma with vein invasion
- Severe dehydration

Respiratory Failure, Hypoventilatory[29]

ABNORMAL RESPIRATORY CAPACITY, NORMAL
RESPIRATORY WORKLOADS

- Acute depression of CNS: various causes
- Chronic central hypoventilation syndromes: obesity-hypoventilation syndrome, sleep apnea syndrome, hypothyroidism, Shy-Drager syndrome (multisystem atrophy syndrome)
- Acute toxic paralysis syndromes: botulism, tetanus, toxic ingestion or bites, organophosphate poisoning
- Neuromuscular disorders (acute and chronic): myasthenia gravis, Guillain-Barré syndrome, drugs, amyotrophic lateral sclerosis (ALS), muscular dystrophies, polymyositis, spinal cord injury, traumatic phrenic nerve paralysis

ABNORMAL PULMONARY WORKLOADS

- Chronic obstructive pulmonary disease (COPD): chronic bronchitis, asthmatic bronchitis, emphysema
- Asthma and acute bronchial hyperreactivity syndromes
- Upper airway obstruction
- Interstitial lung diseases

ABNORMAL EXTRAPULMONARY WORKLOADS

- Chronic thoracic cage disorders: severe kyphoscoliosis, after thoracoplasty, after thoracic cage injury
- Acute thoracic cage trauma and burns
- Pneumothorax
- Pleural fibrosis and effusions
- Abdominal processes

Restless Legs Syndrome

- Periodic limb movement disorder (PLMD), repetitive limb movements (lower extremities or upper extremities) occurring during sleep; associated with arousals from sleep and daytime sleeping; patient is typically unaware, but bed partner reports restlessness or kicking during sleep
- Peripheral neuropathy and radiculopathy
- Anxiety and mood disorders

- Chronic fatigue
- Other sleep disorders
- Neuroleptic-induced akathisia
- Dyskinesias while awake
- Nocturnal leg cramps with or without peripheral artery disease

Reticulocytosis

- Hemolytic anemia (sickle cell crisis, thalassemia major, autoimmune hemolysis)
- Hemorrhage
- Post anemia therapy (folic acid, ferrous sulfate, vitamin B_{12})
- Chronic renal failure

Retinitis Pigmentosa

- Syphilis
- Old inflammatory scars
- Old hemorrhage
- Diabetes
- Toxic retinopathies (phenothiazines, chloroquine)

Retinoblastoma

- Strabismus
- Retinal detachment
- Uveitis
- Other tumors
- Glaucoma
- Coats' disease (pathologic telangiectatic retinal vessels that leak and lead to accumulation of subretinal fluid and lipid)
- Endophthalmitis
- Cataract
- Infectious

Retinopathy, Diabetic

- Retinal inflammatory diseases
- Tumor

- Trauma
- Arteriosclerotic vascular disease

Retinopathy, Hypertensive

- Retinal venous obstruction
- Diabetic retinopathy
- Ocular ischemic syndrome
- Hyperviscosity
- Tortuosity of retinal artery

Retropharyngeal Abscess

- Cervical osteomyelitis
- Pott's disease
- Meningitis
- Calcific tendinitis of the long muscle of the neck

Reye's Syndrome

- Inborn errors of metabolism: carnitine deficiency, ornithine transcarbamylase deficiency
- Salicylate or amiodarone intoxication
- Jamaican vomiting sickness
- Hepatic encephalopathy of any cause

Rhabdomyolysis, Causes

- Exertion (exercise induced)
- Electrical injury
- Drug induced (statins; combination of statins with fibrates or erythromycin; simvastatin and amiodarone; amphetamines, haloperidol)
- Compartment syndrome
- Multiple trauma
- Malignant hyperthermia
- Limb ischemia
- Reperfusion after revascularization procedures for ischemia
- Extensive surgical (spinal) dissection, bariatric surgery
- Tourniquet ischemia

- Prolonged static positioning during surgery
- Infectious and inflammatory myositis
- Metabolic myopathies
- Hypovolemia and urinary acidification are important precipitating causes in the development of acute renal failure.
- Sickle cell trait is a predisposing condition.
- Hypothyroidism
- Alcoholism
- Seizures

Rheumatic Fever

- Rheumatoid arthritis
- Juvenile rheumatoid arthritis (Still's disease)
- Bacterial endocarditis
- Systemic lupus erythematosus (SLE)
- Viral infections
- Serum sickness

Rheumatoid Arthritis

- Systemic lupus erythematosus
- Seronegative spondyloarthropathies
- Polymyalgia rheumatica
- Acute rheumatic fever
- Scleroderma
- Osteoarthritis

Rhinitis

- Allergic rhinitis
- Infectious rhinitis
- Vasomotor rhinitis
- Exercise-induced rhinitis
- Emotional rhinitis
- Rhinitis medicamentosa
- Hormone-mediated rhinitis (menses, pregnancy, oral contraceptives, hypothyroidism)
- GERD
- Chemical- or irritant-induced rhinitis

- Rhinitis mimics:
  - Deviated septum
  - Enlarged adenoids
  - Nasal polyps/tumors
  - Foreign bodies
  - CSF rhinorrhea
  - Sarcoidosis
  - Midline granuloma
  - Wegener's granulomatosis
  - SLE
  - Sjögren's syndrome

Rhinitis, Allergic

- Infections (sinusitis; viral, bacterial, or fungal rhinitis)
- Rhinitis medicamentosa (cocaine, sympathomimetic nasal drops)
- Vasomotor rhinitis (e.g., secondary to air pollutants)
- Septal obstruction (e.g., deviated septum), nasal polyps, nasal neoplasms
- Systemic diseases (e.g., Wegener's granulomatosis, hypothyroidism [rare])

Rhus Dermatitis (Poison Ivy, Poison Oak, Poison Sumac)

- Impetigo
- Lichen simplex chronicus
- Atopic dermatitis
- Nummular
- Seborrheic dermatitis
- Psoriasis
- Scabies

Rickets

- Osteoporosis
- Hyperparathyroidism
- Hyperthyroidism

Right Axis Deviation[23]

- Normal variation
- Right ventricular hypertrophy
- Left posterior fascicular block
- Lateral myocardial infarction
- Pulmonary embolism
- Dextrocardia
- Mechanical shifts or emphysema causing a vertical heart

Rocky Mountain Spotted Fever

- Influenza A
- Enteroviral infection
- Typhoid fever
- Leptospirosis
- Infectious mononucleosis
- Viral hepatitis
- Sepsis
- Ehrlichiosis
- Gastroenteritis
- Acute abdomen
- Bronchitis
- Pneumonia
- Meningococcemia
- Disseminated gonococcal infection
- Secondary syphilis
- Bacterial endocarditis
- Toxic shock syndrome
- Scarlet fever
- Rheumatic fever
- Measles
- Rubella
- Typhus
- Rickettsialpox
- Lyme disease
- Drug hypersensitivity reactions
- Idiopathic thrombocytopenic purpura
- Thrombotic thrombocytopenic purpura

- Kawasaki's disease
- Immune complex vasculitis
- Connective tissue disorders

Rosacea

- Drug eruption
- Acne vulgaris
- Contact dermatitis
- Systemic lupus erythematosus (SLE)
- Carcinoid flush
- Idiopathic facial flushing
- Seborrheic dermatitis
- Facial sarcoidosis
- Photodermatitis
- Mastocytosis

Roseola

- Measles
- Rubella
- Fifth disease
- Drug eruption
- Mononucleosis

Rotator Cuff Syndrome

- Shoulder instability
- Degenerative arthritis
- Cervical radiculopathy
- Avascular necrosis
- Suprascapular nerve entrapment

Rubella

- Other viral infections by enteroviruses, adenoviruses, human parvovirus B19, measles
- Scarlet fever
- Allergic reaction
- Kawasaki's disease

- Congenital syphilis
- Toxoplasmosis
- Herpes simplex
- Cytomegalovirus, enterovirus

Salivary Gland Enlargement

- Neoplasm
- Sialolithiasis
- Infection (mumps, bacterial infection, HIV infection, TB)
- Sarcoidosis
- Idiopathic
- Acromegaly
- Anorexia/bulimia
- Chronic pancreatitis
- Medications (e.g., phenylbutazone)
- Cirrhosis
- Diabetes mellitus

Salivary Gland Secretion, Decreased

- Medications (antihistamines, antidepressants, neuroleptics, antihypertensives)
- Dehydration
- Anxiety
- Sjögren's syndrome
- Sarcoidosis
- Mumps
- Amyloidosis
- CNS disorders
- Head and neck irradiation

Salmonellosis

OTHER CAUSES OF PROLONGED FEVER
- Malaria
- TB
- Brucellosis
- Amebic liver abscess

OTHER CAUSES OF GASTROENTERITIS
- Bacterial: *Shigella, Yersinia, Campylobacter*
- Viral: Norwalk virus, rotavirus
- Parasitic: *Entamoeba histolytica, Giardia lamblia*
- Toxic: enterotoxigenic *Escherichia coli, Clostridium difficile*

Sarcoidosis

- TB
- Lymphoma
- Hodgkin's disease
- Metastases
- Pneumoconioses
- Enlarged pulmonary arteries
- Infectious mononucleosis
- Lymphangitic carcinomatosis
- Idiopathic hemosiderosis
- Alveolar cell carcinoma
- Pulmonary eosinophilia
- Hypersensitivity pneumonitis
- Fibrosing alveolitis
- Collagen disorders
- Parasitic infection

Scabies

- Pediculosis
- Atopic dermatitis
- Flea bites
- Seborrheic dermatitis
- Dermatitis herpetiformis
- Contact dermatitis
- Nummular eczema
- Syphilis
- Other insect infestation

Scarlet Fever

- Viral exanthems
- Kawasaki's disease

- Toxic shock syndrome
- Drug rashes

Schistosomiasis

- Amebiasis
- Bacillary dysentery
- Bowel polyp
- Prostatic disease
- Genitourinary tract cancer
- Bacterial infections of the urinary tract

Schizophrenia

- Any medical condition, medicine, or substance of abuse that can affect brain homeostasis and cause psychosis: distinguished from schizophrenia by its relatively brief course and the alteration in mental status that could suggest an underlying delirium
- Other neurologic conditions (e.g., Huntington's) that have psychosis as the initial presentation
- Other psychiatric disorders: source of greatest confusion
  - Mood disorders with psychosis: indistinguishable from schizophrenia cross-sectionally but have a longitudinal course that includes full recovery
  - Delusional disorder: has nonbizarre delusions and lacks the thought disturbance, hallucinations, and negative symptoms of schizophrenia
  - Autism in the adult: has an early age at onset and lacks significant hallucinations or delusions

Scleroderma

DERMATOLOGIC
- Mycosis fungoides
- Amyloidosis
- Porphyria cutanea tarda
- Eosinophilic fasciitis
- Reflex sympathetic dystrophy

SYSTEMIC
- Idiopathic pulmonary fibrosis
- Primary pulmonary hypertension
- Primary biliary cirrhosis
- Cardiomyopathies
- GI dysmotility problems
- Systemic lupus erythematosus (SLE) and overlap syndromes

Scrotal Pain[29]

- Torsion: appendages, spermatic cord
- Infection: orchitis, abscess, epididymitis
- Neoplasia: benign, malignant
- Incarcerated hernia
- Trauma
- Hydrocele
- Spermatocele
- Varicocele

Scrotal Swelling

- Hydrocele
- Varicocele
- Neoplasm
- Acute epididymitis
- Orchitis
- Trauma
- Hernia
- Torsion of spermatic cord
- Torsion of epididymis
- Torsion of testis
- Insect bite
- Folliculitis
- Sebaceous cyst
- Thrombosis of spermatic vein
- Other: lymphedema, dermatitis, fat necrosis, Henoch-Schönlein purpura, idiopathic scrotal edema

Seasonal Affective Disorder

- Major depressive disorder
- Minor depression or adjustment disorder
- Bipolar affective disorder
- Evaluate for substance use (especially alcohol)
- Medical illness or medications that may contribute to depression (e.g., endocrine disorders, neurologic disease)

Seborrheic Dermatitis

- Psoriasis
- Tinea capitis
- Contact dermatitis
- Atopic dermatitis
- Rosacea
- Erythrasma
- Xerotic eczema
- Candidiasis

Seborrheic Keratosis

- Actinic keratosis
- Melanoma
- Wart
- Lentigo
- Skin tag

Seizure

- Syncope
- Alcohol abuse/withdrawal
- Transient ischemic attack (TIA)
- Hemiparetic migraine
- Psychiatric disorders
- Carotid sinus hypersensitivity
- Hyperventilation, prolonged breath holding
- Hypoglycemia
- Narcolepsy

- Movement disorders (tics, hemiballismus)
- Hyponatremia
- Brain tumor (primary or metastatic)
- Tetanus
- Strychnine, phencyclidine poisoning

Seizures, Absence

- Complex partial seizures
- Daydreaming
- Psychogenic unresponsiveness
- Anxiety disorder

Seizures, Febrile

- Epilepsy
- Meningitis
- Encephalitis
- Brain abscess

Seizures, Partial

- Migraine
- Transient ischemic attack (TIA)
- Presyncope
- Psychogenic phenomena, anxiety disorder

Seizures, Pediatric[2]

FIRST MONTH OF LIFE
First Day
- Hypoxia
- Drugs
- Trauma
- Infection
- Hyperglycemia
- Hypoglycemia
- Pyridoxine deficiency

Day 2–3
- Infection
- Drug withdrawal
- Hypoglycemia
- Hypocalcemia
- Developmental malformation
- Intracranial hemorrhage
- Inborn error of metabolism
- Hyponatremia or hypernatremia

Day >4
- Infection
- Hypocalcemia
- Hyperphosphatemia
- Hyponatremia
- Developmental malformation
- Drug withdrawal
- Inborn error of metabolism

1–6 MONTHS
- As above

6 MONTHS–3 YEARS
- Febrile seizures
- Birth injury
- Infection
- Toxin
- Trauma
- Metabolic disorder
- Cerebral degenerative disease

>3 YEARS
- Idiopathic
- Infection
- Trauma
- Cerebral degenerative disease

Septicemia

- Cardiogenic shock
- Acute pancreatitis

- Pulmonary embolism
- Systemic vasculitis
- Toxic ingestion
- Exposure-induced hypothermia
- Fulminant hepatic failure
- Collagen-vascular diseases

Serotonin Syndrome

- Neuroleptic malignant syndrome
- Substance abuse (e.g., cocaine, amphetamines)
- Thyroid storm
- Infection
- Alcohol and opioid withdrawal

Severe Acute Respiratory Syndrome (SARS)

- *Legionella* pneumonia
- Influenza A and B
- Respiratory syncytial virus
- Acute respiratory distress syndrome (ARDS)

Sexual Precocity[41]

TRUE PRECOCIOUS PUBERTY
- Premature reactivation of LHRH pulse generator

INCOMPLETE SEXUAL PRECOCITY (PITUITARY GONADOTROPIN INDEPENDENT)
Males
- Chorionic gonadotropin–secreting tumor
- Leydig cell tumor
- Familial testotoxicosis
- Virilizing congenital adrenal hyperplasia
- Virilizing adrenal tumor
- Premature adrenarche

Females
- Granulosa cell tumor (follicular cysts may be manifested similarly)
- Follicular cyst

- Feminizing adrenal tumor
- Premature thelarche
- Premature adrenarche
- Late-onset virilizing congenital adrenal hyperplasia

In Both Sexes
- McCune-Albright syndrome
- Primary hypothyroidism

Sexually Transmitted Diseases, Anorectal Region[27]

ULCERATIVE
- Lymphogranuloma venereum
- Herpes simplex virus
- Early (primary) syphilis
- Chancroid (*Haemophilus ducreyi*)
- Cytomegalovirus
- Idiopathic (usually HIV positive)

NONULCERATIVE
- Condyloma acuminatum
- Gonorrhea
- Chlamydia *(C. trachomatis)*
- Syphilis

Sheehan's Syndrome

- Chronic infections
- HIV infection
- Sarcoidosis
- Amyloidosis
- Rheumatoid disease
- Hemochromatosis
- Metastatic carcinoma
- Lymphocytic hypophysitis

Shigellosis

- Bacterial gastroenteritis
- Dysentery caused by *Entamoeba histolytica*

- Enterotoxigenic *Escherichia coli*
- Viral gastroenteritis
- Pseudomembranous colitis

Shoulder Pain

WITH LOCAL FINDINGS IN SHOULDER

- Trauma: contusion, fracture, muscle strain, trauma to spinal cord
- Arthrosis, arthritis, rheumatoid arthritis (RA), ankylosing spondylitis
- Bursitis, synovitis, tendinitis, tenosynovitis
- Aseptic (avascular) necrosis
- Local infection: septic arthritis, osteomyelitis, abscess, herpes zoster, TB

WITHOUT LOCAL FINDINGS IN SHOULDER

- Cardiovascular disorders: ischemic heart disease, pericarditis, aortic aneurysm
- Subdiaphragmatic abscess, liver abscess
- Cholelithiasis, cholecystitis
- Pulmonary lesions: apical bronchial carcinoma, pleurisy, pneumothorax, pneumonia
- GI lesions: peptic ulcer disease (PUD), gastric neoplasm, peptic esophagitis
- Pancreatic lesions: carcinoma, calculi, pancreatitis
- CNS abnormalities: neoplasm, vascular abnormalities
- Multiple sclerosis (MS)
- Syringomyelia
- Polymyositis/dermatomyositis
- Psychogenic
- Polymyalgia rheumatica
- Ectopic pregnancy

Shoulder Pain by Location

TOP OF SHOULDER (C4)

- Cervical source
- Acromioclavicular
- Sternoclavicular
- Diaphragmatic

SUPEROLATERAL (C5)
- Rotator cuff tendinitis
- Impingement
- Adhesive capsulitis
- Glenohumeral arthritis

ANTERIOR
- Bicipital tendinitis and rupture
- Glenoid labral tear
- Adhesive capsulitis
- Glenohumeral arthritis
- Osteonecrosis

AXILLARY
- Neoplasm (Pancoast's, mediastinal)
- Herpes zoster

Sialadenitis

- Salivary gland neoplasm
- Ductal stricture
- Sialolithiasis
- Decreased salivary secretion secondary to medications (e.g., amitriptyline, diphenhydramine, anticholinergics)

Sialolithiasis

- Lymphadenitis
- Salivary gland tumor
- Salivary gland bacterial (staphylococcus or streptococcus), viral (mumps), or fungal infection (sialadenitis)
- Noninfectious salivary gland inflammation (e.g., Sjögren's syndrome, sarcoidosis, lymphoma)
- Salivary duct stricture
- Dental abscess

Sick Sinus Syndrome

- Bradycardia: atrioventricular (AV) block
- Tachycardia: atrial fibrillation

- Atrial flutter
- Paroxysmal atrial tachycardia
- Sinus tachycardia

Silicosis

- Other pneumoconiosis, berylliosis, hard metal disease, asbestosis
- Sarcoidosis
- Tuberculosis
- Interstitial lung disease
- Hypersensitivity pneumonitis
- Lung cancer
- Langerhans cell granulomatosis (histiocytosis X)
- Granulomatous pulmonary vasculitis

Sinusitis

- Temporomandibular joint disease
- Migraine headache
- Cluster headache
- Dental infection
- Trigeminal neuralgia

Sjögren's Syndrome

- Medication-related dryness (e.g., anticholinergics)
- Age-related exocrine gland dysfunction
- Mouth breathing
- Anxiety
- Other: sarcoidosis, primary salivary hypofunction, irradiation injury, amyloidosis

Sleep Apnea

EXCESSIVE DAYTIME SOMNOLENCE
- Inadequate sleep time
- Pulmonary disease
- Parkinsonism
- Sleep-related epilepsy

- Narcolepsy
- Hypothyroidism

SLEEP FRAGMENTATION
- Sleep-related asthma
- Sleep-related gastroesophageal reflux disease (GERD)
- Periodic limb movement disorder
- Parasomnias
- Psychophysiologic insomnia
- Panic disorder
- Narcolepsy

Small Bowel Obstruction[27]

INTRINSIC
- Congenital (atresia, stenosis)
- Inflammatory (Crohn's disease, irradiation enteritis)
- Neoplasms (metastatic or primary)
- Intussusception
- Traumatic (hematoma)

EXTRINSIC
- Hernias (internal and external)
- Adhesions
- Volvulus
- Compressing masses (tumors, abscesses, hematomas)

INTRALUMINAL
- Foreign body
- Gallstones
- Bezoars
- Barium
- *Ascaris* infestation

Small Intestine Ulceration

- Inflammatory bowel disease
- Celiac disease
- Vasculitis, SLE, Behçet's syndrome
- Uremia

- Infections (*Campylobacter*, TB, *Yersinia*, parasites, typhoid, cytomegalovirus [CMV], *Clostridium*)
- Mesenteric insufficiency
- Neoplasms
- Radiation therapy
- Drugs (salicylates, potassium, indomethacin, antimetabolites)
- Meckel's diverticulum
- Zollinger-Ellison syndrome
- Lymphocytic enterocolitis
- Stomal ulceration

Smallpox

- Rash from other viral illnesses (e.g., hemorrhagic chickenpox, measles, coxsackievirus)
- Abdominal pain may mimic appendicitis.
- Meningococcemia
- Insect bites
- Impetigo
- Dermatitis herpetiformis
- Pemphigus
- Papular urticaria

Smell Disturbance

- Upper respiratory tract infection
- Nasal or paranasal sinus disease
- Exposure to noxious vapors
- Head trauma
- Idiopathic
- Dental caries, periodontal disease
- Medications

Somatization Disorder

- Undifferentiated somatoform disorder: one or more physical complaints that cannot be explained by a medical condition are present for at least 6 months. (NOTE: Somatization is more severe and less common.)

- Conversion disorder: there is an alteration or loss of voluntary motor or sensory function with demonstrable physical cause and related to a psychological stress or a conflict. (NOTE: With multiple complaints, the diagnosis of conversion is not made.)
- Pain disorder: distinguished from somatization disorder by the presence of other somatic complaints.
- Munchausen's (factitious disorder) and malingering: the psychological basis of the complaints in somatization disorder is not conscious as in factitious disorder (Munchausen's) and malingering, in which symptoms are produced intentionally.

Sore Throat[34]

WITHOUT PHARYNGEAL ULCERS
- Viral pharyngitis
- Allergic pharyngitis
- Infectious mononucleosis
- Streptococcal pharyngitis
- Gonococcal pharyngitis
- Sinusitis with postnasal drip

WITH PHARYNGEAL ULCERS
- Herpangina
- Herpes simplex
- Candidiasis
- Fusospirochetal infection (Vincent's angina)

Spastic Paraplegias

- Cervical spondylosis
- Friedreich's ataxia
- Multiple sclerosis
- Spinal cord tumor
- HIV infection
- Tertiary syphilis
- Vitamin B_{12} deficiency
- Spinocerebellar ataxias
- Syringomyelia
- Spinal cord arteriovenous (AV) malformations
- Adrenoleukodystrophy

Spinal Cord Compression, Epidural

- Osteoarthritis
- Meningioma
- Spinal epidural abscess
- Spinal epidural hematoma
- Spinal epidural vascular malformations
- RA
- Metastatic cancer (vertebral, intramedullary, leptomeninges)
- Radiation myelopathy
- Neurofibroma
- Sarcoidosis
- Paraneoplastic myelopathy
- Histiocytosis

Spinal Cord Dysfunction

- Trauma
- Multiple sclerosis
- Transverse myelitis
- Neoplasm (primary, metastatic)
- Syringomyelia
- Spinal epidural abscess
- HIV myelopathy
- Diskitis
- Spinal epidural hematoma
- Spinal cord infarction
- Spinal arteriovenous (AV) malformation
- Subarachnoid hemorrhage

Spinal Cord Ischemic Syndromes

- Systemic hypotension
- Venous or arterial occlusion
- Arterial dissection
- Thromboembolism
- Endovascular procedures
- Vasculitis
- Fibrocartilaginous embolism
- Regional hemodynamic compromise

Spinal Epidural Abscess

- Herniated disk
- Vertebral osteomyelitis and diskitis
- Metastatic tumors
- Meningitis

Spinal Stenosis

- Osteoarthritis of the back
- Osteoarthritis of the knee
- Osteoarthritis of the hip
- Osteomyelitis
- Epidural abscess
- Metastatic tumors
- Multiple myeloma
- Intermittent claudication secondary to peripheral vascular disease
- Neuropathy
- Scoliosis
- Herniated nucleus pulposus
- Spondylolisthesis
- Acute cauda equina syndrome
- Ankylosing spondylitis
- Reiter's syndrome
- Fibromyalgia

Spinal Stenosis, Lumbar

- Osteoarthritis of the knee or hip
- Acute cauda equina syndrome, resulting from compression by epidural abscess or tumors
- Pain and weakness caused by multiple myeloma or osteomyelitis
- Intermittent claudication–peripheral vascular disease
- Peripheral neuropathy such as that caused by a herniated nucleus pulposus
- Scoliosis or spondylolisthesis
- Rheumatoid diseases: ankylosing spondylitis, Reiter's syndrome, fibromyalgia

Spinal Tumors[14]

EXTRADURAL
* Metastases
* Primary bone tumors arising in spine

INTRADURAL EXTRAMEDULLARY
* Meningiomas
* Neurofibromas
* Schwannomas
* Lipomas
* Arachnoid cysts
* Epidermoid cysts
* Metastasis

INTRAMEDULLARY
* Ependymoma
* Glioma
* Hemangioblastoma
* Lipoma
* Metastases

Spinocerebellar Ataxia

* Friedreich's ataxia: differs from the SCAs in that inheritance is autosomal recessive, it almost always begins in childhood or adolescence, and it is associated with early lower limb areflexia.
* Sensory ataxias: differ from the SCAs in that the primary defect is not one of cerebellar function but of sensory inputs into the cerebellum. They can be the result of peripheral neuropathies or spinal cord disease that involves the posterior columns.
* Posterior fossa mass lesions
* Acquired vitamin E deficiency: differs from SCAs in that patients almost always have a clinically evident disorder of fat malabsorption.
* Toxin exposure (alcohol, phenytoin, organic mercury)

- Multiple sclerosis, other central nervous system inflammatory diseases: differ from SCAs in that ataxia, when present, usually presents acutely to subacutely.
- Paraneoplastic cerebellar degeneration: differs from SCAs in that the ataxia progresses relatively rapidly.
- Creutzfeldt-Jakob disease: differs from the SCAs in that the ataxia progresses relatively rapidly and is accompanied by dementia and myoclonus.
- Wilson's disease: differs from the SCAs in that there is often accompanying parkinsonism, psychiatric manifestations, and hepatic dysfunction.
- Superficial siderosis: differs from the SCAs in that it also often produces sensorineural hearing loss, anosmia, dementia, and bladder disturbance.
- Mitochondrial encephalomyopathies
- Multiple systems atrophy: differs from the SCAs in that age at onset is usually later and parkinsonism, long tract signs, and orthostatic hypotension are often present.

Splenomegaly

- Hepatic cirrhosis
- Neoplastic involvement: cell-mediated lympholysis (CML), chronic lymphocytic leukemia (CLL), lymphoma, multiple myeloma
- Bacterial infections: TB, infectious endocarditis, typhoid fever, splenic abscess
- Viral infections: infectious mononucleosis, viral hepatitis, HIV infection
- Gaucher's disease and other lipid storage diseases
- Sarcoidosis
- Parasitic infections (malaria, kala-azar, histoplasmosis)
- Hereditary and acquired hemolytic anemias
- Idiopathic thrombocytopenic purpura (ITP)
- Collagen-vascular disorders: systemic lupus erythematosus (SLE), rheumatoid arthritis (RA; Felty's syndrome), polyarteritis nodosa
- Serum sickness, drug hypersensitivity reaction
- Splenic cysts and benign tumors: hemangioma, lymphangioma
- Thrombosis of splenic or portal vein
- Polycythemia vera, myeloid metaplasia

Splenomegaly and Hepatomegaly[39]

Causes of splenomegaly and hepatosplenomegaly:

MASSIVE SPLENOMEGALY
- Hematologic disease (e.g., chronic myeloid leukemia, myelofibrosis)

MODERATE SPLENOMEGALY
- The above causes
- Portal hypertension
- Hematologic disease (e.g., lymphoma, leukemia, thalassemia)
- Storage disease (e.g., Gaucher's disease)

SMALL SPLENOMEGALY
- The above causes
- Infective (hepatitis, leptospirosis, malaria, bacterial endocarditis)
- Hematologic disease (e.g., hemolytic anemias, essential thrombocythemia, polycythemia rubra vera)
- Connective tissue diseases or vasculitis (e.g., rheumatoid arthritis, systemic lupus erythematosus, polyarteritis nodosa)
- Solitary cyst, polycystic syndrome, hydatid cyst
- Infiltration (amyloid, sarcoid)

HEPATOSPLENOMEGALY
- Chronic liver disease with portal hypertension
- Hematologic disease (e.g., myeloproliferative disease, lymphoma)
- Infection (e.g., acute viral hepatitis, infectious mononucleosis)
- Infiltration (e.g., amyloid, sarcoid)
- Connective tissue disease (e.g., systemic lupus erythematosus)

Splenomegaly, Children[21]

DISORDERS OF THE BLOOD
- Hemolytic anemia: congenital/acquired
- Thalassemia
- Sickle cell disease
- Leukemia
- Osteopetrosis
- Myelofibrosis, myeloid metaplasia, thrombocythemia

INFECTIONS: ACUTE AND CHRONIC
Viral
- Congenital (e.g., TORCH association)
- Mononucleosis (e.g., EBV, CMV infection)
- Virus-associated hemophagocytic syndrome
- Human immunodeficiency virus infection

Bacterial
- Sepsis/abscess
- Brucellosis
- Salmonellosis
- Tularemia
- Tuberculosis
- Subacute bacterial endocarditis
- Syphilis
- Lyme disease

Fungal
- Histoplasmosis (disseminated)

Rickettsia
- Rocky Mountain spotted fever
- Cat-scratch disease

Parasitic
- Toxoplasmosis
- Malaria
- Leishmaniasis (kala-azar)
- Schistosomiasis
- Echinococcosis

HEPATIC/PORTAL SYSTEM DISORDERS
- Acute/chronic active hepatitis
- Cirrhosis, hepatic fibrosis, biliary atresia
- Portal or splenic venous obstruction (Banti's syndrome)

AUTOIMMUNE DISEASE
- Juvenile rheumatoid arthritis
- Systemic lupus erythematosus
- Autoimmune lymphoproliferative syndrome (Canale-Smith syndrome)

NEOPLASMS/CYSTS
- Lymphomas (Hodgkin's and non-Hodgkin's)
- Hemangiomas/lymphangiomas
- Hamartomas
- Congenital or acquired (post-traumatic) cysts

STORAGE DISEASES/INBORN ERRORS OF METABOLISM
- Lipidoses: Gaucher's disease, Niemann-Pick disease, others
- Mucopolysaccharidoses
- Defects in carbohydrate metabolism: galactosemia, fructose intolerance
- Sea-blue histiocyte syndrome

MISCELLANEOUS DISORDERS
- Histiocytoses
- Reactive Langerhans cell
- Malignant sarcoidosis
- Congestive heart failure
- Familial Mediterranean fever

Spontaneous Miscarriage

- Normal pregnancy
- Hydatidiform molar gestation
- Ectopic pregnancy
- Dysfunctional uterine bleeding
- Pathologic endometrial or cervical lesions

Sporotrichosis

FIXED, OR PLAQUE, SPOROTRICHOSIS
- Bacterial pyoderma
- Foreign body granuloma
- Tularemia
- Anthrax
- Other mycoses: blastomycosis, chromoblastomycosis

LYMPHOCUTANEOUS SPOROTRICHOSIS
- *Nocardia brasiliensis*
- *Leishmania braziliensis*
- Atypical mycobacterial disease: *Mycobacterium marinum*, *Mycobacterium kansasii*

PULMONARY SPOROTRICHOSIS

- Pulmonary TB
- Histoplasmosis
- Coccidioidomycoses

OSTEOARTICULAR SPOROTRICHOSIS

- Pigmented villonodular synovitis
- Gout
- Rheumatoid arthritis
- Infection with *M. tuberculosis*
- Atypical mycobacteria: *M. marinum*, *M. kansasii*, *M. avium-intracellulare*

MENINGITIS

- Histoplasmosis
- Cryptococcosis
- TB

Squamous Cell Carcinoma

- Keratoacanthomas
- Actinic keratosis
- Amelanotic melanoma
- Basal cell carcinoma
- Benign tumors
- Healing traumatic wounds
- Spindle cell tumors
- Warts

Staphylococcal Scalded Skin Syndrome (SSSS)

- Erythema multiforme
- Scarlet fever
- Kawasaki's disease
- Toxic epidermal necrolysis
- Graft-versus-host disease

Stasis Dermatitis

- Contact dermatitis
- Atopic dermatitis
- Cellulitis

- Tinea dermatophyte infection
- Pretibial myxedema
- Nummular eczema
- Lichen simplex chronicus
- Xerosis
- Asteatotic eczema
- Deep venous thrombosis (DVT)

Status Epilepticus

- Coma
- Encephalopathic states
- Psychogenic unresponsiveness

Steatohepatitis

- Alcohol abuse
- Obesity
- Diabetes mellitus
- Parenteral nutrition
- Medications (high-dose estrogen, amiodarone, corticosteroids, methotrexate, nifedipine)
- Jejunoileal bypass
- Abetalipoproteinemia
- Wilson's disease, Weber-Christian disease

Stevens-Johnson Syndrome

- Toxic erythema (drugs or infection)
- Pemphigus
- Pemphigoid
- Urticaria
- Hemorrhagic fevers
- Serum sickness
- Staphylococcal scalded skin syndrome
- Behçet's syndrome

Stomatitis, Blistery Lesions

- Primary herpetic gingivostomatitis
- Pemphigus and pemphigoid

- Hand-foot-mouth disease: caused by coxsackievirus group A
- Erythema multiforme
- Herpangina: caused by echovirus
- Traumatic ulcer
- Primary syphilis
- Perlèche (or angular cheilitis)
- Recurrent aphthous stomatitis (canker sores)
- Behçet's syndrome (aphthous ulcers, uveitis, genital ulcerations, arthritis, and aseptic meningitis)
- Reiter's syndrome (conjunctivitis, urethritis, and arthritis with occasional oral ulcerations)

Stomatitis, Bullous

- Erythema multiforme
- Erosive lichen planus
- Bullous pemphigoid
- Systemic lupus erythematosus (SLE)
- Pemphigus vulgaris
- Mucous membrane pemphigoid

Stomatitis, Dark Lesions (Brown, Blue, Black)

- Coated tongue: accumulation of keratin; harmless condition that can be treated by scraping
- Melanotic lesions: freckles, lentigines, lentigo, melanoma, Peutz-Jeghers syndrome, Addison's disease
- Varices
- Kaposi's sarcoma: red or purple macules that enlarge to form tumors; seen in patients with AIDS

Stomatitis, Raised Lesions

- Papilloma
- Verruca vulgaris
- Condyloma acuminatum
- Fibroma
- Epulis
- Pyogenic granuloma

- Mucocele
- Retention cyst

Stomatitis, Red Lesions

- Candidiasis may present with red instead of the more frequent white lesion (see Stomatitis, White Lesions). Median rhomboid glossitis is a chronic variant.
- Benign migratory glossitis (geographic tongue): area of atrophic depapillated mucosa surrounded by a keratotic border; benign lesion, no treatment required
- Hemangiomas
- Histoplasmosis: ill-defined irregular patch with a granulomatous surface, sometimes ulcerated
- Allergy
- Anemia: atrophic reddened glossal mucosa seen with pernicious anemia
- Erythroplakia: red patch usually caused by epithelial dysplasia or squamous cell carcinoma
- Burning tongue (glossopyrosis): normal examination; sometimes associated with denture trauma, anemia, diabetes, vitamin B_{12} deficiency, psychogenic problems

Stomatitis, White Lesions

- Candidiasis (thrush)
- Leukoedema: filmy opalescent-appearing mucosa, which can be reverted to normal appearance by stretching. This condition is benign.
- White sponge nevus: thick, white corrugated folds involving the buccal mucosa; appears in childhood as an autosomal dominant trait; benign condition
- Darier's disease (keratosis follicularis): white papules on the gingivae, alveolar mucosa, and dorsal tongue; skin lesions also present (erythematous papules); inherited as an autosomal dominant trait
- Chemical injury: white sloughing mucosa
- Nicotine stomatitis: whitened palate with red papules
- Lichen planus: linear, reticular, slightly raised striae on buccal mucosa; skin is involved by pruritic violaceous papules on forearms and inner thighs

- Discoid lupus erythematosus: lesion resembles lichen planus
- Leukoplakia: white lesions that cannot be scraped off; 20% are premalignant epithelial dysplasia or squamous cell carcinoma
- Hairy leukoplakia: shaggy white surface that cannot be wiped off; seen in HIV infection, caused by Epstein-Barr virus (EBV)

Strabismus

- Refractive errors
- CNS tumors
- Orbital tumors
- Brain and CNS dysfunction

Striae (Stretch Marks)

- Cushing's disease
- Linear focal elastosis
- Trauma
- Anetoderma
- Cutis laxa
- Focal dermal hypoplasia

Stridor, Pediatric Age[4]

RECURRENT
- Allergic (spasmodic) croup
- Respiratory infections in a child with otherwise asymptomatic anatomic narrowing of the large airways
- Laryngomalacia

PERSISTENT
- Laryngeal obstruction
  - Laryngomalacia
  - Papillomas, other tumors
  - Cysts and laryngoceles
  - Laryngeal webs
  - Bilateral abductor paralysis of the cords
  - Foreign body
- Tracheobronchial disease
  - Tracheomalacia
  - Subglottic tracheal webs

- Endotracheal, endobronchial tumors
- Subglottic tracheal stenosis
- Congenital
- Acquired
- Extrinsic masses
- Mediastinal masses
- Vascular ring
- Lobar emphysema
- Bronchogenic cysts
- Thyroid enlargement
- Esophageal foreign body
- Tracheoesophageal fistulas

OTHER

- Gastroesophageal reflux
- Macroglossia, Pierre Robin syndrome
- Cri du chat syndrome
- Hysterical stridor
- Hypocalcemia

Stroke[37]

- Hypoglycemia
- Drug overdose or intoxication
- Hysterical conversion reaction
- Hyperventilation
- Metabolic encephalopathy
- Migraine
- Syncope
- Transient global amnesia
- Seizures
- Vestibular vertigo

Stroke, Pediatric Age[24]

CARDIAC DISEASE

- Congenital: aortic stenosis, mitral stenosis, mitral prolapse, ventricular septal defects, patent ductus arteriosus, cyanotic congenital heart disease involving right-to-left shunt

- Acquired: endocarditis (bacterial, systemic lupus erythematosus [SLE]), Kawasaki's disease, cardiomyopathy, atrial myxoma, arrhythmia, paradoxical emboli through patent foramen ovale, rheumatic fever, prosthetic heart valve

HEMATOLOGIC ABNORMALITIES
- Hemoglobinopathies: sickle cell disease
- Polycythemia
- Leukemia/lymphoma
- Thrombocytopenia
- Thrombocytosis
- Disorders of coagulation: protein C deficiency, protein S deficiency, factor V Leiden, antithrombin III deficiency, lupus anticoagulant, oral contraceptive pill use, pregnancy and the postpartum state, disseminated intravascular coagulation (DIC), paroxysmal nocturnal hemoglobinuria, inflammatory bowel disease (IBD) (thrombosis)

INFLAMMATORY DISORDERS
- Meningitis: viral, bacterial, tuberculosis
- Systemic infection: viremia, bacteremia, local head and neck infections
- Drug-induced inflammation: amphetamine, cocaine

AUTOIMMUNE DISEASE
- SLE
- Juvenile rheumatoid arthritis (JRA)
- Takayasu's arteritis
- Mixed connective tissue disease
- Polyarteritis nodosum
- Primary CNS vasculitis
- Sarcoidosis
- Behçet's syndrome
- Wegener's granulomatosis

METABOLIC DISEASE ASSOCIATED WITH STROKE
- Homocystinuria
- Pseudoxanthoma elasticum
- Fabry's disease
- Sulfite oxidase deficiency

- Mitochondrial disorders: mitochondrial myopathy, encephalopathy, lactic acidosis, and stroke (MELAS); Leigh syndrome
- Ornithine transcarbamylase deficiency

INTRACEREBRAL VASCULAR PROCESSES
- Ruptured aneurysm
- Arteriovenous malformation
- Fibromuscular dysplasia
- Moyamoya disease
- Migraine headache
- Post subarachnoid hemorrhage vasospasm
- Hereditary hemorrhagic telangiectasia
- Sturge-Weber syndrome
- Carotid artery dissection
- Post varicella

TRAUMA AND OTHER EXTERNAL CAUSES
- Child abuse
- Head trauma/neck trauma
- Oral trauma
- Placental embolism
- Extracorporeal membrane oxygenation (ECMO) therapy

Stroke, Young Adult, Causes[1]

- Cardiac factors (atrial septal defect [ASD], mitral valve prolapse [MVP], patent foramen ovale [PFO])
- Inflammatory factors (systemic lupus erythematosus [SLE], polyarteritis nodosa)
- Infections (endocarditis, neurosyphilis)
- Drugs (cocaine, heroin, oral contraceptives, decongestants)
- Arterial dissection
- Hematologic factors (disseminated intravascular coagulation [DIC], thrombotic thrombocytopenic purpura [TTP]; deficiency of protein S, protein C, antithrombin III)
- Migraine
- Postpartum angiopathy
- Others: premature atherosclerosis, fibromuscular dysplasia

ST-Segment Elevations, Nonischemic

- Early repolarization
- Acute pericarditis
- Left ventricular hypertrophy (LVH)
- Normal pattern variant
- Left bundle branch block [LBBB]
- Pulmonary embolism
- Hyperkalemia
- Post cardioversion

Sturge-Weber Syndrome

- Klippel-Trénaunay-Weber syndrome (extensive capillary angiomas associated with dysplastic veins involving the limbs and trunk, often with hypertrophy of the affected extremity)
- von Hippel–Lindau disease (associated with capillary retinal angiomas, in contrast to cavernous angiomas seen in SWS)

Subarachnoid Hemorrhage

- Intraparenchymal hemorrhage
- Subarachnoid extension of an extracranial arterial dissection or intracerebral hemorrhage
- Meningoencephalitis (e.g., hemorrhagic meningoencephalitis caused by herpes simplex virus [HSV])
- Headache associated with sexual activity (e.g., coital/postcoital headache; usually acute onset of severe headache around time of orgasm)

Subclavian Steal Syndrome

- Posterior circulation transient ischemic attack (TIA) and stroke
- Upper extremity ischemia: distal subclavian artery stenosis/occlusion, Raynaud's syndrome, thoracic outlet syndrome

Subdural Hematoma

- Epidural hematoma
- Subarachnoid hemorrhage

- Mass lesion
- Ischemic stroke
- Intraparenchymal hemorrhage

Sudden Death, Pediatric Age[4]

SUDDEN INFANT DEATH SYNDROME (SIDS) AND SIDS "MIMICS"

- SIDS
- Long QT syndromes
- Inborn errors of metabolism
- Child abuse
- Myocarditis
- Duct-dependent congenital heart disease

CORRECTED OR UNCORRECTED CONGENITAL HEART DISEASE

- Aortic stenosis
- Tetralogy of Fallot
- Transposition of great vessels (postoperative atrial switch)
- Mitral valve prolapse
- Hypoplastic left heart syndrome
- Eisenmenger's syndrome

CORONARY ARTERIAL DISEASE

- Anomalous origin
- Anomalous tract
- Kawasaki's disease
- Periarteritis
- Arterial dissection
- Marfan syndrome
- Myocardial infarction

MYOCARDIAL DISEASE

- Myocarditis
- Hypertrophic cardiomyopathy
- Dilated cardiomyopathy
- Arrhythmogenic right ventricular dysplasia

CONDUCTION SYSTEM ABNORMALITY/ARRHYTHMIA

- Long QT syndromes
- Proarrhythmic drugs

- Preexcitation syndromes
- Heart block
- Commotio cordis
- Idiopathic ventricular fibrillation
- Heart tumor

MISCELLANEOUS
- Pulmonary hypertension
- Pulmonary embolism
- Heat stroke
- Cocaine
- Anorexia nervosa
- Electrolyte disturbances

Sudden Death, Young Athlete

- Hypertrophic cardiomyopathy
- Coronary artery anomalies
- Myocarditis
- Ruptured aortic aneurysm (Marfan syndrome)
- Arrhythmias
- Aortic valve stenosis
- Asthma
- Trauma (cerebral, cardiac)
- Drug and alcohol abuse
- Heat stroke
- Cardiac sarcoidosis
- Atherosclerotic coronary artery disease
- Dilated cardiomyopathy

Swollen Limb

- Trauma
- Insect bite
- Abscess
- Lymphedema
- Thrombophlebitis
- Lipoma
- Neurofibroma
- Postphlebitic syndrome

- Myositis ossificans
- Nephrosis, cirrhosis, congestive heart failure (CHF)
- Hypoalbuminemia
- Varicose veins

Syncope

- Seizure
- Recreational drugs/alcohol
- Psychological stress
- Vertebrobasilar transient ischemic attack (TIA) (usually manifested as diplopia, vertigo, ataxia but not loss of consciousness)

Syndrome of Inappropriate Antidiuresis

- Hyponatremia associated with hypervolemia (congestive heart failure, cirrhosis, nephrotic syndrome)
- Factitious hyponatremia (hyperglycemia, abnormal proteins, hyperlipidemia)
- Hyponatremia associated with hypovolemia (e.g., burns, GI fluid loss)

Syringomyelia

- Amyotrophic lateral sclerosis (ALS)
- Multiple sclerosis (MS)
- Spinal cord tumor
- Tabes dorsalis
- Progressive spinal muscular atrophy

Systemic Lupus Erythematosus

- Other connective tissue disorders (e.g., rheumatoid arthritis [RA], mixed connective tissue disease [MCTD], progressive systemic sclerosis)
- Metastatic neoplasm
- Infection

Tabes Dorsalis

- Vitamin B_{12} deficiency (subacute combined degeneration of the spinal cord)
- Vitamin E deficiency
- Chronic nitrous oxide abuse
- Spinal cord neoplasm (involving conus medullaris)
- Lyme disease

Takayasu's Arteritis

- Giant cell arteritis
- Syphilis
- TB
- Systemic lupus erythematosus (SLE)
- Rheumatoid arthritis (RA)
- Buerger's disease
- Behçet's disease
- Cogan's syndrome
- Kawasaki's disease
- Spondyloarthropathy

Tall Stature[28]

CONSTITUTIONAL (FAMILIAL OR GENETIC)
Most common cause

ENDOCRINE CAUSES
- Growth hormone excess: gigantism
- Sexual precocity (tall as children, short as adults): true sexual precocity, pseudosexual precocity
- Androgen deficiency: Klinefelter's syndrome, bilateral anorchism

GENETIC CAUSES
- Klinefelter's syndrome
- Syndromes of XYY, XXYY

MISCELLANEOUS SYNDROMES AND DISORDERS
- Cerebral gigantism or Sotos syndrome: prominent forehead, hypertelorism, high arched palate, dolichocephaly, mental

retardation, large hands and feet, and premature eruption of teeth; large at birth, with most rapid growth in first 4 years of life
- Marfan syndrome: disorder of mesodermal tissues, subluxation of the lenses, arachnodactyly, aortic aneurysm
- Homocystinuria: same phenotype as Marfan syndrome
- Obesity: tall as infants, children, and adolescents
- Total lipodystrophy: large hands and feet, generalized loss of subcutaneous fat, insulin-resistant diabetes mellitus, hepatomegaly
- Beckwith-Wiedemann syndrome: neonatal tallness, omphalocele, macroglossia, neonatal hypoglycemia
- Weaver-Smith syndrome: excessive intrauterine growth, mental retardation, megalocephaly, widened bifrontal diameter, hypertelorism, large ears, micrognathia, camptodactyly, broad thumbs, limited extension of elbows and knees
- Marshall-Smith syndrome: excessive intrauterine growth, mental retardation, blue sclerae, failure to thrive, early death

Tardive Dyskinesia[13]

- Medications (antidepressants, anticholinergics, amphetamines, lithium, levodopa, phenytoin)
- Brain neoplasms
- Ill-fitting dentures
- Huntington's disease
- Idiopathic dystonias (tics, blepharospasm, aging)
- Wilson's disease
- Extrapyramidal syndrome (postanoxic or postencephalitic)
- Torsion dystonia

Tarsal Tunnel Syndrome

- Plantar fasciitis
- Peripheral neuropathy
- Proximal radiculopathy
- Local tendinitis
- Peripheral vascular disease
- Morton's neuroma

Taste and Smell Loss[1]

TASTE
- Local: radiation therapy
- Systemic: cancer, renal failure, hepatic failure, nutritional deficiency (vitamin B_{12}, zinc), Cushing's syndrome, hypothyroidism, diabetes mellitus (DM), infection (influenza), drugs (antirheumatic and antiproliferative)
- Neurologic: Bell's palsy, familial dysautonomia, multiple sclerosis

SMELL
- Local: allergic rhinitis, sinusitis, nasal polyposis, bronchial asthma
- Systemic: renal failure, hepatic failure, nutritional deficiency (vitamin B_{12}), Cushing's syndrome, hypothyroidism, DM, infection (viral hepatitis, influenza), drugs (nasal sprays, antibiotics)
- Neurologic: head trauma, multiple sclerosis (MS), Parkinson's disease, frontal brain tumor

Telangiectasia

- Oral contraceptive agents
- Pregnancy
- Rosacea
- Varicose veins
- Trauma
- Drug induced (corticosteroids, systemic or topical)
- Spider telangiectases
- Hepatic cirrhosis
- Mastocytosis
- Systemic lupus erythematosus (SLE), dermatomyositis, systemic sclerosis

Tendinopathy[27]

INTRINSIC FACTORS
Anatomic Factors
- Malalignment
- Muscle weakness or imbalance

- Muscle inflexibility
- Decreased vascularity

Systemic Factors
- Inflammatory conditions (e.g., systemic lupus erythematosus [SLE])
- Pregnancy
- Quinolone-induced tendinopathy

Age-Related Factors
- Tendon degeneration
- Increased tendon stiffness
- Tendon calcification
- Decreased vascularity

EXTRINSIC FACTORS
Repetitive Mechanical Load
- Excessive duration
- Excessive frequency
- Excessive intensity
- Poor technique
- Workplace factors

Equipment Problems
- Footwear
- Athletic field surface
- Equipment factors (e.g., racquet size)
- Protective gear

Testicular Failure[10]

PRIMARY
- Klinefelter's syndrome (XXY)
- XYY
- Vanishing testes syndrome (in utero or early postnatal torsion)
- Noonan's syndrome
- Varicocele
- Myotonic dystrophy
- Orchitis (mumps, gonorrhea)
- Cryptorchidism
- Chemical exposure
- Irradiation to testes

- Spinal cord injury
- Polyglandular failure
- Idiopathic oligospermia or azoospermia
- Germinal cell aplasia (Sertoli cell–only syndrome)
- Idiopathic testicular failure
- Testicular torsion
- Testicular trauma
- Diethylstilbestrol (maternal use during pregnancy resulting in estrogen exposure in utero)
- Testicular tumor with subsequent radiation therapy, chemotherapy, or surgery (retroperitoneal lymph node dissection or orchiectomy)

SECONDARY
- Delayed puberty
- Kallmann's syndrome
- Isolated gonadotropin deficiency
- Prader-Labhart-Willi syndrome
- Lawrence-Moon-Biedl syndrome
- CNS irradiation
- Prepubertal panhypopituitarism
- Postpubertal panhypopituitarism
- Hypogonadism secondary to hyperprolactinemia
- Adrenogenital syndrome
- Chronic liver disease
- Chronic renal failure/uremia
- Hemochromatosis
- Cushing's syndrome
- Malnutrition
- Massive obesity
- Sickle cell anemia
- Hyperthyroidism/hypothyroidism
- Anabolic steroid use

Testicular Neoplasm

- Spermatocele
- Varicocele
- Hydrocele
- Epididymitis

- Epidermoid cyst of the testicle
- Epididymis tumors

Testicular Pain

- Testicular torsion
- Trauma
- Epididymitis
- Orchitis
- Neoplasm
- Urolithiasis
- Inguinal hernia
- Infection (cellulitis, abscess, folliculitis)
- Anxiety

Testicular Size Variations[10]

SMALL TESTES
- Normal variant
- Hypothalamic-pituitary dysfunction
- Gonadotropin deficiency
- Growth hormone deficiency
- Primary hypogonadism
- Autoimmune destruction, chemotherapy, cryptorchidism, irradiation, Klinefelter's syndrome, orchitis, testicular regression syndrome, torsion, trauma

LARGE TESTES
- Adrenal rest tissue
- Compensatory
- Fragile X syndrome
- Idiopathic
- Tumor

Testicular Torsion

- Torsion of the testicular appendages
- Testicular tumor
- Epididymitis
- Incarcerated inguinoscrotal hernia

- Orchitis
- Spermatocele
- Hydrocele

Tetanus[27]

- Acute abdomen
- Black widow spider bite
- Dental abscess
- Dislocated mandible
- Dystonic reaction
- Encephalitis
- Head trauma
- Hyperventilation syndrome
- Hypocalcemia
- Meningitis
- Peritonsillar abscess
- Progressive fluctuating muscular rigidity (stiff-man syndrome)
- Psychogenic
- Rabies
- Sepsis
- Subarachnoid hemorrhage
- Status epilepticus
- Strychnine poisoning
- Temporomandibular joint syndrome

Tetralogy of Fallot

- Asthma
- Isolated ventricular septal defect (VSD)
- Pulmonary atresia
- Patent ductus arteriosus
- Aortic stenosis
- Pneumothorax

Thoracic Outlet Syndrome

- Carpal tunnel syndrome
- Cervical radiculopathy
- Brachial neuritis

- Ulnar nerve compression
- Reflex sympathetic dystrophy
- Superior sulcus tumor

Thromboangiitis Obliterans

- Limb ischemia resulting from emboli or atherosclerotic occlusive disease
- Antiphospholipid antibody syndrome
- Autoimmune disorders
- Acrocyanosis
- Carpal tunnel syndrome
- CREST (calcinosis cutis, Raynaud's phenomenon, esophageal motility disorder, sclerodactyly, and telangiectasia) syndrome
- Systemic lupus erythematosus
- Diabetes mellitus
- Repetitive vibratory equipment use
- Hypothenar hammer syndrome
- Raynaud's phenomenon
- Ergotamine intoxication
- Polyarteritis nodosa
- Cannabis arteritis
- Peripheral neuropathy

Thrombocytopenia

INCREASED DESTRUCTION
Immunologic

- Drugs: quinine, quinidine, digitalis, procainamide, thiazide diuretics, sulfonamides, phenytoin, aspirin, penicillin, heparin, gold, meprobamate, sulfa drugs, phenylbutazone, nonsteroidal anti-inflammatory drugs (NSAIDs), methyldopa, cimetidine, furosemide, isoniazid (INH), cephalosporins, chlorpropamide, organic arsenicals, chloroquine, platelet glycoprotein IIb/IIIa receptor inhibitors, ranitidine, indomethacin, carboplatin, ticlopidine, clopidogrel
- Idiopathic thrombocytopenic purpura (ITP)
- Transfusion reaction: transfusion of platelets with plasminogen activator (PLA) in recipients without PLA-1
- Fetal/maternal incompatibility

- Collagen-vascular diseases (e.g., systemic lupus erythematosus [SLE])
- Autoimmune hemolytic anemia
- Lymphoreticular disorders (e.g., chronic lymphocytic leukemia [CLL])

Nonimmunologic
- Prosthetic heart valves
- Thrombotic thrombocytopenic purpura (TTP)
- Sepsis
- Disseminated intravascular coagulation (DIC)
- Hemolytic-uremic syndrome (HUS)
- Giant cavernous hemangioma

DECREASED PRODUCTION
- Abnormal marrow
- Marrow infiltration (e.g., leukemia, lymphoma, fibrosis)
- Marrow suppression (e.g., chemotherapy, alcohol, irradiation)
- Hereditary disorders
  - Wiskott-Aldrich syndrome: X-linked disorder characterized by thrombocytopenia, eczema, and repeated infections
  - May-Hegglin anomaly: increased megakaryocytes but ineffective thrombopoiesis
- Vitamin deficiencies (e.g., vitamin B_{12}, folic acid)

HYPERSPLENISM; SPLENIC SEQUESTRATION; DILUTIONAL, AS A RESULT OF MASSIVE TRANSFUSION

Thrombocytopenia, Inherited Disorders[21]

- Amegakaryocytic thrombocytopenia
- Thrombocytopenia absent radii
- *MYH9*-related thrombocytopenia
- May-Hegglin anomaly
- Fechtner syndrome
- Epstein syndrome
- Sebastian syndrome
- X-linked macrothrombocytopenia
- Wiskott-Aldrich syndrome
- X-linked thrombocytopenia
- Thrombocytopenia and radioulnar synostosis

- Familial platelet disorder–AML
- Familial dominant thrombocytopenia
- Paris-Trousseau thrombocytopenia
- Bernard-Soulier syndrome
- Bernard-Soulier carrier/Mediterranean
- Macrothrombocytopenia

Thrombocytopenia, in Pregnancy[21]

- Incidental thrombocytopenia of pregnancy (gestational thrombocytopenia)
- Preeclampsia/eclampsia
- Disseminated intravascular coagulation (DIC) secondary to
  - Abruptio placentae
  - Endometritis
  - Amniotic fluid embolism
  - Retained fetus
  - Preeclampsia/eclampsia*
  - Peripartum/postpartum thrombotic microangiopathy
  - Thrombotic thrombocytopenic purpura
  - Hemolytic-uremic syndrome

Thrombocytosis

- Iron deficiency
- Post hemorrhage
- Neoplasms (GI tract)
- Cell-mediated lympholysis (CML)
- Polycythemia vera
- Myelofibrosis with myeloid metaplasia
- Infections
- After splenectomy
- Postpartum
- Hemophilia
- Pancreatitis
- Cirrhosis
- Idiopathic

---

*Preeclampsia/eclampsia is usually not associated with overt DIC.

Thrombophlebitis, Superficial

- Lymphangitis
- Cellulitis
- Erythema nodosum
- Panniculitis
- Kaposi's sarcoma

Thrombosis, Deep Venous

- Postphlebitic syndrome
- Superficial thrombophlebitis
- Ruptured Baker's cyst
- Cellulitis, lymphangitis, Achilles tendinitis
- Hematoma
- Muscle or soft tissue injury, stress fracture
- Varicose veins, lymphedema
- Arterial insufficiency
- Abscess
- Claudication
- Venous stasis

Thrombotic Thrombocytopenic Purpura

- Disseminated intravascular coagulation (DIC)
- Malignant hypertension
- Vasculitis
- Eclampsia or preeclampsia
- Hemolytic-uremic syndrome (typically encountered in children, often after a viral infection)
- Gastroenteritis as a result of a serotoxin-producing serotype of *Escherichia coli*
- Medications: clopidogrel, ticlopidine, penicillin, antineoplastic chemotherapeutic agents, oral contraceptives

Thyroid Carcinoma

- Multinodular goiter
- Lymphocytic thyroiditis
- Ectopic thyroid

- Thyroglossal duct cyst
- Epidermoid cyst
- Laryngocele
- Nonthyroid neck neoplasm
- Branchial cleft cyst
- Benign thyroid cyst

Thyroid Nodule

- Thyroid carcinoma
- Multinodular goiter
- Thyroglossal duct cyst
- Epidermoid cyst
- Laryngocele
- Nonthyroid neck neoplasm
- Branchial cleft cyst

Thyroid Storm

- Psychiatric disorders
- Alcohol or other drug withdrawal
- Pheochromocytoma
- Metastatic neoplasm

Thyroiditis

- The hyperthyroid phase of Hashimoto's, subacute, or silent thyroiditis can be mistaken for Graves' disease.
- Riedel's thyroiditis can be mistaken for carcinoma of the thyroid.
- Painful subacute thyroiditis can be mistaken for infections of the oropharynx and trachea or for suppurative thyroiditis.
- Factitious hyperthyroidism can mimic silent thyroiditis.

Thyromegaly

- Goiter
- Graves' disease
- Thyroiditis (lymphocytic, granulomatous, suppurative)
- Toxic adenoma
- Neoplasm (primary, metastatic)

Tick-Related Infections

- Lyme disease
- Rocky Mountain spotted fever
- Babesiosis
- Tularemia
- Q fever
- Colorado tick fever
- Ehrlichiosis
- Relapsing fever

Tics

- Tourette's syndrome
- Physiologic tic
- Anxiety disorder
- Huntington's disease
- Medications (e.g., antipsychotics, carbamazepine, phenytoin, phenobarbital)
- Encephalitis
- Head trauma
- Schizophrenia
- Carbon monoxide poisoning
- Stroke
- Sydenham's chorea
- Creutzfeldt-Jakob disease

Tinea Barbae and Tinea Faciei

- Folliculitis
- Furunculosis
- Actinomycosis
- Acne

Tinea Capitis

- Alopecia areata
- Impetigo
- Pediculosis
- Trichotillomania

- Traction alopecia
- Folliculitis
- Pseudopelade
- Seborrhea/atopic
- Dermatitis
- Psoriasis
- Carbuncles
- Pyoderma
- Lichen ruber planus
- Lupus erythematosus

Tinea Corporis

- Pityriasis rosea
- Erythema multiforme
- Psoriasis
- Systemic lupus erythematosus (SLE)
- Syphilis
- Nummular eczema
- Eczema
- Granuloma annulare
- Lyme disease
- Tinea versicolor
- Contact dermatitis

Tinea Cruris

- Intertrigo
- Psoriasis
- Seborrheic dermatitis
- Erythrasma
- Candidiasis
- Tinea versicolor

Tinea Pedis

- Contact dermatitis
- Toe web infection
- Eczema
- Psoriasis

- Keratolysis exfoliativa
- Juvenile plantar dermatosis

Tinea Versicolor (Pityriasis Versicolor)

- Vitiligo
- Pityriasis alba
- Secondary syphilis
- Pityriasis rosea
- Seborrheic dermatitis

Tinnitus

- Pulsatile sounds: carotid stenosis, aortic valve disease, high cardiac output, arteriovenous malformations
- Muscular sounds: palatal myoclonus, spasm of stapedius or tensor tympani muscle
- Spontaneous autoacoustic emissions
- Auditory hallucinations
- Anxiety disorder

Torsades de Pointes[23]

- Antiarrhythmics known to increase the QT interval (e.g., quinidine, procainamide, amiodarone, disopyramide, sotalol)
- Tricyclic antidepressants and phenothiazines
- Histamine (H_1) antagonists (e.g., astemizole, terfenadine)
- Antiviral and antifungal agents and antibiotics
- Hypokalemia
- Hypomagnesemia
- Insecticide poisoning
- Bradyarrhythmias
- Congenital long QT syndrome
- Subarachnoid hemorrhage
- Chloroquine, pentamidine
- Cocaine abuse

Tourette's Syndrome

- Sydenham's chorea: occurs after infection with group A streptococcus

- Pediatric autoimmune neuropsychiatric disorder associated with streptococcal infection (PANDAS)
- Sporadic tic disorders: these tend to be motor or vocal but not both.
- Head trauma
- Drug intoxication: many drugs are known to induce or to exacerbate tic disorder, including methylphenidate, amphetamines, pemoline, anticholinergics, and antihistamines.
- Postinfectious encephalitis
- Inherited disorders: these include Huntington's disease, Hallervorden-Spatz disease, and neuroacanthocytosis. All of these should have other abnormalities on neurologic examination.

Toxic Epidermal Necrolysis

- Toxic erythema (drugs or infection)
- Pemphigus
- Pemphigoid
- Urticaria
- Hemorrhagic fevers
- Serum sickness
- Staphylococcal scalded skin syndrome
- Behçet's syndrome

Toxic Shock Syndrome

- Staphylococcal food poisoning
- Septic shock
- Mucocutaneous lymph node syndrome
- Scarlet fever
- Rocky Mountain spotted fever
- Meningococcemia
- Toxic epidermal necrolysis
- Kawasaki's disease
- Leptospirosis
- Legionnaires' disease
- Hemolytic-uremic syndrome
- Stevens-Johnson syndrome
- Scalded skin syndrome
- Erythema multiforme
- Acute rheumatic fever

Toxoplasmosis

LYMPHADENOPATHY
* Infectious mononucleosis
* Cytomegalovirus (CMV) mononucleosis
* Cat-scratch disease
* Sarcoidosis
* Tuberculosis
* Lymphoma
* Metastatic cancer

CEREBRAL MASS LESIONS IN IMMUNOCOMPROMISED HOST
* Lymphoma
* Tuberculosis
* Bacterial abscess

PNEUMONITIS IN IMMUNOCOMPROMISED HOST
* *Pneumocystis jiroveci* pneumonia
* Tuberculosis
* Fungal infection

CHORIORETINITIS
* Syphilis
* Tuberculosis
* Histoplasmosis (competent host)
* CMV
* Syphilis
* Herpes simplex
* Fungal infection
* TB (AIDS patient)

MYOCARDITIS
* Organ rejection in heart transplant recipients

CONGENITAL INFECTION
* Rubella
* CMV
* Herpes simplex
* Syphilis
* Listeriosis
* Erythroblastosis fetalis
* Sepsis

Tracheitis

- Viral croup
- Epiglottitis
- Diphtheria
- Necrotizing herpes simplex infection in the elderly
- Cytomegalovirus (CMV) in immunocompromised patients
- Invasive aspergillosis in immunocompromised patients
- Transient ischemic attack (TIA)
- Hypoglycemia
- Seizures
- Migraine
- Subdural hemorrhage
- Mass lesions
- Vestibular disease

Tremor

TREMOR PRESENT AT REST
- Parkinsonism
- CNS neoplasms
- Tardive dyskinesia

POSTURAL TREMOR (PRESENT DURING
MAINTENANCE OF A POSTURE)
- Essential senile tremor

ACTION TREMOR (PRESENT WITH MOVEMENT)
- Anxiety
- Medications (e.g., bronchodilators, caffeine, corticosteroids, lithium)
- Endocrine disorders (hyperthyroidism, pheochromocytoma, carcinoid)
- Withdrawal from substance abuse

Trichinosis

- Early illness may resemble gastroenteritis.
- Later symptoms may be confused with measles, dermatomyositis, or glomerulonephritis.

Trichotillomania

* Iron deficiency
* Malnutrition
* Hypothyroidism
* Telogen effluvium
* Traction alopecia
* Alopecia areata
* Anagen effluvium
* Tinea capitis

Tricuspid Stenosis

* Congenital tricuspid atresia
* Endomyocardial fibrosis
* Right atrial thrombi
* Constrictive pericarditis

Trigger Finger

* Dupuytren's contracture
* de Quervain's tenosynovitis
* Acute digital tenosynovitis
* Proliferative tenosynovitis
* Carpal tunnel syndrome
* Flexion tendon rupture
* Trauma

Trochanteric Bursitis

* Osteoarthritis of the hip
* Osteonecrosis of the hip
* Stress fracture of the hip
* Osteoarthritis of the lumbar spine
* Fibromyalgia
* Iliopsoas bursitis
* Trochanteric tendinitis
* Gout
* Pseudogout

- Trauma
- Neuropathy

Tropical Sprue

- Celiac disease
- Parasitic infestation
- Inflammatory bowel disease (IBD)
- Other causes of malabsorption (e.g., Whipple's disease)

Tuberculosis, Miliary

- Widespread sites of possible dissemination associated with myriad differential diagnostic possibilities
- Lymphoma
- Typhoid fever
- Brucellosis
- Neoplasms
- Collagen-vascular disease

Tuberculosis, Pulmonary

- Necrotizing pneumonia (anaerobic, gram-negative)
- Histoplasmosis
- Coccidioidomycosis
- Melioidosis
- Interstitial lung diseases (rarely)
- Cancer
- Sarcoidosis
- Silicosis
- Paragonimiasis
- Rare pneumonias: *Rhodococcus equi* (cavitation), *Bacillus cereus* (50% hemoptysis), *Eikenella corrodens* (cavitation)

Tubulointerstitial Disease, Acute[14]

DRUGS
- Antibiotics, penicillins, cephalosporins, rifampin
- Sulfonamides: cotrimoxazole, sulfamethoxazole

- Nonsteroidal anti-inflammatory drugs (NSAIDs): propionic acid derivatives
- Miscellaneous: phenytoin, thiazides, allopurinol, cimetidine, ifosfamide

INFECTIONS
- Invasion of renal parenchyma
- Reaction to systemic infections: streptococcal, diphtheria, hantavirus

SYSTEMIC DISEASES
- Immune mediated: lupus, transplanted kidney, cryoglobulinemias

METABOLIC
- Urate, oxalate

NEOPLASTIC
- Lymphoproliferative diseases

IDIOPATHIC

Tubulointerstitial Kidney Disease[14]

- Ischemic and toxic acute tubular necrosis
- Allergic interstitial nephritis
- Interstitial nephritis secondary to immune complex–related collagen-vascular disease (e.g., systemic lupus erythematosus [SLE], Sjögren's syndrome)
- Granulomatous diseases (sarcoidosis, uveitis)
- Pigment-related tubular injury (myoglobinuria, hemoglobinuria)
- Hypercalcemia with nephrocalcinosis
- Tubular obstruction (drugs such as indinavir, uric acid in tumor lysis syndrome)
- Myeloma kidney or cast nephropathy
- Infection-related interstitial nephritis: *Legionella*, *Leptospira*
- Infiltrative diseases (e.g., lymphoma)

Tularemia

- Rickettsial infections
- Meningococcal infections

- Cat-scratch disease
- Infectious mononucleosis
- Atypical pneumonia
- Group A streptococcal pharyngitis
- Typhoid fever
- Fungal infection: sporotrichosis
- Anthrax
- Bacterial skin infections

Tumor Markers Elevation[39]

Causes of elevated levels of tumor markers:

CARCINOEMBRYONIC ANTIGEN (CEA)
- Colonic cancer (higher levels if the tumor is more differentiated or is extensive or has spread to the liver)
- Lung or breast cancer; seminoma
- Cigarette smokers
- Cirrhosis, inflammatory bowel disease, rectal polyps, pancreatitis
- Advanced age

ALPHA-FETOPROTEIN
- Hepatocellular cancer: very high titers or a rising titer is strongly suggestive, but >10% of patients do not have an elevated level
- Hepatic regeneration (e.g., cirrhosis, alcoholic or viral hepatitis)
- Cancer of the stomach, colon, pancreas, or lung
- Teratocarcinoma or embryonal cell carcinoma (testis, ovary, extragonadal)
- Pregnancy
- Ataxia-telangiectasia
- Normal variant

PROSTATE-SPECIFIC ANTIGEN
- Prostate carcinoma (localized disease)
- Prostatic hyperplasia
- Prostatitis
- Prostatitic infarction

CANCER-ASSOCIATED ANTIGEN (CA19-9)*
- Pancreatic carcinoma (80% with advanced, well-differentiated cancer have an elevated level)
- Other gastrointestinal cancers: colon, stomach, bile duct
- Acute or chronic pancreatitis
- Chronic liver disease
- Biliary tract disease

Turner's Syndrome

- Noonan's syndrome, an autosomally dominant inherited disorder also characterized by loose nuchal skin, midface hypoplasia, canthal folds, and stenotic cardiac valvular defects and affecting males and females equally; also have normal chromosome constitutions
- Other conditions in the differential diagnosis of loose skin, whether or not associated with edema:
  - Fetal hydantoin syndrome (loose nuchal skin, midface hypoplasia, distal digital hypoplasia)
  - Disorders of chromosome constitution (trisomy 21, tetrasomy 12p mosaicism)
  - Congenital lymphedema (Milroy's edema)

Typhoid Fever

- Malaria
- TB
- Brucellosis
- Amebic liver abscess

Ulcerative Colitis

- Crohn's disease
- Bacterial infections
- Acute: *Campylobacter, Yersinia, Salmonella, Shigella, Chlamydia, Escherichia coli, Clostridium difficile*, gonococcal proctitis

---

*Patients who cannot synthesize Lewis blood group antigens (~5% of the population) do not produce CA19-9 antigen.

- Chronic: Whipple's disease, TB, enterocolitis
- Irritable bowel syndrome
- Protozoal and parasitic infections (amebiasis, giardiasis, cryptosporidiosis)
- Neoplasm (intestinal lymphoma, carcinoma of colon)
- Ischemic bowel disease
- Diverticulitis
- Celiac sprue, collagenous colitis, irradiation enteritis, endometriosis, gay bowel syndrome

Urethral Discharge and Dysuria

- Urethritis (gonococcal, chlamydial, trichomonal)
- Cystitis
- Prostatitis
- Vaginitis (candidiasis, chemical)
- Meatal stenosis
- Interstitial cystitis
- Trauma (foreign body, masturbation, horseback or bike riding)

Urethritis, Gonococcal

- Nongonococcal urethritis
- Herpes simplex virus

Urethritis, Nongonococcal

- Gonococcal urethritis
- Herpes simplex virus
- Trichomoniasis

Uric Acid Stones

- Hyperuricemia
- Excessive dietary purine
- Medications (salicylates, allopurinol, probenecid)
- Urine pH < 5.5 (e.g., diarrhea, high animal protein diet)
- Decreased urine output (dehydration, malabsorption, diarrhea, inadequate fluid intake)
- Tumor lysis

- Hemolytic anemia
- Myeloproliferative disorders

Urinary Retention, Acute

- Mechanical obstruction: urethral stone, foreign body, urethral stricture, benign prostatic hyperplasia (BPH), prostate carcinoma, prostatitis, trauma with hematoma formation)
- Neurogenic bladder
- Neurologic disease (multiple sclerosis [MS], parkinsonism, tabes dorsalis, cerebrovascular accident [CVA])
- Spinal cord injury
- CNS neoplasm (primary or metastatic)
- Spinal anesthesia
- Lower urinary tract instrumentation
- Medications (antihistamines, antidepressants, narcotics, anticholinergics)
- Abdominal or pelvic surgery
- Alcohol toxicity
- Pregnancy
- Anxiety
- Encephalitis
- Postoperative pain
- Spina bifida occulta

Urinary Tract Infection

- Interstitial cystitis
- Vaginitis
- Urethritis (gonococcal, nongonococcal, *Trichomonas*)
- Frequency-urgency syndrome, prostatitis (acute and chronic)
- Obstructive uropathy
- Infected stones
- Fistulas
- Papillary necrosis
- Vesicoureteral reflux

Urine Casts

- Normal finding
- Pyelonephritis

- Chronic renal disease
- Nephrotic syndrome
- Acute tubular necrosis
- Interstitial nephritis
- Nephritic syndrome
- Glomerulonephritis
- Eclampsia
- Heavy metal ingestion
- Allograft rejection
- Hypothyroidism

Urine, Red[30]

WITH A POSITIVE DIPSTICK
- Hematuria
- Hemoglobinuria: negative urinalysis
- Myoglobinuria: negative urinalysis

WITH A NEGATIVE DIPSTICK
Drugs
- Aminosalicylic acid
- Deferoxamine mesylate
- Ibuprofen
- Phenacetin
- Phenolphthalein
- Phensuximide
- Rifampin
- Anthraquinone laxatives
- Doxorubicin
- Methyldopa
- Phenazopyridine
- Phenothiazine
- Phenytoin

Dyes
- Azo dyes
- Eosin

Foods
- Beets, berries, maize
- Rhodamine B

Metabolic
- Porphyrins
- *Serratia marcescens* (red diaper syndrome)
- Urate crystalluria

Urolithiasis

- Urinary tract infection
- Pyelonephritis
- Diverticulitis
- Pelvic inflammatory disease (PID)
- Ovarian pathology
- Factitious (drug addicts)
- Appendicitis
- Small bowel obstruction
- Ectopic pregnancy

Uropathy, Obstructive[37]

INTRINSIC CAUSES
- Intraluminal: intratubular deposition of crystals (uric acid, sulfas), stones, papillary tissue, blood clots
- Intramural
- Functional: ureter (ureteropelvic or ureterovesical dysfunction); bladder (neurogenic): spinal cord defect or trauma, diabetes, multiple sclerosis (MS), Parkinson's disease, cerebrovascular accidents (CVA), bladder neck dysfunction
- Anatomic: tumors, infection, granuloma, strictures

EXTRINSIC CAUSES
- Originating in the reproductive system
  - Prostate: benign hypertrophy or cancer
  - Uterus: pregnancy, tumors, prolapse, endometriosis
  - Ovary: abscess, tumor, cysts
- Originating in the vascular system: aneurysms (aorta, iliac vessels), aberrant arteries (ureteropelvic junction), venous (ovarian veins, retrocaval ureter)
- Originating in the gastrointestinal tract: Crohn's disease, pancreatitis, appendicitis, tumors
- Originating in the retroperitoneal space: inflammations, fibrosis, tumor, hematomas

Urticaria (Hives)

- Erythema multiforme
- Erythema marginatum
- Erythema infectiosum
- Urticarial vasculitis
- Herpes gestationis
- Drug eruption
- Multiple insect bites
- Bullous pemphigoid

Uterine Bleeding, Abnormal[12]

PREGNANCY

- Threatened abortion
- Incomplete abortion
- Complete abortion
- Molar pregnancy
- Ectopic pregnancy
- Retained products of conception

OVULATORY

- Vulva: infection, laceration, tumor
- Vagina: infection, laceration, tumor, foreign body
- Cervix: polyps, cervical erosion, cervicitis, carcinoma
- Uterus: fibroids (submucous fibroids most likely to cause abnormal bleeding), polyps, adenomyosis, endometritis, intrauterine device, atrophic endometrium
- Pregnancy complications: ectopic pregnancy; threatened, incomplete, complete abortion; retained products of conception
- Abnormality of clotting system
- Midcycle bleeding
- Halban's disease (persistent corpus luteum)
- Menorrhagia
- Pelvic inflammatory disease (PID)

ANOVULATORY

- Physiologic causes
  - Puberty
  - Perimenopausal

- Pathologic causes
  - Ovarian failure (follicle-stimulating hormone [FSH] >40 IU/ml)
  - Hyperandrogenism
  - Hyperprolactinemia
  - Obesity
  - Hypothalamic dysfunction (polycystic ovaries); luteinizing hormone (LH)/FSH ratio >2 : 1
  - Hyperplasia
  - Endometrial carcinoma
  - Estrogen-producing tumors
  - Hypothyroidism

Uterine Myoma

- Leiomyosarcoma
- Ovarian mass (neoplastic, non-neoplastic, endometrioma)
- Inflammatory mass
- Pregnancy

Uveitis

- Glaucoma
- Conjunctivitis
- Retinal detachment
- Retinopathy
- Keratitis
- Scleritis
- Episcleritis

Vaginal Bleeding

ANY GESTATIONAL AGE
- Cervical lesions: polyps, decidual reaction, neoplasia
- Vaginal trauma
- Cervicitis/vulvovaginitis
- Postcoital trauma
- Bleeding dyscrasias

GESTATION <20 WEEKS
- Spontaneous abortion
- Presence of intrauterine device
- Ectopic pregnancy
- Molar pregnancy
- Implantation bleeding
- Low-lying placenta

GESTATION >20 WEEKS
- Molar pregnancy
- Placenta previa
- Placental abruption
- Vasa previa
- Marginal separation of the placenta
- Bloody show at term
- Preterm labor

Vaginal Bleeding, Pregnancy[7]

FIRST TRIMESTER
- Implantation bleeding
- Abortion
  - Threatened
  - Complete
  - Incomplete
  - Missed
- Ectopic pregnancy
- Neoplasia
- Hydatidiform mole
- Cervix

THIRD TRIMESTER
- Placenta previa
- Placental abruption
- Premature labor
- Choriocarcinoma

Vaginal Discharge, Prepubertal Girls[20]

- Irritative (bubble baths, sand)
- Poor perineal hygiene

- Foreign body
- Associated systemic illness (group A streptococci, chickenpox)
- Infections
  - *Escherichia coli* with foreign body
  - *Shigella* organisms
  - *Yersinia* organisms
- Infections (consider sexual abuse)
  - *Chlamydia trachomatis*
  - *Neisseria gonorrhoeae*
  - *Trichomonas vaginalis*
- Tumor (rare)

Varicocele

- Hydrocele
- Spermatocele
- Epididymal orchitis
- Testicular tumor

Varicose Veins

CONDITIONS THAT CAN LEAD TO SUPERFICIAL VENOUS STASIS OTHER THAN PRIMARY VALVULAR INSUFFICIENCY
- Arterial occlusive disease
- Diabetes
- Deep vein thrombophlebitis
- Peripheral neuropathies
- Unusual infections
- Carcinoma

Vasculitis, Classification[27]

LARGE-VESSEL DISEASE
Arteritis
- Giant cell arteritis
- Takayasu's arteritis
- Arteritis associated with Reiter's syndrome, ankylosing spondylitis

MEDIUM- AND SMALL-VESSEL DISEASE

Polyarteritis Nodosa

- Primary (idiopathic)
- Associated with viruses (hepatitis B or C, cytomegalovirus [CMV], HIV, herpes zoster)
- Associated with malignant disease (hairy cell leukemia)
- Familial Mediterranean fever

Granulomatous Vasculitis

- Wegener's granulomatosis
- Lymphomatoid granulomatosis
- Behçet's syndrome
- Kawasaki's disease (mucocutaneous lymph node syndrome)

PREDOMINANTLY SMALL-VESSEL DISEASE

Hypersensitivity Vasculitis (Leukocytoclastic Vasculitis)

- Henoch-Schönlein purpura
- Mixed cryoglobulinemia
- Serum sickness
- Vasculitis associated with connective tissue diseases (systemic lupus erythematosus [SLE], Sjögren's syndrome)
- Vasculitis associated with specific syndromes: primary biliary cirrhosis, Lyme disease, chronic active hepatitis, drug-induced vasculitis
- Churg-Strauss syndrome
- Goodpasture's syndrome
- Erythema nodosum
- Panniculitis
- Buerger's disease (thrombophlebitis obliterans)

Vasculitis, Diseases That Mimic Vasculitis[29]

EMBOLIC DISEASE

- Infectious or marantic endocarditis
- Cardiac mural thrombus
- Atrial myxoma
- Cholesterol embolization syndrome

NONINFLAMMATORY VESSEL WALL DISRUPTION

- Atherosclerosis
- Arterial fibromuscular dysplasia

- Drug effects (vasoconstrictors, anticoagulants)
- Irradiation
- Genetic disease (neurofibromatosis, Ehlers-Danlos syndrome)
- Amyloidosis
- Intravascular malignant lymphoma

DIFFUSE COAGULATION
- Disseminated intravascular coagulation (DIC)
- Thrombotic thrombocytopenic purpura
- Hemolytic-uremic syndrome
- Protein C and S deficiencies, factor V Leiden mutation
- Antiphospholipid syndrome

Venous Lake

- Hemangioma
- Melanoma
- Blue nevus
- Angiokeratoma
- Melanosis of buccal mucosa

Venous Leg Ulcers

- Peripheral arterial disease (with ischemia and necrosis)
- Diabetic ulceration (often secondary to neuropathy)
- Decubitus ulceration (due to pressure over a bone prominence)
- Vasculitis (with erythema and bullae)
- Necrotic ulceration from infection
- Basal cell carcinoma or squamous cell carcinoma

Ventricular Failure

LEFT VENTRICULAR FAILURE
- Systemic hypertension
- Valvular heart disease (aortic stenosis [AS], atrial regurgitation [AR], mitral regurgitation [MR])
- Cardiomyopathy, myocarditis
- Bacterial endocarditis
- Myocardial infarction
- Idiopathic hypertrophic subaortic stenosis

RIGHT VENTRICULAR FAILURE
- Valvular heart disease (mitral stenosis)
- Pulmonary hypertension
- Bacterial endocarditis (right sided)
- Right ventricular infarction

BIVENTRICULAR FAILURE
- Left ventricular failure
- Cardiomyopathy
- Myocarditis
- Arrhythmias
- Anemia
- Thyrotoxicosis
- Arteriovenous fistula
- Paget's disease
- Beriberi

Ventricular Septal Defect

OTHER CAUSES OF SYSTOLIC MURMURS
- Mitral regurgitation
- Aortic stenosis
- Asymmetric septal hypertrophy
- Pulmonary stenosis

Vertebral Compression Fractures

- Hyperparathyroidism
- Osteomalacia
- Granulomatous diseases (e.g., tuberculosis)
- Hematologic/oncologic diseases (e.g., multiple myeloma, malignant neoplasm)

Vertigo

PERIPHERAL
- Otitis media
- Acute labyrinthitis
- Vestibular neuronitis
- Benign positional vertigo

- Meniere's disease
- Ototoxic drugs: streptomycin, gentamicin
- Lesions of the eighth nerve: acoustic neuroma, meningioma, mononeuropathy, metastatic carcinoma
- Mastoiditis

CNS OR SYSTEMIC
- Vertebrobasilar artery insufficiency
- Posterior fossa tumor or other brain tumors
- Infarction/hemorrhage of cerebral cortex, cerebellum, or brainstem
- Basilar migraine
- Metabolic: drugs, hypoxia, anemia, fever
- Hypotension/severe hypertension
- Multiple sclerosis (MS)
- CNS infections: viral, bacterial
- Temporal lobe epilepsy
- Arnold-Chiari malformation, syringobulbia
- Psychogenic: ventilation, hysteria

Vesiculobullous Diseases[14]

- Immunologically mediated diseases
  - Bullous pemphigoid
  - Herpes gestationis
  - Mucous membrane pemphigoid
  - Epidermolysis bullosa acquisita
  - Dermatitis herpetiformis
  - Pemphigus (vulgaris, foliaceus, paraneoplastic)
- Hypersensitivity diseases
  - Erythema multiforme minor
  - Erythema multiforme major (Stevens-Johnson syndrome)
  - Toxic epidermal necrolysis
- Metabolic diseases
  - Porphyria cutanea tarda
  - Pseudoporphyria
  - Diabetic blisters
- Inherited genetic disorders
  - Epidermolysis bullosa: simplex, junctional, dystrophic
- Infectious diseases

- Impetigo
- Staphylococcal scalded skin syndrome
- Herpes simplex
- Varicella
- Herpes zoster

Vesiculopustules, Newborn Infants[16]

- Congenital cutaneous candidiasis
- Congenital herpes simplex
- Erythema toxicum neonatorum
- Genodermatosis
- Impetigo
- Miliaria
- Scabies
- Syphilis
- Transient neonatal pustulosis

Vestibular Neuronitis

- Labyrinthitis: similar cause but includes hearing loss
- Labyrinthine infarction
- Perilymph fistula
- Brainstem and cerebellar infarction
- Migraine-associated vertigo
- Multiple sclerosis

Vision Loss, Acute, Painful

- Acute angle-closure glaucoma
- Corneal ulcer
- Uveitis
- Endophthalmitis
- Factitious
- Somatization syndrome
- Trauma

Vision Loss, Acute, Painless

- Retinal artery occlusion
- Optic neuritis

- Retinal vein occlusion
- Vitreous hemorrhage
- Retinal detachment
- Exudative macular degeneration
- Cerebrovascular accident (CVA)
- Ischemic optic neuropathy
- Factitious
- Somatization syndrome, anxiety reaction

Vision Loss, Chronic, Progressive

- Cataract
- Macular degeneration
- Cerebral neoplasm
- Refractive error
- Open-angle glaucoma

Vision Loss, Monocular, Transient

- Thromboembolism
- Vasculitis
- Migraine (vasospasm)
- Anxiety reaction
- CNS tumor
- Temporal arteritis
- Multiple sclerosis (MS)

Vitiligo

ACQUIRED
- Chemical induced
- Halo nevus
- Idiopathic guttate hypomelanosis
- Leprosy
- Leukoderma associated with melanoma
- Pityriasis alba
- Postinflammatory hypopigmentation
- Tinea versicolor
- Vogt-Koyanagi syndrome (vitiligo, uveitis, deafness)

CONGENITAL
* Albinism, partial (piebaldism)
* Albinism, total
* Nevus anemicus
* Nevus depigmentosus
* Tuberous sclerosis

Vocal Cord Paralysis

* Neoplasm: primary or metastatic (e.g., lung, thyroid, parathyroid, mediastinum)
* Neck surgery (parathyroid, thyroid, carotid endarterectomy, cervical spine)
* Idiopathic
* Viral, bacterial, or fungal infection
* Trauma (intubation, penetrating neck injury)
* Cardiac surgery
* Rheumatoid arthritis
* Multiple sclerosis (MS)
* Parkinsonism
* Toxic neuropathy
* Cerebrovascular accident (CVA)
* CNS abnormalities: hydrocephalus, Arnold-Chiari malformation, meningomyelocele

Volume Depletion[1]

* Gastrointestinal losses
  * Upper: bleeding, nasogastric suction, vomiting
  * Lower: bleeding, diarrhea, enteric or pancreatic fistula, tube drainage
* Renal losses
  * Salt and water: diuretics, osmotic diuresis, postobstructive diuresis, acute tubular necrosis (recovery phase), salt-losing nephropathy, adrenal insufficiency, renal tubular acidosis
  * Water loss: diabetes insipidus
* Skin and respiratory losses: sweat, burns, insensible losses
* Sequestration without external fluid loss: intestinal obstruction, peritonitis, pancreatitis, rhabdomyolysis, internal bleeding

Volume Excess[1]

PRIMARY RENAL SODIUM RETENTION (INCREASED EFFECTIVE CIRCULATING VOLUME)

- Renal failure, nephritic syndrome, acute glomerulonephritis
- Primary hyperaldosteronism
- Cushing's syndrome
- Liver disease

SECONDARY RENAL SODIUM RETENTION (DECREASED EFFECTIVE CIRCULATING VOLUME)

- Heart failure
- Liver disease
- Nephrotic syndrome (minimal change disease)
- Pregnancy

Vomiting

- GI disturbances
  - Obstruction: esophageal, pyloric, intestinal
  - Infections: viral or bacterial enteritis, viral hepatitis, food poisoning, gastroenteritis
  - Pancreatitis
  - Appendicitis
  - Biliary colic
  - Peritonitis
  - Perforated bowel
  - Diabetic gastroparesis
  - Other: gastritis, peptic ulcer disease (PUD), inflammatory bowel disease (IBD), GI tract neoplasms
- Drugs: morphine, digitalis, cytotoxic agents, bromocriptine
- Severe pain: myocardial infarction (MI), renal colic
- Metabolic disorders: uremia, acidosis/alkalosis, hyperglycemia, diabetic ketoacidosis (DKA), thyrotoxicosis
- Trauma: blows to the testicles, epigastrium
- Vertigo
- Reye's syndrome
- Increased intracranial pressure
- CNS disturbances: trauma, hemorrhage, infarction, neoplasm, infection, hypertensive encephalopathy, migraine

- Radiation sickness
- Nausea and vomiting of pregnancy, hyperemesis gravidarum
- Motion sickness
- Bulimia, anorexia nervosa
- Psychogenic: emotional disturbances, offensive sights or smells
- Severe coughing
- Pyelonephritis
- Boerhaave's syndrome
- Carbon monoxide poisoning

Vulvar Cancer

- Lymphogranuloma inguinale
- TB
- Vulvar dystrophies
- Vulvar atrophy
- Paget's disease

Vulvar Lesions[12]

RED LESION
Infection/Infestation

- Fungal infection: *Candida*, tinea cruris, intertrigo, pityriasis versicolor
- *Sarcoptes scabiei*
- Erythrasma: *Corynebacterium minutissimum*
- Granuloma inguinale: *Calymmatobacterium granulomatis*
- Folliculitis: *Staphylococcus aureus*
- Hidradenitis suppurativa
- Behçet's syndrome

Inflammation

- Reactive vulvitis
- Chemical irritation: detergent, dyes, perfume, spermicide, lubricants, hygiene sprays, podophyllum, topical 5-fluorouracil, saliva, gentian violet, semen
- Mechanical trauma: scratching
- Vestibular adenitis
- Essential vulvodynia
- Psoriasis
- Seborrheic dermatitis

Neoplasm
- Vulvar intraepithelial neoplasia (VIN): mild dysplasia, moderate dysplasia, severe dysplasia, carcinoma in situ
- Vulvar dystrophy
- Bowen's disease
- Invasive cancer: squamous cell carcinoma, malignant melanoma, sarcoma, basal cell carcinoma, adenocarcinoma, Paget's disease, undifferentiated

WHITE LESION
- Vulvar dystrophy: lichen sclerosus, vulvar dystrophy, vulvar hyperplasia, mixed dystrophy
- VIN
- Vitiligo
- Partial albinism
- Intertrigo
- Radiation treatment

DARK LESION
- Lentigo
- Nevi (mole)
- Neoplasm (vulvar)
- Reactive hyperpigmentation
- Seborrheic keratosis
- Pubic lice

ULCERATIVE LESION
Infection
- Herpes simplex
- Vaccinia
- *Treponema pallidum*
- Granuloma inguinale
- Pyoderma
- Tuberculosis

Noninfectious
- Behçet's syndrome
- Crohn's disease
- Pemphigus
- Pemphigoid
- Hidradenitis suppurativa

Neoplasm
- Basal cell carcinoma
- Squamous cell carcinoma
- Vulvar tumor <1 cm: condyloma acuminatum, molluscum contagiosum, epidermal inclusion, vestibular cyst, mesonephric duct, VIN, hemangioma, hidradenoma, neurofibroma, syringoma, accessory breast tissue, acrochordon, endometriosis, Fox-Fordyce disease, pilonidal sinus
- Vulvar tumor >1 cm: Bartholin's cyst or abscess, lymphogranuloma venereum, fibroma, lipoma, verrucous carcinoma, squamous cell carcinoma, hernia, edema, hematoma, acrochordon, epidermal cysts, neurofibromatosis, accessory breast tissue

Vulvovaginitis, Bacterial

- Fungal vaginitis
- Trichomonas vaginitis
- Atrophic vaginitis
- Cervicitis

Vulvovaginitis, Estrogen Deficient

- Infectious vulvovaginitis
- Squamous cell hyperplasia
- Lichen sclerosus
- Vulvar malignant neoplasm
- Vaginal malignant neoplasm
- Cervical and endometrial malignant neoplasm

Vulvovaginitis, Fungal

- Bacterial vaginosis
- *Trichomonas* vaginitis
- Atrophic vaginitis

Vulvovaginitis, Prepubescent

- Physiologic leukorrhea
- Foreign body

- Bacterial vaginosis
- Gonorrhea
- Fungal vulvovaginitis
- *Trichomonas* vulvovaginitis
- Sexual abuse
- Pinworms

Vulvovaginitis, *Trichomonas*

- Bacterial vaginosis
- Fungal vulvovaginitis
- Cervicitis
- Atrophic vulvovaginitis
- Waldenström's macroglobulinemia
- Monoclonal gammopathy of unknown significance (MGUS)
- Multiple myeloma
- Chronic lymphocytic leukemia
- Hairy cell leukemia
- Lymphoma

Warts

- Molluscum contagiosum
- Condyloma latum
- Acrochordon (skin tags) or seborrheic keratosis
- Epidermal nevi
- Hypertrophic actinic keratosis
- Squamous cell carcinomas
- Acquired digital fibrokeratoma
- Varicella zoster virus in patients with AIDS
- Recurrent infantile digital fibroma
- Plantar corns (may be mistaken for plantar warts)

Weakness, Acute, Emergent[27]

- Demyelinating disorders (Guillain-Barré, chronic inflammatory demyelinating polyneuropathy [CIDP])
- Myasthenia gravis
- Infectious (poliomyelitis, diphtheria)

- Toxic (botulism, tick paralysis, paralytic shellfish toxin, puffer fish, newts)
- Metabolic (acquired or familial hypokalemia, hypophosphatemia, hypermagnesemia)
- Metals poisoning (arsenic, thallium)
- Porphyria

Weakness, Gradual Onset

- Depression
- Malingering
- Anemia
- Hypothyroidism
- Medications (e.g., sedatives, antidepressants, narcotics)
- Congestive heart failure (CHF)
- Renal failure
- Liver failure
- Respiratory insufficiency
- Alcoholism
- Nutritional deficiencies
- Disorders of motor unit
- Basal ganglia disorders
- Upper motor neuron lesions

Wegener's Granulomatosis

- Other granulomatous lung diseases (e.g., lymphomatoid granulomatosis, Churg-Strauss syndrome, necrotizing sarcoid granulomatosis, bronchocentric granulomatosis, sarcoidosis)
- Neoplasms
- Goodpasture's syndrome
- Bacterial or fungal sinusitis
- Midline granuloma
- Viral infections

Weight Gain

- Sedentary lifestyle
- Fluid overload
- Discontinuation of tobacco abuse

- Endocrine disorders (hypothyroidism, hyperinsulinism associated with maturity-onset diabetes mellitus [DM], Cushing's syndrome, hypogonadism, insulinoma, hyperprolactinemia, acromegaly)
- Medications (e.g., nutritional supplements, oral contraceptives, glucocorticoids)
- Anxiety disorders with compulsive eating
- Laurence-Moon-Biedl syndrome, Prader-Willi syndrome, other congenital diseases
- Hypothalamic injury (rare; <100 cases reported in medical literature)

Weight Loss

- Malignant disease
- Psychiatric disorders (depression, anorexia nervosa)
- New-onset diabetes mellitus (DM)
- Malabsorption
- Chronic obstructive pulmonary disease (COPD)
- AIDS
- Uremia, liver disease
- Thyrotoxicosis, pheochromocytoma, carcinoid syndrome
- Addison's disease
- Intestinal parasites
- Peptic ulcer disease (PUD)
- Inflammatory bowel disease (IBD)
- Food faddism
- Postgastrectomy syndrome

Wernicke's Encephalopathy

- Thiamine deficiency, including alcohol abuse, malnutrition, and iatrogenic cause
- Stroke, mass lesion, or trauma affecting upper brainstem, thalamus, and associated structures

West Nile Virus Infection

- Meningitis or encephalitis caused by more common viruses (e.g., enteroviruses, herpes simplex)
- Bacterial meningitis

- Vasculitis
- Fungal meningitis (e.g., cryptococcal infection)
- Tuberculous meningitis

Wheezing

- Asthma
- Chronic obstructive pulmonary disease (COPD)
- Interstitial lung disease
- Infections (pneumonia, bronchitis, bronchiolitis, epiglottitis)
- Cardiac asthma
- Gastroesophageal reflux disease (GERD) with aspiration
- Foreign body aspiration
- Pulmonary embolism
- Anaphylaxis
- Obstruction airway (neoplasm, goiter, edema or hemorrhage from trauma, aneurysm, congenital abnormalities, strictures, spasm)
- Carcinoid syndrome

Wheezing, Pediatric Age[4]

- Reactive airways disease
  - Atopic asthma
  - Infection-associated airway reactivity
  - Exercise-induced asthma
  - Salicylate-induced asthma and nasal polyposis
  - Asthmatic bronchitis
  - Other hypersensitivity reactions: hypersensitivity pneumonitis, tropical eosinophilia, visceral larva migrans, allergic bronchopulmonary aspergillosis
- Aspiration
  - Foreign body
  - Food, saliva, gastric contents
- Laryngotracheoesophageal cleft
- Tracheoesophageal fistula, H type
- Pharyngeal incoordination or neuromuscular weakness
- Cystic fibrosis
- Primary ciliary dyskinesia
- Cardiac failure

- Bronchiolitis obliterans
- Extrinsic compression of airways
  - Vascular ring
  - Enlarged lymph node
  - Mediastinal tumor
  - Lung cysts
  - Tracheobronchomalacia
  - Endobronchial masses
- Gastroesophageal reflux
- Pulmonary hemosiderosis
- Sequelae of bronchopulmonary dysplasia
- "Hysterical" glottic closure
- Cigarette smoke, other environmental insults

Whiplash

- Osteoarthritis
- Cervical disk disease
- Fibrositis
- Neuritis
- Torticollis
- Spinal cord tumor
- Temporomandibular joint (TMJ) syndrome
- Tension headache
- Migraine headache

Whipple's Disease

MALABSORPTION/MALDIGESTION

- Celiac disease
- *Mycobacterium avium-intracellulare* intestinal infection in patients with AIDS
- Intestinal lymphoma
- Abetalipoproteinemia
- Amyloidosis
- Systemic mastocytosis
- Irradiation enteritis
- Crohn's disease
- Short bowel syndrome
- Pancreatic insufficiency

- Intestinal bacterial overgrowth
- Lactose deficiency
- Postgastrectomy syndrome
- Other cause of diarrhea

SERONEGATIVE INFLAMMATORY ARTHRITIS

PERICARDITIS AND PLEURITIS

LYMPHADENITIS

NEUROLOGIC DISORDERS

Wrist Pain

MECHANICAL
- Osteoarthritis
- Ligament tear
- Fracture
- Ganglion
- de Quervain's tenosynovitis
- Avascular necrosis (scaphoid, lunate)
- Nonunion of scaphoid or lunate
- Neoplasm

METABOLIC
- Pregnancy
- Diabetes
- Gout
- Pseudogout
- Paget's disease
- Acromegaly
- Hypothyroidism
- Hyperparathyroidism

INFECTIOUS
- Osteomyelitis
- Septic arthritis
- Cat-scratch disease
- Tick bite (Lyme disease, babesiosis)
- Tuberculosis

NEUROLOGIC
- Peripheral neuropathy
- Nerve injury (median, ulnar, radial nerve)
- Thoracic outlet compression syndrome
- Distal posterior interosseous nerve syndrome

RHEUMATOLOGIC
- Psoriasis
- RA
- SLE, mixed connective tissue disorder (MCTD)
- Scleroderma

MISCELLANEOUS
- Granulomatous (sarcoidosis)
- Amyloidosis
- Multiple myeloma
- Leukemia

Wrist and Hand Pain, in Different Age Groups[8]

Common causes of wrist and hand pain in different age groups:

CHILDHOOD (2–10 YEARS)
Intra-articular
- Infection

Periarticular
- Fracture
- Osteomyelitis

ADOLESCENCE (10–18 YEARS)
Intra-articular
- Infection

Periarticular
- Trauma
- Osteomyelitis
- Tumors
- Ganglion
- Idiopathic wrist pain

EARLY ADULTHOOD (18–30 YEARS)
Intra-articular
- Inflammatory arthritis
- Infection

Periarticular
- Peripheral nerve entrapment
- Tendinitis
- Ganglion

Referred
- Cervical

ADULTHOOD (30–50 YEARS)
Intra-articular
- Inflammatory arthritis
- Infection
- Osteoarthritis
- Periarticular
- Peripheral nerve entrapment
- Tendinitis

Referred
- Cervical
- Chest
- Cardiac

OLD AGE (>50 YEARS)
Intra-articular
- Inflammatory arthritis
- Osteoarthritis

Periarticular
- Peripheral nerve entrapment
- Tendinitis

Referred
- Cervical
- Chest
- Cardiac

Xanthoma

- Necrobiosis lipoidica
- Rheumatoid nodules
- Neurofibromas
- Nodular elastoidosis
- Granuloma annulare
- Giant tumor of tendon sheath
- Erythema elevatum diutinum
- Histiocytoses

Xerophthalmia[29]

MEDICATIONS
- Tricyclic antidepressants: amitriptyline, doxepin
- Antihistamines: diphenhydramine, chlorpheniramine, promethazine, and many cold and decongestant preparations
- Anticholinergic agents: antiemetics such as scopolamine, antispasmodic agents such as oxybutynin chloride

ABNORMALITIES OF EYELID FUNCTION
- Neuromuscular disorders
- Aging
- Thyrotoxicosis

ABNORMALITIES OF TEAR PRODUCTION
- Hypovitaminosis A
- Stevens-Johnson syndrome
- Familial diseases affecting sebaceous secretions

ABNORMALITIES OF CORNEAL SURFACES
- Scarring from past injuries and herpes simplex infection

Xerosis

- Ichthyosis
- Stasis dermatitis
- Asteatotic eczema
- Nummular eczema
- Eczema craquelé

Xerostomia[29]

MEDICATIONS
- Tricyclic antidepressants: amitriptyline, doxepin
- Antihistamines: diphenhydramine, chlorpheniramine, promethazine, and many cold and decongestant preparations
- Anticholinergic agents: antiemetics such as scopolamine, antispasmodic agents such as oxybutynin chloride

DEHYDRATION
- Debility
- Fever

POLYURIA
- Alcohol intake
- Arrhythmia
- Diabetes

PREVIOUS HEAD AND NECK IRRADIATION

SYSTEMIC DISEASES
- Sjögren's syndrome
- Sarcoidosis
- Amyloidosis
- HIV infection
- Graft-versus-host disease

Yellow Fever

- Viral hepatitis
- Leptospirosis
- Malaria
- Typhoid fever
- Hemorrhagic fevers (HF) with jaundice
- Dengue (HF)
- Valley fever
- Crimean-Congo (HF)

Yellow Urine

- Normal coloration
- Concentrated urine

- Use of multivitamin supplements
- Diet rich in carrots
- Use of cascara
- Urinary tract infection

Zenker's Diverticulum

- Achalasia
- Esophageal spasm
- Esophageal carcinoma
- Esophageal webs
- Peptic stricture
- Lower esophageal (Schatzki's) ring
- Foreign bodies
- CNS disorders (stroke, Parkinson's disease, amyotrophic lateral sclerosis [ALS], multiple sclerosis [MS], myasthenia gravis, muscular dystrophies)
- Dermatomyositis
- Infection

References

1. Andreoli TE, ed: Cecil Essentials of Medicine, 5th ed. Philadelphia, WB Saunders, 2001.
2. Barkin RM, Rosen P: Emergency Pediatrics: A Guide to Ambulatory Care, 5th ed. St. Louis, Mosby, 1998.
3. Baude AI: Infectious Diseases and Medical Microbiology, 2nd ed. Philadelphia, WB Saunders, 1986.
4. Behrman RE: Nelson Textbook of Pediatrics, 16th ed. Philadelphia, WB Saunders, 2000.
5. Canoso J: Rheumatology in Primary Care. Philadelphia, WB Saunders, 1997.
6. Callen JP: Color Atlas of Dermatology, 2nd ed. Philadelphia, WB Saunders, 2000.
7. Carlson KJ: Primary Care of Women, 2nd ed. St. Louis, Mosby, 2003.
8. Carr A, Hamilton W: Orthopedics in Primary Care, 2nd ed. Philadelphia, Elsevier, 2005.
9. Conn R: Current Diagnosis, 9th ed. Philadelphia, WB Saunders, 1997.
10. Copeland LJ: Textbook of Gynecology, 2nd ed. Philadelphia, WB Saunders, 2000.
11. Custer JW, Rau RE: The Harriet Lane Handbook, 18th ed. St. Louis, Mosby, 2009.

12. Danakas G, ed: Practical Guide to the Care of the Gynecologic/Obstetric Patient. St. Louis, Mosby, 1997.

13. Goldberg RJ: The Care of the Psychiatric Patient, 2nd ed. St. Louis, Mosby, 1998.

14. Goldman L, Bennet JC: Cecil Textbook of Medicine, 22nd ed. Philadelphia, WB Saunders, 2004.

15. Goldman L, Braunwauld E, eds: Primary Cardiology. Philadelphia, WB Saunders, 1998.

16. Goldstein BG, Goldstein AO: Practical Dermatology, 2nd ed. St. Louis, Mosby, 1997.

17. Gorbach SL: Infectious Diseases, 2nd ed. Philadelphia, WB Saunders, 1998.

18. Harrington J: Consultation in Internal Medicine, 2nd ed. St. Louis, Mosby, 1997.

19. Henry JB: Clinical Diagnosis and Management by Laboratory Methods, 20th ed. Philadelphia, WB Saunders, 2001.

20. Hoekelman R: Primary Pediatric Care, 3rd ed. St. Louis, Mosby, 1997.

21. Hoffman R, Benz EJ, Shattil SJ, Furie B, Silberstein LE, Mc Glave P, Heslop H: Hematology, Basic Principles and Practice, 5th ed. Philadelphia, Churchill Livingstone, 2009.

22. Kassirer J, ed: Current Therapy in Adult Medicine, 4th ed. St. Louis, Mosby, 1998.

23. Khan MG: Rapid ECG Interpretation, Philadelphia, WB Saunders, 2003.

24. Kliegman R: Practical Strategies in Pediatric Diagnosis and Therapy. Philadelphia, WB Saunders, 1996.

25. Klippel J, ed: Practical Rheumatology. London, Mosby, 1995.

26. Mandell GL: Mandell, Douglas, and Bennett's Principles and Practice of Infectious Diseases, 5th ed. New York, Churchill Livingstone, 2000.

27. Marx J, ed: Rosen's Emergency Medicine: Concepts and Clinical Practice, 5th ed. St. Louis, 2002, Mosby.

28. Moore WT, Eastman RC: Diagnostic Endocrinology, 2nd ed. St. Louis, Mosby, 1996.

29. Noble J, ed: Primary Care Medicine, 3rd ed. St. Louis, Mosby, 2001.

30. Nseyo UO: Urology for Primary Care Physicians. Philadelphia, WB Saunders, 1999.

31. Palay D, ed: Ophthalmology for the Primary Care Physician. St. Louis, Mosby, 1997.

32. Rakel RE: Principles of Family Practice, 6th ed. Philadelphia, WB Saunders, 2002.

33. Schwarz MI: Interstitial Lung Disease, 2nd ed. St. Louis, Mosby, 1993.

34. Seller RH: Differential Diagnosis of Common Complaints, 4th ed. Philadelphia, WB Saunders, 2000.

35. Siedel HM, ed: Mosby's Guide to Physical Examination, 4th ed. St. Louis, Mosby, 1999.

36. Specht N: Practical Guide to Diagnostic Imaging. St. Louis, Mosby, 1998.
37. Stein JH, ed: Internal Medicine, 5th ed. St. Louis, Mosby, 1998.
38. Swain R, Snodgrass S: Managing groin pain: even when the source is not obvious. Phys Sportsmed 1995;23:55–66.
39. Talley NJ, Martin CJ: Clinical Gastroenterology, 2nd ed. Sidney, Churchill Livingstone, 2006.
40. Wiederholt WC: Neurology for Non-neurologists, 4th ed. Philadelphia, WB Saunders, 2000.
41. Wilson JD: Williams Textbook of Endocrinology, 9th ed. Philadelphia, WB Saunders, 1998.

Index

519